Healing Minds

Comprehensive Approaches to Mental Health Care and Policy

snova
New York

Mental Illnesses and Treatments Series

Understanding Youth Mental Health: Causes, Interventions, and Policy Perspectives
Michael A. Post (Editor)
ISBN: 979-8-89530-700-7
eBook ISBN: 979-8-89530-874-5

Mental Health and Substance Use Disorders: A Growing Crisis
Darren D. Stewart (Editor)
ISBN: 979-8-89530-699-4
eBook ISBN: 979-8-89530-825-7

Hoarding Disorder: Insights and Implications for Health and Safety
Paul M. Singleton (Editor)
ISBN: 979-8-89530-506-5
eBook ISBN: 979-8-89530-521-8

A Desperate Asylum: Crisis in a Canadian Psychiatric Hospital During Wartime
Anne Marie Creamer, PhD
ISBN: 979-8-88697-696-0
eBook ISBN: 979-8-88697-863-6

The Training and Practice of Psychotherapy in Post-Apartheid South Africa: Case Studies, Controversies and Contemplations
Zelda G. Knight
ISBN: 979-8-88697-782-0
eBook ISBN: 979-8-88697-974-9

More information about this series can be found at
https://novapublishers.com/product-category/series/mental-illnesses-and-treatments/

Wilburn M. Conner
Editor

Healing Minds

Comprehensive Approaches to Mental Health Care and Policy

snova
New York

Library of Congress Cataloging-in-Publication Data

ISBN: 979-8-89530-893-6 (Hardcover)
ISBN: 979-8-90134-002-8 (eBook)

Published by Nova Science Publishers, Inc. † New York

Contents

Preface

Mental health encompasses our emotional, psychological, and social well-being. It affects how we think, feel, and act, and helps determine how we cope with stress, relate to others, and make healthy choices. Mental health is important at every stage of life, from childhood and adolescence to adulthood.

Every American must have access to mental health care when they need it. Several laws mandate that mental health care should be on equal footing with physical health care. However, in practice, the system still reflects the dangerous, outdated stigma against identifying and treating mental illness. This disparity in treatment underscores the urgent need for policy reform and societal change.

This book delves into the complexities of mental health care in America, examining the root causes of current issues and exploring policy solutions. Through detailed analysis and expert insights, we aim to shed light on the importance of mental health parity and provide a strategic framework for addressing mental health disparities, especially among youth. Additionally, we explore the role of telemental health, legislative efforts, and the impact of genetic research on mental health care.

Chapter 1

Mental Health Care in America: Addressing Root Causes and Identifying Policy Solutions*

Committee on Finance

Tuesday, June 15, 2021

U.S. Senate, Committee on Finance,
Washington, DC.

The hearing was convened, pursuant to notice, at 10:10 a.m., via Webex, in Room SD–215, Dirksen Senate Office Building, Hon. Ron Wyden (chairman of the committee) presiding.

Present: Senators Stabenow, Cantwell, Carper, Cardin, Bennet, Casey, Warner, Whitehouse, Hassan, Warren, Crapo, Grassley, Thune, Portman, Cassidy, Daines, Young, and Sasse.

Also present: Democratic staff: Eva DuGoff, Senior Health Advisor; Marisa Dowling, Health Policy Fellow; and Kristen Lunde, Health Policy Advisor. Republican staff: Kellie McConnell, Health Policy Director; Gregg Richard, Staff Director; and Stuart Portman, Senior Health Policy Advisor.

* This is an edited, reformatted and augmented version of Hearing Before the Committee on Finance United States Senate One Hundred Seventeenth Congress, First Session, Publication No. S. HRG. 117–628, dated June 15, 2021.

In: Healing Minds
Editor: Wilburn M. Conner
ISBN: 979-8-89530-893-6

Opening Statement of Hon. Ron Wyden, a U.S. Senator from Oregon, Chairman, Committee on Finance

The CHAIRMAN. The Senate Finance Committee will come to order. The Finance Committee meets this morning to discuss mental health care in America, and this issue certainly ought to bring Democrats and Republicans together, starting with a single, clear lodestar. That lodestar is: every American must have mental health care when they need it.

The shameful reality is, the United States does not come close to meeting that bar today. Multiple Federal laws say that mental health care is supposed to be on a level playing field with physical health care. In practice, however, the system still reflects the dangerous, outdated stigma against recognizing and treating mental illness. And that is why millions of Americans are now falling between the cracks.

For someone with a mental illness, it can often be nearly impossible to find a provider who can meet your needs, or one who accepts insurance, particularly in rural communities or communities of color. Insurance claims often get denied or cut off too quickly, particularly for those experiencing homelessness. The outcome of a mental health crisis is often incarceration instead of treatment.

Prior to the pandemic, one in five Americans was living with mental illness. All the evidence suggests that the pandemic is adding to that crisis. The proportion of Americans reporting symptoms of anxiety or depression has nearly quadrupled.

On Friday, the Centers for Disease Control and Prevention released a new report finding that, over the last year, suicide attempts among teenaged girls were up more than 50 percent. Meanwhile, studies that the Government Accountability Office conducted at our request found that many provider offices closed or cut staff during the pandemic, and then too many patients were turned away.

So, there is a lot for this committee to work on on a bipartisan basis. There are a few key challenges.

First, the country clearly needs a larger mental health workforce. There simply are not enough providers, whether psychiatrists or therapists or staff in inpatient facilities. For example, due to a major staffing shortage, the psychiatric hospital in my home State of Salem, OR, is currently being staffed by members of the Oregon National Guard. That is in the State Capitol where there are people and resources to focus on the issue. Many other communities have it far worse. More than one in three Americans lives in an area with a serious shortage of mental healtcare professionals.

Second, insurance companies must not be allowed to cut corners when it comes to mental health coverage. I hear about this issue constantly at town hall meetings. People describe having their claims denied. In other cases, insurance only covers a portion of the treatment that people need. Furthermore, it does not make any sense to leave somebody experiencing a true mental health crisis waiting for a green light from an insurance company before they can get treated.

Third, clearly the committee has a big challenge to address racial inequities in mental health care. Black and Latino Americans are roughly half as likely as white Americans to receive treatment for mental illness. Suicide rates are much higher among black kids. There are not enough black, Latino, and Native American mental health providers. So, this is a question of equity, and we have a long way to go.

Finally, the committee ought to build on recent telehealth. For example, early in the pandemic this committee led the fight to get Medicare to cover mental health services via telehealth. In December, the Congress made that permanent. I believe that is going to be a game changer, particularly for seniors who live in rural areas, and it is going to work in traditional Medicare as well.

My colleagues all know that so many of our reforms have helped, particularly with Medicare Advantage and other programs where there is coordinated care, but we have to make sure traditional Medicare is afforded these benefits as well.

Finally, Senator Stabenow has been a champion of mental healtcare treatment, and I have watched for years as she has led the effort to bring Certified Community Behavioral Health Clinics, a program that she battled for and created, to American communities. These clinics are up and running now in 40 States, including Oregon. It is an approach that works and meets major needs.

I believe the Congress ought to look at ways to build on the success that my colleague has led, and we should also note again the bipartisan route, because I cannot tell Senators how often I have seen Senator Stabenow and Senator Blunt huddled in intense discussions about how they are going to expand this.

Finally, the Congress also passed a big down payment for pioneering a new approach on mental health services and law enforcement. It is called the CAHOOTS program. It originally comes from Eugene—Eugene, OR—where I went to law school. But it is expanding now all over the country.

Essentially what happens with this approach is, you have a 911 call with somebody experiencing a mental health crisis. And at that point, the mental healthcare professionals and the law enforcement in these communities have essentially teamed up and figured out a way to actually meet the needs of the patient and the community.

So, in many instances, these are joint efforts of the mental health professionals and law enforcement—a team, a coalition approach. In Oregon, I have talked to the police officials in Eugene, the mental health professionals in Eugene, and very often the response— and they both have kind of worked up a system to do the right thing—is to use mental health professionals rather than law enforcement. And law enforcement, to their credit, is saying that they want to do that, and often the mental health professionals are the right response.

The American Rescue Plan included a billion-dollar payment to help States build on their own programs, and I think we ought to look at what else ought to be done.

The last point I will make—and Dr. Cassidy is here, and he has great expertise in this area. Colleagues, this is an enormous challenge, and I think it is natural for Democratic and Republican members of this committee to step up and shape a major response that we can take to the full Senate. I look forward to working with all my colleagues.

Senator Crapo?

[The prepared statement of Chairman Wyden appears in the appendix.]

Opening Statement of Hon. Mike Crapo, a U.S. Senator from Idaho

Senator CRAPO. Thank you very much, Mr. Chairman. I appreciate you holding this hearing, and I agree with your comments that this is an issue that deeply needs good solutions, and on which we can build strong bipartisan solutions that work. And I look forward to working with you, Senator Stabenow, and all the others that you have mentioned, on these issues.

Ensuring access to high-quality mental health services has been and must continue to be a priority. Far too often, individuals with mental health, addiction, or substance abuse disorders find themselves isolated from their communities and separated from their providers. While Congress has taken decisive steps to address addiction, bolster behavioral health care, and curb substance abuse disorders, challenges remain. This committee has the ability to turn the tide. We can begin by empowering States to craft innovative, targeted solutions. Medicaid functions most effectively when States have the flexibilities they need to address patients' unique care needs and adapt to unforeseen circumstances.

As the Nation's largest payer of mental health and substance abuse disorder services, Medicaid must support rather than subvert State efforts to serve communities in need. Unfortunately, the COVID–19 pandemic has highlighted and exacerbated the mental and behavioral health challenges we continue to confront.

Loss of loved ones, increased isolation, and delayed treatment prompted a spike in anxiety, depression, and other debilitating conditions. While many are returning to their pre-pandemic lives, we should not be content to allow our mental healthcare delivery system to revert to its pre-pandemic ways.

Whether for rural communities, urban areas, or tribes, telehealth has undoubtedly increased access to care. Through emergency flexibilities and permanent legislation authored by this committee late last year, we have taken crucial first steps toward modernizing telehealth coverage. I look forward to working with you, Mr. Chairman, and the other members of this committee to build on those efforts in the months ahead.

Further, by partnering with State and local leaders, we can spur care coordination, strengthen the mental health workforce, and drive value through delivery system reforms. While there is no silver bullet here, I am confident we can tackle all of these challenges while upholding core principles of fiscal responsibility and program integrity.

Before concluding, it bears emphasizing that we must continue to make progress in improving understanding of mental health so that people in need are not afraid or ashamed to seek treatment. We cannot discount the impact of stigma on preventing those in need of treatment from receiving care.

I look forward to hearing our witnesses' testimony today, and I appreciate each of you coming here to share your expertise and ideas about how we can achieve these objectives.

Thank you very much.

[The prepared statement of Senator Crapo appears in the appendix.]

The CHAIRMAN. Thank you, Senator Crapo.

We have four terrific witnesses. The one who will testify first— and I think we will do the introductions, because colleagues are juggling a lot this morning—is Dr. Miller. And Senator Bennet will give the introduction for Dr.

Miller. And we will introduce all our witnesses, and then we will hear their testimony.

Opening Statement of Hon. Michael F. Bennet, A U.S. Senator from Colorado

Senator BENNET. Thank you, Mr. Chairman. I would like to thank you and Senator Crapo for holding this important hearing. From the perspective of Colorado, it could not come soon enough. In my calls with parents and teachers over the past year, the number one issue has been mental health.

Over the years, the person my office has turned to for advice on these issues is Dr. Benjamin Miller, one of our witnesses today. Dr. Miller is one of the country's foremost experts on mental health. Today he serves as the chief strategy officer for Well Being Trust, a national foundation dedicated to advancing a more holistic approach to the health of every American.

In his early training, which included a doctorate from Spalding University and post-doctoral roles at the University of Colorado and the University of Massachusetts, Dr. Miller saw firsthand how America's inattention to mental health inflicts a terrible cost on our society, from our schools to our foster care, healthcare, and criminal justice systems.

Dr. Miller has not just studied these issues in the academy, he has worked on them firsthand in our communities. He has helped emotionally disturbed children make it through school, cancer patients cope with difficult diagnoses, and prisoners plan their reintegration into society. He has also trained physicians to better handle their patients' mental health. These issues are not abstractions for him, they are real people whose lives have directly benefited from greater attention to their mental health.

I know Dr. Miller from his time at the University of Colorado, where he led the University's Health Policy Center for 6 years and was an invaluable resource to my team. During his time at the Center, Dr. Miller led a breakthrough project demonstrating the cost savings of integrating mental health with primary care. That project saved over $1 million for Medicare and Medicaid beneficiaries in Colorado by significantly reducing hospitalizations and other medical needs down the road.

As healthcare costs in this country continue to rise, I think the committee has a lot to learn from Dr. Miller's experience and expertise. I could spend the next 5 minutes listing the numerous awards and appointments he has earned over the years, but let me instead conclude by thanking Dr. Miller for joining us today, especially since he is supposed to be on vacation right now with his wife and two daughters. We are grateful for Dr. Miller's time, and for his service to Colorado and the country.

Thank you, Mr. Chairman.

The CHAIRMAN. Thank you, Senator Bennet.

The next witness will be from Oregon, Chantay Jett, who is the executive director of Wallowa Valley Center for Wellness in Enterprise, OR. It is a small community—I have been there often—in rural eastern Oregon. And as is the case for so many people I have the honor to represent, she is the bionic woman. She is basically everywhere, colleagues.

She has worked in the Wallowa River House, a residential treatment facility for folks in Oregon afflicted with severe mental illness. She has been an outpatient mental health clinician. She is a pillar of the community. I remember recently—we have sessions in schools called ''Listening to the Future.'' Chantay was there. And she holds a master's degree in psychology with a child, couple, and family emphasis; a bachelor's degree in business administration; and she also worked with children in the inpatient psychiatric unit at Children's Hospital.

Chantay, thank you for making the long journey from rural Oregon. We are so glad you are here. I know the committee is going to appreciate hearing from you.

Next, we will have Dr. Durham, a great advocate for patients and those facing health challenges. Senator Elizabeth Warren is, I believe, online and she can introduce Dr. Durham.

Senator Warren, are you out there in cyberspace?

Opening Statement of Hon. Elizabeth Warren, a U.S. Senator from Massachusetts

Senator WARREN. I am. Thank you very much, Chairman Wyden, Ranking Member Crapo. Thank you for having this hearing today. I have the privilege of introducing Dr. Michelle Durham of Massachusetts. She has agreed to speak to the committee today about the importance of expanding access to mental health services all across our country.

Dr. Durham currently works as a pediatric and adult psychiatrist at Boston Medical Center. Now, BMC is the largest safety-net hospital in New England,

and it is also an academic medical center that is located in the heart of Boston. And it is an amazing place. Most of BMC's patients are low-income or from underserved populations. About half are covered by Medicaid. Throughout the COVID–19 pandemic, providers at Boston Medical Center, including Dr. Durham, have gone above and beyond to get patients the healthcare services that they need. Our communities owe a great debt to the folks at BMC.

At BMC, Dr. Durham serves as the vice chair of education in the Department of Psychiatry. She also has a joint appointment as assistant professor of psychiatry at Boston University School of Medicine, and she runs the training program for BMC's general psychiatry residency program.

As you say, Chair Wyden, this is another woman who is everywhere. Throughout her career, Dr. Durham has been a tireless advocate of health, equity, and mental health. And she is the associate director of BMC's Global and Local Center for Mental Health Disparities. She also co-leads the TEAM UP for Children initiative at BMC, which works to expand pediatric mental health care at Federally Qualified Community Health Centers.

Dr. Durham was an expert on mental health long before the coronavirus, and she also worked on the front lines of the pandemic. Her testimony today will offer significant insight into how Congress should be considering reforming and improving our mental health system to both build back from the pandemic, and to fix problems that existed long before that pandemic hit.

So, Dr. Durham, I am deeply grateful for the work you do for patients, for students, and for the people of the Commonwealth of Massachusetts. I look forward to having a great discussion today.

Thank you, Mr. Chairman.

The CHAIRMAN. Thank you very much, Senator Warren. Thanks for your help in assisting us in making sure Dr. Durham could be with us today.

Our last witness will be Tom Betlach, a partner at Speire Healthcare Strategies. Prior to joining Speire, Mr. Betlach served the State of Arizona for 27 years under five different Governors in three different cabinet positions. For 10 years he served as Director of the Arizona Health Care Cost Containment System. That is, as I understand it, Arizona's Medicaid program. He has a bachelor's and a master's in public administration from the University of Arizona, and a bachelor of arts in political science from the University of Wisconsin. So, we are very glad you are here as well.

Let's begin, and we will start with Dr. Miller.

Statement of Benjamin F. Miller, PSY.D., Chief Strategy Officer, Well Being Trust, Oakland, CA

Dr. MILLER. Well, thank you for that wonderful introduction, Senator Bennet.

Chairman Wyden, Ranking Member Crapo, and members of the committee, my name is Dr. Benjamin F. Miller, and I am the chief strategy officer for Well Being Trust, a national foundation started in 2016 through a gift by the Providence Health System that is focused on advancing the mental, social, and spiritual health of the Nation.

I am a clinical psychologist by training and have spent most of my adult life pursuing strategies that can advance mental health to a place of priority within our society. This goal has guided much of my work during my time as the founding director of the University of Colorado's Farley Health Policy Center, and is continuing today in my capacity as an adjunct professor at Stanford School of Medicine and at Well Being Trust.

It is an honor to be able to speak to you today about an issue that every American is experiencing, an issue that we need to aggressively pursue, and which COVID–19 has all but exacerbated, especially among communities of color and other marginalized people: their mental health.

Several government reports highlight how broken our mental health system is. The 2020 DoD Inspector General report found over 52 percent of service members and their families who needed mental health care did not receive it. SAMHSA found that over 56 percent of adults with mental illness did not receive any treatment in the past year, nor did 35 percent of those with serious mental illness. And a recent GAO report highlighted a multitude of issues at multiple levels for mental health, including ongoing challenges with health insurance, enforcing laws like mental health parity, and finding the right clinician who can help. In one survey, almost 30 percent of people reported not seeking care because they did not know where to go.

The need to solve these and other existing problems is real and immediate. Clear pathways do not exist for people seeking mental health care. There are not obvious doors to enter, and we have no system that routinely is able to identify and treat people in a timely manner. This is perhaps our greatest challenge as we emerge from the devastating COVID–19 pandemic.

With broad majorities of both parties now understanding the importance of addressing mental health, I believe it is time to enact immediate fixes for people in need, as well as to begin to lay the foundation for a reimagined mental health system, a mental health system that is grounded in community and is an integral part of a broader healthcare infrastructure.

There are three key priorities I believe this committee should consider as it pursues both short- and long-term reforms for mental health. First and foremost, we need to bring mental health care to where people are. This includes schools and even our work places. But to most immediately meet this moment, the best place to start is primary care, the largest platform of healthcare delivery. In one poll, 70 percent of adults agreed that it would be more convenient if their mental health and substance use services were integrated into their primary care doctor's office.

To do this, we must create more global and flexible funding mechanisms for primary care practices that are working to integrate mental health. Our payment mechanisms often reinforce a siloed delivery model, and this must change. By first using existing payment structures like those found in Medicaid managed care organizations, Medicare Accountable Care Organizations, and Medicare Advantage Plans to expand mental health integration work, primary care practices would have the flexible financial resources to onboard mental health clinicians as a part of their integrated team.

Second, we must reconsider the design and capabilities of our workforce. Demand for care has far outpaced the supply of mental health clinicians, and it is inconceivable to rely upon clinician recruitment strategies alone to meet our ever-growing need.

There are two things we can do simultaneously to address this workforce issue. First, we can map out mental health utilization gaps to better determine where services are needed, and for whom. Without this, we run the risk of widening disparities, or putting money into places or programs that people are not using for their mental health. Second, we can invest in our community workforce, those like peer support specialists, community health workers, or more broadly, lay people in our communities. We can train them in mental health skills to help become the first line of mental health support, complementing our clinical enterprise and enhancing the overall capacity for communities to address mental health needs.

Finally, we must modernize and connect our Federal programs and systems to collaboratively solve our common mental health problems. I realize it is hard to ask committees to work across jurisdictional boundaries, but so many aspects of our mental health need to be understood together, and implemented together, at both the State and community level. Because there are multiple agencies, funding streams, and programs that support mental health, performing a landscape analysis can create a strategy for synergistic efficiencies by breaking down silos across Federal agencies and departments, and allowing for a more cohesive plan for mental health.

In closing, I thank this committee again for holding this hearing on mental health. This is our moment to be bold in what we can do to boost our Nation's mental health and ultimately save lives.

Thank you, Mr. Chairman.

[The prepared statement of Dr. Miller appears in the appendix.]

The CHAIRMAN. Thank you very much, Dr. Miller.

Okay, I think next we will go to—Dr. Miller has gotten us off to a strong start, and now we will hear from Ms. Jett. [Pause.]

Statement of Chantay Jett, MA, Mft, Executive Director, Wallowa Valley Center For Wellness, Enterprise, OR

Ms. JETT. Good morning, Chairman Wyden, Ranking Member Crapo, and members of the Senate Finance Committee. Thank you for the opportunity to appear before the committee to discuss policy solutions to address both the mental health and substance use crises impacting the United States, and in particular the rural and frontier areas of our Nation. My name is Chantay Jett, and I am executive director of Wallowa Valley Center for Wellness (WVCW), which provides community-based mental health and substance use treatment services in the most remote region of the great State of Oregon.

We represent a truly frontier area of our Nation where the cows outnumber the people and our closest major airport is in Boise, ID, nearly 4 hours away. We are literally at the end of the road, where everyone knows everyone, which unfortunately contributes to the stigma and lack of access for people seeking treatment services.

I am here to tell you that the Certified Community Behavioral Health Clinic model has truly made a difference in our frontier communities. I hope every State in the near future has an opportunity to use the resources this model has made available to us to meet the specific needs of our community.

The State of Oregon participates in the 10-State demonstration of the Excellence in Mental Health and Addiction Treatment Act that this committee helped to establish in 2014 through the bipartisan leadership of Senators Stabenow and Blunt. The Center for Wellness is one of 12 CCBHCs that operate within our State. We provide high-quality integrated community-based mental health and substance use services to individuals, while also screening for possible co-morbid conditions like heart disease, diabetes, HIV, and AIDs.

Among the most important services that CCBHCs provide, both in Oregon and Nationwide, are immediate access to medication-assisted treatment services for substance use and 24-hour psychiatric services. Please permit me to provide some very brief context of CCBHCs within rural and frontier counties in the State of Oregon.

According to the Oregon Health Authority, our State reports higher rates of mental health conditions, including severe and persistent mental illness and suicidal ideation. The COVID–19 pandemic has only exacerbated an ongoing mental health and substance use crisis in rural Oregon.

OHA also detailed the lack of access to mental health and substance use care, especially in frontier communities. To give you a sense, there is no stop light within this 76-mile radius of Wallowa County. OHA reports an average wait time of as much as 6 months Statewide due to a lack of providers. However, we are the lucky ones, because the CCBHC model helped create an internal reorganization of service delivery which resulted in same-day access to care.

Prior to becoming a CCBHC, the Center for Wellness was heavily reliant upon grants. Grant funding is crucially important, but it carries limitations. Grants typically end every 2 to 3 years. They all have different reporting requirements and different program specifications, which ultimately result in more time spent filling out paperwork rather than treating our patients.

By contrast, the CCBHC prospective payment system allows us to do three major things. First, the Center for Wellness contracts with more skilled clinicians, including psychiatrists and medical professionals, to prescribe medication-assisted treatment for patients with opioid use disorder. This directly results in decreased wait times and reduced emergency department visits.

Secondly, the CCBHC program is designed to expand access to underserved populations. In our communities, the CCBHC really opened the door for mental health care to veterans. According to our local VSO in our county, there are at least 1,000 community members who have donned the uniform out of 7,000 residents. Becoming a CCBHC has allowed us to increase our services to 23 veterans in our community. This may not seem significant to you, but it is a 300-percent increase in services.

Thirdly, consistent CCBHC resources are a fundamental driver of integrated care. In Oregon, the CCBHC demonstration financing has made it possible to integrate with a local Federally Qualified Health Center, allowing primary care and behavioral health services all under the same roof.

We also share a single electronic health record to permit immediate care coordination. Patients often tell me that it is such a relief to not have to retell their stories with every provider they meet. We are lucky that we have a great neighbor in the State of Idaho when we have no acute psychiatric beds available. This component of care coordination in partnership with primary care in hospitals, even across State lines, is imperative because patients with severe mental illness and substance abuse challenges have shockingly high rates of medical conditions. The CCBHC model allows us to have these partnerships and get patients the services they deserve in a timely manner.

In closing, I strongly believe that this model represents the future of community-based mental health and substance abuse treatment in the United States. This is why I am asking you to make this model available to every State Nationwide. As a Nation, we can do better than first treating mental health and substance abuse in hospitals, homeless shelters, and our county jails. Investing in CCBHCs is streamlining services in efficient ways that drive costs down over the entire continuum of care.

Despite being from a tiny frontier community at the end of the road in northeast Oregon, I hope you can see that CCBHCs make an enormous impact. Again, thank you for the opportunity to testify, and I am happy to answer any questions.

[The prepared statement of Ms. Jett appears in the appendix.] The CHAIRMAN. Thank you very much, Ms. Jett. You make Oregonians proud this morning. I would also note you mentioning the Idaho-Oregon alliance. Senator Crapo's ears perked up when he heard that. And on all these incredible efforts, we have talked about a lot of them. And I just want you to know that it is a tremendous honor to really be your wing man in some of these causes, because we have a lot of work to do, and you have laid out a very powerful case about some of the most important elements. So, thank you. And thank you for making the long trip.

Okay; next will be Dr. Durham.

Statement of Michelle P. Durham, M.D., Mph, Fapa, Dfaacap, Assistant Professor of Psychiatry, Boston University School of Medicine; and Vice Chair of Education, and Psychiatry Residency Training Director, Department of Psychiatry, Boston Medical Center, Boston, MA

Dr. DURHAM. Thank you, Chairman Wyden, Ranking Member Crapo, and distinguished members of the Senate Committee on Finance, for holding this hearing and providing me with the opportunity to speak today about the state of the mental healthcare system in America—where it is working, where it falls short, and how the Federal Government can play a role in helping to fill the gaps. Thank you, Senator Warren, for the kind introduction.

Boston Medical Center is an academic medical center and the largest safety-net hospital in New England. The patients we serve are predominantly low-income, with approximately half of our patients covered by Medicaid or the Children's Health Insurance Program—the highest percentage of any acute care hospital in Massachusetts, and one of the highest in the country.

Mental illnesses are all too common among the patients BMC treats in our emergency department and across our continuum of mental healthcare services, which include outpatient integrated mental health care within our pediatric and adult primary care clinics, and at local community health center partners. A mental health urgent care clinic, a crisis stabilization unit, and our Boston Emergency Services Team (BEST) provide community-based evaluations and a jail-diversion program. At present, BMC does not own or operate a locked inpatient psychiatric unit.

The patients we see at BMC who present with mental illness frequently have co-occurring substance use disorders, homelessness, malnutrition, and other health-related social needs linked to poverty. The current COVID–19 pandemic, structural racism, and economic crisis have further exacerbated the mental illness and trauma experienced by our patients.

In my 10 years at BMC, I have never seen our mental healthcare services stretched so far beyond their capacity as they are now. Just the other day we had 25 patients in our psychiatric emergency department, more than triple its capacity, presenting with much higher level of acuity, some waiting for evaluations, and others boarding, awaiting placement in an inpatient psychiatric unit.

It is widely understood and well documented that America has a dearth of licensed mental health professionals in general, and that particular areas of the country, largely rural and outside of the Northeast, are disproportionately impacted. Even where I practice in Boston, which has one of the highest numbers of child and adolescent psychiatrists per capita in the country, the capacity is insufficient to meet the mental health needs of the community.

Increased Medicare graduate medical education funding for psychiatry residency slots can help increase the physician workforce. Increased funding for loan forgiveness programs for those who work in underserved areas can help alleviate the over $250,000 of debt that the average medical student has accumulated by the time their residency education is completed. The need to pay off medical school loan burdens is also likely to cause physicians to pursue practice in more affluent areas, adversely impacting access to care for low-income populations.

Beyond the shortage of providers, the mental health workforce is not diverse—for instance, only 2 percent of psychiatrists identify as black—and not representative or reflective of the U.S. population. In order to address this, we must understand that the issue at its root is a pipeline issue that requires holistic solutions.

Just as we say in medicine that a person's ZIP code is more influential than their genetic code in determining life trajectory and long-term health, where a person lives, the color of their skin, and the language they speak is highly determinative of quality of education and resources available, the level of exposure to the mental health field, and the stigma associated with mental illness.

In terms of access to mental health services, COVID–19 led to an accelerated adoption of telemedicine. At peak, over 90 percent of our outpatient psychiatric visits were conducted via telehealth, which enabled BMC to maintain and exceed our pre-pandemic volume of service. That said, while telehealth is an important tool for ensuring patient access to mental health care, it does not work for everyone, due to digital inequities that exist related to Internet access and digital literacy, especially among low-income communities. The social determinants of mental health and structural vulnerabilities inherently involved with treating low-income patients require more dedicated time with patients to provide appropriate care. Insufficient Medicaid reimbursement acts as a deterrent for providers to see Medicaid patients, producing a cascade effect in which the more oppressed, marginalized populations have limited to no access to mental health professionals.

At BMC, we have developed some innovative models to improve access to mental health services, which are ripe for replication and scaling.

Transforming and Expanding Access to Mental Health Care in Urban Pediatrics, otherwise known as TEAM UP for Children, a pediatric integrated model in Federally Qualified Health Centers in Massachusetts, builds the capacity of health centers to deliver high-quality, evidence-informed care to children and families. The model includes behavioral health clinicians and community health workers working with pediatric primary care providers to provide timely mental health treatment.

The Wellness and Recovery After Psychosis program is tailored for people experiencing psychotic symptoms using a team-based approach and providing individual, group, and family therapy; medication management; case management; and peer support.

In addition, Massachusetts is home to some other models in which BMC participates. The Massachusetts Child Psychiatry Access Program, known as MCPAP, improves access to treatment for children with behavioral health needs and their families by making child psychiatry services accessible to primary care providers across Massachusetts via remote consultation and education. This model has been expanded to other States such as Connecticut, where I completed my fellowship. The Metro Boston Recovery Learning Community offers peer-to-peer services for people in recovery from mental health and/or substance use issues through peer support, advocacy, and career coaching.

We are at a pivotal time in our country. Over a year into the COVID–19 pandemic, every person's mental well-being has been impacted in some way. The need for a more robust mental healthcare system has never been more clear or pronounced.

Treatment for mental health issues should be accessible, no matter who you are, where you live, or your ability to pay. Appropriate investment along the care continuum and for the mental health workforce can improve access to care and retention and recruitment of mental health professionals. The time is now to invest in a 21st-century mental healthcare system in America.

Thank you for your time, and I look forward to the discussion. [The prepared statement of Dr. Durham appears in the appendix.]

The CHAIRMAN. Very good, Dr. Durham. I know that we will have questions for you in just a couple of minutes.

Mr. Betlach, welcome.

Statement of Thomas Betlach, MPA, Partner, Speire Healthcare Strategies, Phoenix, AZ

Mr. BETLACH. Thank you, Chairman Wyden, Ranking Member Crapo, and members of the Senate Finance Committee. Thank you for the opportunity to testify today on policy solutions for addressing mental health.

I had the privilege of serving as the Arizona Medicaid Director for almost a decade and, for a portion of that time, as the Mental Health Commissioner. Medicaid serves over 70 million members, offering comprehensive mental health benefits to some of the country's most complex populations. As you formulate health policy options, State Medicaid programs should be a critical component of the discussion. Understanding the system and the forces prevailing on it should be at the core of the discussion.

The last year brought to light the extreme fragmentation of our healthcare delivery system at all levels. Our policy and program structures are in silos. Funding streams to support these populations follow those siloed program and policy structures. Providers gravitate towards these funding streams, creating more complexity at the point of care, and the very beneficiary the system is designed to serve is forced to navigate the maze we have created.

Today's environment has challenges, but States and Medicaid programs now have access to considerable Federal investments to address these challenges. Examples include the 5-percent set-aside for mental health block grants used for crisis, 85-percent enhanced match in Medicaid for the CAHOOTS program, 10-percent increase in Federal funding for home and community-based services for the rehab option services, and the expansion of Certified Community Behavioral Health Clinics.

In February 2021, the National Association of Medicaid Directors published ''Medicaid Forward: Behavioral Health,'' outlining a series of strategies Medicaid programs are pursuing to advance mental health services for members. The strategies vary based on the unique population served by Medicaid. This report highlighted initiatives such as expanding access and improving timeliness to care, integrating physical health and behavioral health, and expanding access for the full continuum of care, including crisis services.

Further, a March 2021 Bipartisan Policy Council report concluded that integrating primary and behavioral health care is necessary and would ensure that individuals with behavioral health conditions and co-morbid physical health problems receive high- quality access to care. Arizona provides a strong example of this. In 2011, we pursued a multiyear strategy to better integrate services for individuals with serious mental illness. This strategy was focused on driving integration at three levels: policy integration, payer integration, provider integration. In 2018, Mercer consulting conducted an analysis of the integration efforts. Their final report for individuals with serious mental illness found that all measures of ambulatory care, preventative care, and chronic disease management demonstrated improvement. Just as important, all indicators of patient experience improved, with 5 of 11 measures exhibiting double-digit increases.

Another opportunity highlighted by NAMD is to strengthen crisis systems. This issue is front and center with the implementation of 988. SAMHSA provided extensive thought leadership with the development of the Crisis Now model to serve anyone, anywhere, at any time.

The Crisis Now model is based on three critical components: call center capability, 24-by-7 community mobile response teams, and 23-hour crisis receiving and stabilization units.

In Arizona, the system has been developed over the past 20 years and serves all Arizonans. The financing for the system comes from creative multiple funding streams, while leveraging Medicaid for support. While we have seen improvement, there is clearly much more to do.

To that end, Congress and the executive branch need to develop and implement strategies holistically by ensuring Medicaid and behavioral health collaborate and partner in a meaningful manner. On several occasions, Congress has leveraged the mental health expertise of SAMHSA to advance policy initiatives. However, there do not appear to be sufficient expectations established by Congress that these important planning and investment dollars are to be linked to the Medicaid program. Unfortunately, the dollars often get siloed, and the opportunity is suboptimal. At the end of the day, Medicaid beneficiaries may or may not benefit from these forward-looking investments.

Congress should provide more flexibility with block grant funds for States to address social determinants of health, as States look at ways to support these investments. Congress should look at legislation to establish parity between Medicare and Medicaid. Where Medicaid has led the way in developing paraprofessional staff such as peer support services and systems to support broader populations like Crisis, Medicare should follow.

Congress should continue to provide financial incentives for States to modernize mental health infrastructure, like the investments made in CAHOOTS and CCBHCs. Congress should continue to evaluate the impact of the IMD 16-bed limit. While there have been efforts made to allow for some payments in select instances, some States have not been able to avail themselves of these opportunities.

Congress should rectify the fact that behavioral health providers were excluded from the electronic health record incentive program provided through the HITECH Act. And finally, as was mentioned by Dr. Durham, Congress should revisit the GME funding that is made available through Medicare and the 1996 caps.

We are at a critical moment in time to advance the delivery of mental health services, not only with Medicaid, but for our entire country. Thank you for your time and interest in these topics.

[The prepared statement of Mr. Betlach appears in the appendix.]

The CHAIRMAN. Thank you very much, Mr. Betlach.

We will start with you, Ms. Jett. I think what you and your colleagues are saying is, you cannot expand mental health care without expanding a trained workforce. And this is especially true in rural areas. And your eloquent words, I believe, spoke for a lot of providers from rural areas. And it seems to me you have a big challenge filling key slots like licensed clinical social workers who serve Medicare and Medicaid patients, nurses who do so many things well, starting with health screening and recovering patients, who play a key role in terms of peer support. In listening to you over the years, you have convinced me the professionals are essentially the glue holding the mental health system together.

Now I would like to get your thoughts with respect to the workforce, and particularly on the question of having enough people, and then preventing burnout. Because my understanding is that the pandemic just made things a lot more treacherous for so many professionals who just wanted to step up and help people.

Deaths from opioids are 30 percent higher than last year. The number of emergency department visits for suicide and drug overdoses are up more than 25 percent. Three to four times as many people are identifying as facing depression today than before the pandemic.

Why don't you tell the committee—because I have heard you speak to this in the past. It was always a challenge before the pandemic. Tell us what you think is really happening now with how the pandemic has made it much harder for you and your colleagues to do the terrific advocacy you do.

Ms. JETT. Sure. I am happy to speak to that. Crisis burnout is at an all-time high. Every single one of our crisis clinicians will— well, clinicians in general that we hire have to take a crisis rotation. The crisis numbers since the pandemic started have tripled. And the acuity level of those crises has gone from a very simple ''I have a lot of anxiety''; ''my cat is stuck in a tree for the past 2 days, and I am not sure what to do''; ''I am having a panic attack''; to the most recent crisis call that we had, which was, ''I have a loaded shotgun, and I intend to use it as soon as we get off this call.''

I have never, in my 15 years of being part of a mental health system, ever experienced the acuity level of crises, the burnout with clinicians, and crisis acuity levels with the patients that we see now.

The CHAIRMAN. Well, thank you for giving us a case example. I have heard you speak to this challenge of facing cases that are so much more serious—I guess the technical lingo is the greater level of acuity—but what a wake-up call, to go from having lots of calls where people are facing anxiety with cats in the trees and the like, to people with loaded shotguns saying that they are prepared to use them. So, thank you very much for that, and for coming.

Dr. Durham, I want to talk to you about our challenges with parity. As you know, we got a Government Accountability Office report documenting all the barriers people face in trying to get behavioral health. The Federal laws have been on the books. I remember the day my Dad and I talked about the parity law. We said, ''This could help Jeff Wyden, a schizophrenic.'' We rejoiced. And yet, what I hear is that there are still all kinds of barriers to patients getting the care they need.

And I would like to have you describe what you think is really going on out there with the parity law. And I gather your patients are facing a lot of barriers, and you still do not think the spirit of the law that would treat mental health like physical health is being honored.

I would like to hear your words.

Dr. DURHAM. Thank you for the question, Senator Wyden. I completely agree that we have not made any headway with parity for mental health and physical health. We have a long way to go.

A really concrete example is that I work in the psychiatric emergency room at Boston Medical Center. As I mentioned in my oral testimony, we have people who—we have like tripled, quadrupled the capacity during the pandemic. One of the things that slows the process for us as a team of psychiatrists, licensed clinical social workers, psychologists, is that we evaluate the patient, we decide that they need inpatient psychiatric level of care, and then we start talking to the insurer.

And that takes a lot of time, where we could be seeing other patients that are acutely in need of services by us, and we have to go back and forth faxing paperwork. Then you have to do a bed search and see what psych unit will accept your patient. And if it is Medicaid or Medicare, generally they want to know for Medicare, ''Well, have they met their capacity of days they can be in a psych unit?'' And then if they have, total lifetime days, then we are stuck with a patient boarding with us until we can figure out what else we can do.

And for Medicaid, it is a lot of back and forth for our folks. And around 50 percent of our patients are on Medicaid. So that is a huge amount of time when we are in the emergency room spent going back and forth for, essentially, a prior authorization

And I like to use the example that when a patient comes into the emergency room in acute stroke, or having a heart attack, the physician in that moment makes a decision that they need inpatient hospitalization, and they go to the medical floor without having to go back and forth with an insurer deciding if that is actually the appropriate level of care.

The CHAIRMAN. Thank you. And you know, obviously it was not the spirit of this bipartisan law from Senator Wellstone and Senator Domenici, to have patients and providers having to go into what is almost armed battle to try to navigate just a fair shake for patients and their providers. So I really appreciate your being here.

I am over my time.

Senator Crapo?

Senator CRAPO. Thank you, Mr. Chairman.

This question is for you, Mr. Betlach. There is bipartisan interest in expanding opportunities for integration of physical and mental health services across all payers. While some approaches prioritize payment, others use co-location services, or the use of case managers under a medical home model, to achieve this goal.

What are some of the examples of integration that could be a road map for Medicare or Medicaid in the near future? And how could waivers be used in State Medicaid programs to enhance access to care?

Mr. BETLACH. Senator, thank you for the question. I think there are a lot of different approaches States can take, and certainly it depends upon the ecosystem of each unique State.

I think the first thing it starts with is, States need a strategy. What is your integration strategy? So as States think about this, they should be able to develop a plan in terms of a multiyear strategy that they are going to be implementing around integration.

And as I mentioned in my testimony, there are really three levels to integration. There is how you think about it at the policy level. And for us in Arizona, it was thinking about some simple things like, what are the regulations that we have in place for providers to help build integration? Do we require some silly things like—we had two separate entryways and challenges around billing; and so, making sure that, as a State, we were clearing out some of those regulatory burdens that existed for integration.

States may or may not want to integrate and braid funding sources like we did in Arizona at the payer level, but States should certainly have a strategy around maximizing care coordination between payers. So, if you are going to have a carve-out of behavioral health services, how are you going to ensure that there is care coordination for individuals who require both physical health and behavioral health services?

And then finally, States need a strategy in terms of how they are supporting providers in terms of integration. It may be opening up things like the collaborative care model codes in terms of being able to pay for services that are done at the primary care site, like Dr. Miller talked about. There may be other incentives.

We leveraged, in Arizona, an 1115 waiver to create provider payments for milestones that were achieved in terms of advancing integration strategies like connecting to our health information exchange and other areas like that.

So, States need a plan, and the plan needs to address each of those three critical areas: policy, pay integration, and provider support of integration.

Senator CRAPO. Thank you.

Ms. Jett, you have very well described the issues that you face in a rural community in providing the needed services we are discussing today. Unfortunately, the stigma around receiving mental health treatment can be even higher in rural areas.

Can you speak to these challenges? And what approaches has your clinic taken to combat them?

Ms. JETT. I can. Thank you for the question.

We have been integrated with primary care since 2012 through a series of SAMHSA and HRSA grants. We are partnered, as I said in my testimony, with a local Federally Qualified Health Center. And together we have built a 20,000-square-foot building to provide primary care, dental services, VA services, and behavioral health, all under one roof.

We are moving in, hopefully in August, and we are hoping that this destigmatizes your car from being in the parking lot, because people will not understand why you are there or what services you are receiving. So this is one way that we thought, in a frontier community, we could reduce the stigma of people receiving services.

Senator CRAPO. Well, thank you very much.

And, Dr. Durham, one of the positive outcomes of the pandemic has been, as we have discussed here, the significant expansion of telehealth, which is an important tool to expand access.

Have you found any limitations to tele-mental health for treating your patients, and particularly the younger ones?

Dr. DURHAM. Thank you for the question. Absolutely, I think telehealth has been critical to meeting our patients' needs during this time. But there is a subset of the population where I think we need more research and understanding of how it is going to work fundamentally.

I am a child psychiatrist who practices in a child clinic, and we went to telehealth pretty quickly as well. And I think it was difficult with some of our families too, because when we practice, we want a place where someone can speak to us directly. We want the parents to be separate from the room so that we can engage with the kid, whether that is a 5-year-old, or a 12-year-old, or a 16-year old.

And it was very hard for some of the families who are in lowincome communities, who are in multigenerational homes, to have that private place to have a session. And so that was some of the difficulty we saw.

I think for little ones, especially kids who have early intervention services as well, so that 0 to 5 age range, we are also thinking about how we come back now to the office space again. And some of those kids we probably will need to see in person at some point and then maybe go back to telehealth once we have established a relationship. For the little ones, it is a little bit more challenging. And I think for the adult population, some of our folks who have substance use disorders in particular, and are homeless, really did not have the technology necessary to always engage with that support. So, throughout the pandemic as well, what we did was, every day of the week we always had somebody who was there in person in our clinics to make sure that people could get the care they needed and did not have to rely on tele-technology to get the services they wanted.

So, I think there is work to do. And I would also say that the audio-only was critical during this time as well. And so, any way we can expand that and make sure post-COVID, if you will, that we still get reimbursement for that, especially in some of our integrated care models—it was critical to have the audio-only be reimbursed at the same rate.

Senator CRAPO. Thank you. I am out of time.

The CHAIRMAN. Thank you, Senator Crapo. Senator Stabenow?

Senator STABENOW. Well, thank you very much, Mr. Chairman and Senator Crapo. I really want to thank you for this hearing. It has been a while since we have had a hearing focus on mental health and substance abuse services, and I really appreciate your leadership. And to all of you, you have all raised issues that are so incredibly important.

I want to speak specifically to what I think is foundational in the community. And, Ms. Jett, you were talking about the Certified Community Behavioral Health Clinics that go to the core of integrating funding and really treating mental health and substance abuse as part of the healthcare system. I always say we should treat health care above the neck the same as health care below the neck, and not just through a focus on grants that stop and start. It needs to be integrated in Medicaid, and it needs to be prospective payment so we can have the full opportunity for professionals being funded.

So today I am really pleased to say that Senator Blunt and I— along with our chairman, Senators Daines, Cortez Masto, Smith, and Tester—welcome all the members of the committee to be cosponsors in the next step. We have 10 States that have been doing a demonstration of how this can work with high-quality standards, and today we introduced legislation that would allow States across the country to be able to do this, which is incredibly important.

We have, through our startup grants, through the COVID process, we have been able to bring in dollars, as has been indicated, to over 300 communities across the country, 40 States plus DC, to do startup grants. But what we need is comprehensive community care. And this all really started, I have to say, because Senator Blunt and I worked together on Federally Qualified Health Centers, which are widely supported on a bipartisan basis. And the idea, as you said, is quality standards. If the community clinic can meet the high quality standards, they get full reimbursement in the healthcare system. And so that is what this is. The idea is to integrate those payments.

So, Ms. Jett, no surprise, I have a question for you to expand on CCBHCs. You really were one of the very first in the country and have done just a marvelous job in showing what can be done. But I wonder if you could expand more on the issue of permanent funding.

You know, I have always said to colleagues that it is like having someone having a heart attack, and they go to the hospital and they are going to immediately get treated. Right now, in too many places around the country, if somebody walks into a mental health center, it is the equivalent of saying, ''I am sorry, the grant ran out, can you come back in a few months?'' when somebody is in crisis, which obviously is ridiculous.

So, could you talk a little bit more about the importance of integrating funding and permanent funding in the mental health and substance abuse system?

Ms. JETT. Of course. I would like to give a couple of examples first about how the system is currently funded, which presents a variety of challenges for us.

For example, on the Medicare side, only licensed clinical social workers or medical doctors can treat Medicare patients for mental health services. What this means in a frontier county is, if we only have one or two licensed clinical social workers on staff, then the remainder of those services being delivered to Medicare patients are being written off.

In our CCBHC, we write off upwards of $500,000 a year for Medicare-delivered services. Our growing population is over 65 and under 17. We have the under-17 covered, but the over-65 population is underserved. And really the reason is, we do not have the licenses available to treat those people.

So, the funding for CCBHCs allows that wrap-around payment to bridge the gap of services not being currently financed. It is vital, and it is important that we fund the business of mental health. People just want to fund the services, but there is an actual infrastructure that is required to provide this high level of integrated care.

Senator STABENOW. Thank you so much. And in the limited time I have left, let me ask you to speak a little bit more to integrating care. Again, the financing model really is about integrating primary care for individuals. It is a whole person, and we segregate them when we are talking about various ways to provide health care. But could you talk about the delivery of behavioral health services and what you do in the context of providing primary care for people?

Ms. JETT. Sure. Well, the CCBHC model in Oregon allows for 20 hours or more of primary care to be delivered, as we say, on our turf in the behavioral health system. This building, co-located with our local FQHC, works both sides of that equation, right? Because we understand that there are many people who want to access behavioral health services—specifically those with persistent and severe mental illness—on the behavioral health side.

Conversely, there are people on the primary care side who only want to access behavioral health services from their primary care doc. And so, having both an FQHC and a CCBHC in one location allows for multiple access to services in the integration.

Senator STABENOW. Thank you very much. Thank you, Mr. Chairman.

The CHAIRMAN. I thank my colleague.

Senator Crapo and I will be working very closely with you and Senator Daines as we go forward on these issues in a bipartisan way.

Let's see. What we are going to do, because I think a couple of our hearings have been a challenge with so many Senators having hectic schedules, I am just going to call the names in order of appearance.

So, Senator Grassley would be next. I am not sure he is available, but I thought we ought to check. Senator Grassley?

[No response.]

The CHAIRMAN. Okay. Senator Cantwell is of course here and has been a longstanding leader in terms of healthcare advocacy, so let's recognize Senator Cantwell.

Senator CANTWELL. Thank you, Mr. Chairman. And thank you and the ranking member for holding this important hearing, and my colleague Senator Stabenow for her leadership on this.

Many of you have mentioned—well, a big theme this morning is the integration of mental and physical health. I appreciate everybody honing in on what we could do about that. To me, this is— you know, when I look at 20 to 25 percent of the homeless population having mental health problems, I think there are costs. These are just continued costs to the system that we have not taken care of. And if we had an integrated system, and I think even better case management, because—who is managing the situation? If the person has mental health problems, who is managing the situation? And if no one can talk to any of the people, how could you possibly integrate the physical and mental health?

I am sure I am not telling you anything. The drugs that people are taking for mental health cause a lot of physical problems. So, this has to be fixed.

So what do you think we can do to get our colleagues to understand that we are losing money that we could save now if we would just fix this integration? So either Dr. Miller, since you were very big on this, or Dr. Durham—either one.

Dr. MILLER. Well, Senator, thank you for the question. I will just begin by saying that I think you put your finger right in the center of the biggest problem that we have, which is how we have bifurcated, trifurcated, and split apart health. When you talk about services for the unhoused, or you begin to look at our children versus adults, we have fragmentation in almost every level. So, to integrate requires us to have really thoughtful strategies that look at the issue at multiple levels simultaneously. And I will give you one example of that.

If we simply look at how we clinically integrate care, without paying attention to how we financially support that integration, it usually falls apart. If we do not look at the administrative or operational functions that also provide oversight, it means that a lot of well-intended folks out there trying to bring these integration services together usually fall apart because there is not a structure for them to ultimately be grabbed by and supported.

So, when we look at health, it is an opportunity to really think about that integration at multiple levels. So, thank you for the question.

Senator CANTWELL. Dr. Durham?

Dr. DURHAM. Sure. Thank you for that question. I am very aligned with what you said about case management and those services needed for families that present with a lot of issues besides just the mental health issue.

In our model for TEAM UP for Children, which is in FQHCs in the greater Boston area, we have a community health worker as part of the model for just that: to do some of that care coordination not only between the schools, but thinking about housing insecurity, food insecurity, and what other services are needed.

I think what happens many times, though, is that the case management service, the community health worker, or even a peer coach, are not usually reimbursed by the system. And so it does end up being a lot of grant funding. And I appreciated what Ms. Jett said as well, that the grant funding ends and then all those services that helped support families and patients also go away.

And so, ways that we can embed that more into the system from a reimbursement perspective would be fantastic.

Senator CANTWELL. Well, I just go back to an example of the— as the chairman knows, I am a big supporter of affordable housing too, but hospitals are now helping to finance affordable housing so you can have a roof over somebody's head so that they do not keep coming to the emergency room. And while you are talking about helping families, I am talking about the cost to the system when people have no support or no help.

I do not think we have a clue about how much we are running up the bills that we could do a better job with if we just had integration and case management for these people. Then we could make better decisions and lower the costs.

And so, I hope we come to understand this, because a lot of our— I think what we are seeing in homelessness is people who just literally fall through the cracks. They do not have anybody advocating for them. They have bounced in between these things. They do not have the issue taken care of, and the next thing you know, they are out on the street.

This is then costing all of us in all sorts of other ways. So to me, let's understand that this is a task certainly about helping people, but it is also a task about fixing the system that is costing us way more than it needs to cost us at this point.

Thank you, Mr. Chairman.

The CHAIRMAN. Thank you, Senator Cantwell. And as usual, you go right to the heart of the case, which is, who manages a lot of these cases? Who is, in effect, in charge? And as I saw with my late brother, as he suffered from schizophrenia, he got good care in a number of instances, but too often we could not figure out who was in charge. And I said to myself continually through this odyssey, if this is what an elected official who has tried to specialize in health care faces—and I spent years and years in those communities playing basketball—what is it like for the typical person? So, thank you. Thank you for hitting the question of who is going to manage these cases, and Senator Cantwell said it so well, as always.

Senator Thune, I believe you are out there on the web.

Senator THUNE. Yes, I am.

The CHAIRMAN. Are you available?

Senator THUNE. Yes, sir. Thank you, Mr. Chairman. And thanks to our panelists for being with us today.

I think most everyone can agree that telehealth has proven to be an important tool on our tool belt for increasing access to mental health services. And once we get past this pandemic, I have concerns about a policy enacted last year that will require an in- person visit for Medicare to pay for tele-mental health.

One of the things I hear everywhere in South Dakota is, it does not matter what the provider setting is, whether it is Indian Health Service or the VA or our public hospitals in South Dakota, our schools, we cannot find, recruit, and retain providers. And so, as we are talking about the need to increase access, it seems to me that this arbitrary and inconsistent barrier does not make sense.

In fact, in rural America it stands to make access even more inequitable.

Ms. Jett, can you share some perspectives on how telehealth has helped rural patients overcome the stigma of seeking mental health services and the potential challenge an in-person requirement can have moving forward?

Ms. JETT. Of course. Thank you for the question. Of course, there are both pros and cons to receiving telehealth services. I am happy to say that our clinic provided services nearly seamlessly through the pandemic because of the use of telehealth.

However, as Dr. Durham has pointed out, those in underprivileged or underserved communities often struggle with technology, as well as appropriate hot spots or Wi-Fi capability.

And so, what we have done as a community is, we took some of the FEMA crisis money that we received, and we bought 10 iPads and 10 hot spots to deliver to children and families and community members who were without Wi-Fi or technology services that were available to them.

We would often have them drive into the clinic and park in the parking lot. We would walk out an iPad, and they would hook up to our system right there in the parking lot and have their psychiatrist appointment or therapist appointment right there in the parking lot.

So, telehealth services have certainly expanded the access, but also have prevented some people from accessing services too, specifically the population with severe and persistent mental illness. This has been a great barrier to them, unfortunately.

It is very difficult to explain to someone with severe and persistent mental illness that their therapist is on the TV. That is a little odd. So it has been a bit of a challenge with that particular population. But overall, I think it has improved access.

Senator THUNE. Well, thank you. And I guess I would direct this to anybody on the panel. The in-person requirement passed last year is not consistent with multiple telehealth policies previously enacted by this committee, like the eTREAT Act for substance use disorder, and the FAST Act for stroke.

Would you support legislation to remove the face-to-face requirement for mental health, like Senator Cassidy has introduced along with Senators Cardin, Smith, and I? And keep in mind that there is nothing to stop an individual provider from requiring their patient to have an in-person visit. And to Ms. Jett's earlier comment, I serve on another committee, the Commerce, Science, and Transportation Committee, which is working on the Wi-Fi issue and trying to make those services available to more people across the country.

But with respect to this issue, this piece of legislation that Senator Cassidy is leading, and some of us are co-sponsoring, does anybody want to talk about that particular legislation, whether or not you think that is something that you all could support and that makes sense as we look at better solutions to deal with mental health challenges facing this country?

Dr. DURHAM. Yes, I can take that. I think that having a 6-month in-person provision will really be an unnecessary barrier to folks getting care. And I think it should be at the discretion of the clinician or physician seeing the patient whether or not they need to see them again for an in-person visit. And I think we would go down this road again of, it is a parity issue of why, for certain illnesses or disorders you do not need it, and for mental health you would need it.

So, I would be very aligned with not having this provision and just using the discretion of the clinician on whether or not they need an in-person evaluation.

Senator THUNE. Great. Anybody else?

Ms. JETT. Well, I think the bottom line is, we just have to be a flexible system that is amenable to serving all people of all populations at any time they request access for services.

So, requiring these barriers seems sort of silly to me. And I hope that we can think twice about something like that.

Mr. BETLACH. Especially if the beneficiaries have now seen the value in receiving services through this mode of treatment.

Senator THUNE. Okay. Great. My time has expired. Thank you, Mr. Chairman. Thank you, panel.

The CHAIRMAN. Thank you, Senator Thune. And I think you are making very important points with respect to these various issues requiring a previous appointment in order to get to telehealth. We have to work through those issues, and we are going to do it in a bipartisan way Senator Grassley would be next.

Senator GRASSLEY. Thank you, Mr. Chairman.

In 2019, I passed the bipartisan ACE Kids Act, with the help of Senator Bennet, that will align Medicaid rules and payments to incentivize coordination and improve health outcomes. This Congress, I am working with Senator Bennet to build onto the ACE Kids Act with the Accelerating Kids Access to Care Act. A key aspect of this effort is to enable the pediatric health home to coordinate care with children, including the prevention and treatment of mental illness and substance abuse.

So, for Mr. Betlach and Dr. Durham, you both discussed in your written testimony the importance of care coordination to addressing fragmentations in the healthcare system. The ACE Kids Act requires States to ensure mental healthcare coordination is included when establishing a pediatric health home. What lessons can be learned from both your experience as a provider and a State Medicaid Director with upcoming implementation of the ACE Kids Act in 2022?

Dr. DURHAM. Thank you for the question, Senator Grassley. I think the more we can coordinate care for kids and families, the better, at any opportunity. Kids are in many different systems: school systems, their community, their family network, and all of their providers, especially as kids have more complex medical conditions. And so, I would be in great support—any time we can provide the services to coordinate care, the better it is. And I think what we have seen in some of our models that have focused on pediatric and mental health integration in FQHCs is that, the more members of the team that are involved with every system that the kid is in, the better it is for the kid. Their mental health gets better. Their physical health gets better. And then of course, where they thrive is at school and at home, ultimately. So, thank you for that question.

Mr. BETLACH. Senator Grassley, what we have seen in Arizona is that States need to have a strategy around the different silos that exist in terms of where complex kids may be, whether it is working with the foster care system, whether it is working with kids who may be receiving services through a waiver for individuals with developmental disabilities. Really, the State needs to be looking at the delivery of behavioral health services holistically and how it is going to serve those populations and reduce the fragmentation.

And so, it is leveraging the investments that SAMHSA has made, for example, with first-episode psychosis to make sure that Medicaid is plugging into the infrastructure that is being created, and looking at that. So, if it is using managed care or fee-for-service, the State needs a plan in terms of how it is going to take kids with these complex needs and get them the services that they need.

Senator GRASSLEY. In the last Congress, we made mental health services via telehealth a permanent benefit of Medicaid. So, for Dr. Durham and Dr. Miller: as healthcare providers, how best can Congress support this expansion of mental telehealth while ensuring improved health outcomes for individuals served by the expansion of access?

Dr. DURHAM. Access has been greatly improved with telehealth. We have seen that throughout the pandemic, and with our patients. You know, as we discussed previously, I do think there are certain populations where it is more difficult.

And so, audio-only has been very helpful throughout the pandemic. We have seen that a lot in some of our integrated care settings, whether that is pediatric integrated care, or internal medicine integrated care for primary care—at least at Boston Medical Center.

And so, I hope that the provision would still continue to allow audio-only visits at the same reimbursement rates, because it has significantly impacted and helped many of the homeless population, folks who do not always have access to the technology.

Dr. MILLER. I agree with Dr. Durham. And, Senator Grassley, thank you for the question.

The uptick in telehealth utilization for mental health has been a very helpful sign. The people like it when care is able to come to them. And if we are really going to put the patients and families first, we do have to consider policies like the in-person requirement we just discussed and consider whether or not these things are good or bad for people. Does it restrict their access? Does it restrict where they are going to be able to ultimately use these services? So, making permanent the audio-only, having payment parity, and allowing this for all forms of outpatient care, is a tremendous benefit for so many people across our country.

Senator GRASSLEY. I will yield.

The CHAIRMAN. Thank you, Senator Grassley.

Next would be Senator Carper. Is he available on the web? Senator CARPER. Senator Carper is right here.

The CHAIRMAN. Okay, and we can hear you. Go ahead.

Senator CARPER. Thank you, sir. I welcome each of our witnesses today.

My staff and I have heard from pediatricians from across the country, including in the Nemours Children's Hospital, the fabled children's hospital that we are very proud of. And we hear from any number of sources that our country is experiencing a mental health crisis among our children. And I do not think it is just in Delaware, I think it is throughout our country.

But during the pandemic, children have experienced major disruptions as a result of public health safety measures, including school closures, social isolation, financial hardships, and gaps in healthcare access. It has become clear that COVID–19 has significantly exacerbated the health stress on our children and youth, highlighting our Nation's acute shortage of mental health services and the need to reinforce and expand the pediatric mental health delivery systems and infrastructure.

A question for Dr. Durham, if I could. Dr. Durham, what more can those of us in the Congress do to address root causes and support effective approaches to prevention and early identification of mental and behavioral health issues? Dr. Durham?

Dr. DURHAM. Thank you very much for that question. As you mentioned, many of our kids have experienced a lot of loss. And when we think of loss, it is not only death within their family, but also thinking of not being able to see their friends or do the social activities and other things that fulfill and support their livelihood. I do think one thing that we need to think through from a prevention/promotion standpoint is that many of our schools, even in the Boston area, do not have school therapists that they have access to. So, we do not want people to always get treatment once there is a severe level of illness and they need to be in a hospital or an emergency room, but how can we start thinking in a prevention and promotion framework of just touches, if you will? So, meaning that something is going on. A teacher notes it, or a principal, or someone in the school or the family, and they have the services right there within the school system before we get to the point where you are calling the emergency services or a crisis line. There are not enough supports within the school system to do any of that sort of prevention and promotion framework. Teachers are doing a lot. They are doing their job. But we do not have therapists embedded in many of our schools, even when we think about a resource-rich place like Massachusetts. And so, I think it is critical that we think about it in that framework.

I do think pediatric integrated care is another way to think more about prevention and promotion; so, seeing children and families at their well-child visit, which we do in Massachusetts, and start thinking and asking those questions about what stresses are happening in their lives and getting care for immediate needs—whether it is a mild behavioral health need, depression or anxiety that is not to the point where maybe they are thinking about harming themselves or harming anyone else.

So, using that framework of prevention and promotion, I think, is critical. And sometimes that is not necessarily reimbursable from a mental health standpoint as it is for physical health. Kids are supposed to go get their visits quite early in life for a check-in. And the more we can think about even like a mental health check-in with their primary care provider or therapist in the school, I think the better we would all be in the long run.

Senator CARPER. Thanks.

A question for the record, if I could, for all of our witnesses. Several months ago I was in the Bay Area in California visiting a number of promising technology companies. One was called Ginger, G-i-n-g-e-r, in the Bay Area. And they focus on coverage for—or they focus on mental health screenings, and behavioral health coaching. And I have a question regarding the coverage for those screenings and coaching. And I would just ask you if any of you find virtual behavioral health coaching to be an efficient means of preventing serious mental illness? And if so, should Congress consider mandating coverage for virtual mental health screenings and behavioral health coaching in plans offered on the health insurance marketplace? That is a question for the record for each of you.

Thank you, very much. Thank you, Mr. Chairman and Ranking Member.

The CHAIRMAN. Thank you, Senator Carper.

So, colleagues, we are going to keep this going. Our guests will, I am sure, find this somewhat entertaining, because we have all these votes, and Senators are coming in and going, but we are going to keep it going.

The next four questioners from the committee will be Senator Cardin, Senator Cassidy, Senator Bennet, and Senator Daines.

So, Senator Cardin, if he is available on the web, would be next. And as I say, we are just going to keep this going.

Senator Cardin, are you out there in cyberspace? [No response.]

The CHAIRMAN. Okay. Senator Cassidy has been sitting here all morning.

Senator CASSIDY. Thank you, Mr. Chairman.

Dr. Durham, I think I may have given you a lecture in medical school.

Dr. DURHAM. I think you may have. [Laughter.]

Senator CASSIDY. You may recall, it was on diarrhea and hepatitis. I was famous on those lectures. There will be a quiz as to hepatitis A and how it is transmitted, but we will do that off the record. Thank you, very much.

It is incredibly gratifying to me to see you and how your career has gone.

Dr. DURHAM. Thank you very much.

Senator CASSIDY. Let me echo Senator Thune's endorsement of the bill that we have introduced as regards telehealth, tele-mental health. And, Mr. Chair, I would like to submit two letters which support this legislation that we are putting forward with Senator Thune, as you mentioned, but also Senators Smith and Cardin— and I have lost the list. And so, this letter is from the American Telemedicine Association, and this is a group of folks with the Health Innovation Alliance of the American Telemedicine Association.

The CHAIRMAN. Without objection, so ordered, Senator Cassidy. And Senator Crapo and I will be working very closely with you and the coalition on this very important idea.

[The letters appear in the appendix on p. 54.]

Senator CASSIDY. Thank you.

Mr. Betlach, good to see you.

Mr. BETLACH. Senator Cassidy, good to see you, sir.

Senator CASSIDY. Your hair is a little longer—— [Laughter.]

Listen, several questions for you. You and I both know, in fact we all know, dual-eligibles are just a terrible mess, very expensive to care for, with terrible outcomes. We are spending incredible amounts of money to get terrible outcomes. It is the worst of all. Now SAMHSA has a lot of grants out there in order to address the issues of the mentally ill, as well as those who have substance abuse, and yet there seems to be poor coordination with Medicaid.

You have experience. Can you give some ideas as to how we could better coordinate those programs?

Mr. BETLACH. Sure, Senator Cassidy. That is an incredibly important question. In Arizona, roughly 40 percent of the population of individuals with serious mental illness are dual-eligible members, which actually leads to incredible fragmentation, as you described.

When I first became the Medicaid Director, if you were an individual with a serious mental illness, you had a plan for physical health for Medicaid, a plan for behavioral health for Medicaid, Medicare fee-for-service, Medicare Part D—four different organizations that were potentially involved in paying for your services, none of them coordinated.

As you said, it has led to just terrible results. On average, an individual with serious mental illness dies 25 years younger than peers, and oftentimes it is from untreated chronic diseases.

And so, in Arizona, it all comes back to the system design issue. Who is accountable in this? And it is very challenging with dual-eligible members. But we created and built off some of the Federal regulations that exist that said the managed care organization that was responsible for providing services for individuals with serious mental illness not only had to deliver Medicaid services but Arizona Medicaid programs, the third largest housing authority, so there were rental subsidies that were flowing through the Medicaid program—employment support services. Very importantly, the plan had to be a dual special needs plan, which meant that it offered the Medicare services, which meant it was then accountable for delivering Medicare services to that population.

Senator CASSIDY. Let me stop you.

Mr. BETLACH. Yes.

Senator CASSIDY. Great ideas: aligning incentives, a point of authority, everything that checks the boxes. What were your outcomes? Were you able to improve outcome for the duals?

Mr. BETLACH. Yes. In the independent third-party study that was done by Mercer, we saw an increase in terms of all the HEDIS scores for ambulatory and chronic management, and an increase in all of the CAHPS scores.

Senator CASSIDY. Now let me ask, because sometimes those are process-oriented as opposed to outcomes-oriented——

Mr. BETLACH. Right.

Senator CASSIDY. And so, to what degree did you see emergency room visits decrease? Return to workforce? Longer life span, et cetera?

Mr. BETLACH. We do not have the indicator yet on longer life- span. We are only a few years into this, right? So that is going to be a lagging measure as we look at the different indicators. But we did see a decrease in emergency department utilization and an increased use of primary care. Again, not necessarily outcome measures, right, but it is a start.

Senator CASSIDY. Well, let me ask, then—because I am almost out of time—specifically, integrating SAMHSA grants in there, were you able to do that as well?

Mr. BETLACH. We did. We flowed all of the SAMHSA block grant dollars to that organization. They were responsible for those as well. So again, a single accountable organization that had all those dollars braided in it.

Senator CASSIDY. Gotcha. I thank you all for your good work. I really appreciate it.

And again, Dr. Durham, it is great to see your success.

Dr. DURHAM. Thank you.

Senator CASSIDY. And I yield back.

The CHAIRMAN. Thank you, Senator Cassidy. We are going to be working very closely with you as we go forward on this committee effort.

Senator Bennet is next.

Senator BENNET. Thank you, Mr. Chairman. And again, thank you very much for holding this hearing. I hope that it is only the start of a larger effort to address the mental health issues in our country. I, like my colleagues, am deeply concerned about the issue of parity and how insurance companies and providers often erect barriers to adequate mental health coverage.

Senator Kaine and I were working on developing our Medicare- X Choice Act to create a public option, and mental health access was at the top of our mind. We viewed this as an opportunity to improve access to people, especially in rural areas. And a key provision in this proposal provides primary care to patients with a public option without cost sharing—and this should absolutely include mental health care.

Dr. Miller—and anybody else on the panel who would like to answer—can you speak to how a public option could be designed to integrate mental health and primary care? How should this elevate the standards on parity that currently do not exist in the private health insurance market?

Dr. MILLER. Thank you for the question, Senator Bennet, and thanks for your ongoing leadership in this space.

First, from a coverage perspective, any public option should incorporate some of the key lessons that we are learning from landmark Federal cases like Wit vs. United Behavioral Health. This includes things like requiring coverage to be consistent with generally accepted standards of care that ensure the inclusion of civil enforcement provisions.

Second, a public option can actually create a standard for integrating care. A public option can determine the scope of services, and it can actually raise the bar on expectations for integrated practices. This is needed, and overnight it could create a new mechanism to support integrated primary care.

And then finally, a public option could expand the scope of services and the range of providers to make sure that it pays for critical services that augment the onsite delivery, like peer support specialists. Hence really, if you bake it into a public option, you are beginning to change the game from how people have experienced mental health and primary care on the ground.

Senator BENNET. Anybody else? [No response.]

Senator BENNET. I am deeply concerned with the increased rates of mental illness that young people are experiencing, leading to death by suicide, substance use, or other mental and behavioral health challenges.

In Colorado, it has been 5 years since suicide became the leading cause of death for kids aged 10 and older. And at the same time, we have seen a reduction in beds for youth suffering from mental illness. We have seen that decreased by 1,000 in the past decade. A few weeks ago, our children's hospital declared, quote, ''a pediatric mental health state of emergency,'' as emergency mental health visits were up 90 percent in April of 2021 compared to April 2019.

What gaps exist in the tools needed to address the mental health challenges facing our children and young adults across the continuum of mental health care, particularly for the Medicaid population? I know a lot of our colleagues are working on improving home and community-based services. How can we ensure that kids and families are receiving mental health services at home or in their communities? I don't know, Dr. Durham, whether you might want to get us started?

Dr. DURHAM. Sure, I can get us started. I think it is a fantastic and great question, so I appreciate it. I think it also has a lot to do with the care continuum. I think what we have seen is, everything has been exacerbated. What we knew pre-pandemic was that we do not have enough services for kids. I think a State like Massachusetts has done a good job. Senator Cassidy is from Louisiana, which is my home State, which is very different. And my family and friends are still there, and I can compare Massachusetts and Louisiana.

And so, we do have a continuum for care. We have in-home services for kids on State Medicaid in Massachusetts with different language capacities. And I think that model should be replicated in other States similar to the State of Louisiana, where I come from, where there are very limited resources for kids on the State Medicaid.

And that care continuum has day programs in Massachusetts. We have crisis units for kids so we do not have to go all the way to the highest level of care, which is a locked psychiatric unit for kids. And you know, as previously stated, I do think we need to do something to expand school-based therapists at schools.

We do not have enough. That is where kids are most of the day. That is what gets noticed quickly by teachers and other people who see them day in and day out. And so, these are ways that we can work from a prevention and promotion framework. Kids as young as 12, 13, and 14 will tell you when they are in their early 20s, ''I knew when I was 12 that something was going on.'' And either maybe a parent or a caregiver did not recognize, but also there was no one to go to.

So, the more that we can invest in that, all the way from prevention and promotion along the care continuum, I think the better for all of our kids.

Senator BENNET. Thank you, Mr. Chairman.

I am out of time, but I appreciate that answer very much.

Senator CRAPO [presiding]. Thank you, Senator Bennet. The chairman has gone over to vote. I don't know if it has been explained that we have two votes going right now, so we are kind of rotating back and forth. Plus, we have a lot of members who may or may not be available because of that. But I am just going to go down the list.

I am told that Senator Daines is on his way here, but let me just ask. Is Senator Daines on the Internet?

[No response.]

Senator CRAPO. All right. I am just going to call out some names, and if nobody answers, I am going to—did I just hear somebody? If nobody answers, I will ask a few of my own additional questions.

Senator Casey? [No response.]

Senator CRAPO. Senator Young? [No response.]

Senator CRAPO. Senator Warner? [No response.]

Senator CRAPO. Senator Whitehouse? [No response.]

Senator CRAPO. Senator Hassan? Here is Senator Daines. You are up. [Pause.]

Senator DAINES. Mr. Chairman, thank you. And truly, I am very glad that we are holding this hearing today on such an important topic.

Last month, Senator Stabenow and I hosted our first Finance Health Care Subcommittee hearing of the year, since May was mental health month. We focused on the importance of improving access to mental health services and how the COVID crisis has im- pacted patients as well as providers.

We were fortunate to have Lenette Kosovich as our Montana witness. She is the CEO of the largest behavioral health organization in Montana, and she was able to highlight the challenges our rural communities face when it comes to accessing mental health care. She also discussed the benefits of the Certified Community Behavioral Health Clinic model, known as the CCBHC model, which brings the reimbursement for behavioral health services on par with that for physical healthcare services.

In fact, following that hearing, Senator Stabenow and I decided to team up in this legislation to allow States, including Montana, to adopt the CCBHC model. In fact, we are introducing it today. Our bipartisan bill will integrate the physical and the mental health care and provide patients with access to treatment more quickly.

Ms. Jett, how can the CCBHC model help rural communities like those in Montana that face access challenges and have a shortage of mental health professionals?

Ms. JETT. Thank you for your question. We really believe in the CCBHC model. In fact, we have been one of the first to adopt it and have been using the model for about 4 years now.

We find that integrating the services, or creating what we like to call the neck in between the head and the body, really helps improve outcomes for patients that we serve. It also improves access to underserved populations, specifically veterans in our community who have really benefited from us becoming a CCBHC, primarily because Oregon wrote a waiver with the CCBHC model that would allow veterans to access care from non-veteran clinics.

So, where we live in northeast Oregon is about a 2-hour drive for any veteran receiving any sort of services, medical or mental health services. And so, by becoming a CCBHC, and along with that Oregon waiver, we are able to treat local veterans for behavioral health issues. It has been really powerful.

Senator DAINES. As the son of a veteran, thank you.

I recently introduced legislation with Senator Cortez Masto to make permanent a CARES Act policy that I championed allowing first-dollar coverage of virtual care under these high-deductible health plans. Our bipartisan bill would allow Montanans and Americans across our country to continue accessing essential care like mental health and primary care services, without the burden of first meeting a deductible. With more than 50 percent of American workers now receiving their healthcare coverage through the high-deductible healthcare plans, I believe this policy should be made permanent.

A question for Dr. Miller. Do you agree that limiting barriers to telehealth services, after the public health emergency, would benefit patients seeking mental health services?

Dr. MILLER. Senator Daines, thank you for the question. As we have discussed today, there is such power in being flexible with how we are able to deliver services to where people are. And so, what we need to do is continue to explore how these services have added value to people's lives, and how they have improved outcomes.

Many of the changes that we have seen through the emergency order have made a difference in countless lives. And I think to take that away would not only be to the detriment of those families that have become dependent on it, it would also hurt our Nation's overall health.

And so, we have to be very thoughtful and very considerate when it comes to these issues of telehealth. I would recommend that this group, this committee and this Congress, really consider ways to either make some of these changes permanent, or to consider an extension that goes on for the next year to 2 years to allow for us to continue to maximize on what many folks have benefited from.

Senator DAINES. Thank you.

I want to shift gears and talk about a problem we are facing in Montana, and that is meth. In Montana, meth is taking a devastating toll on our families and our communities. I had a briefing with our Guard in Montana on Friday, their Counter-Drug Task Force, and we were talking about significant increases year over year in 2020 versus 2019 on drug seizures in our State—meth and heroin.

In fact, in 2020 drug overdose deaths hit a record high. We are now looking at a disturbing increase in meth-related violent crime. While medications can be effective in treating some substance use disorders, there are currently no FDA-approved medications to help meth addiction.

According to the National Institute of Drug Abuse, contingency management, which involves giving patients incentives to not use drugs, is an effective treatment for some individuals suffering with addiction. Mr. Betlach, in your experience, are there any Federal barriers that prevent States from implementing effective contingency management?

Mr. BETLACH. Senator, thank you for the question. I would say, I am not aware of any, but we can do some further research and get back to you.

Senator DAINES. Okay. Thank you. Thanks, Mr. Chairman.

Senator CRAPO. Thank you very much.

And I do understand that Senator Young is on the web. Senator Young, are you there?

Senator YOUNG. I am, Mr. Chairman. Thank you so much for holding this hearing. I think this is a really important topic.

The coronavirus outbreak has created an unprecedented mental health challenge for our country. I know it has certainly created challenges back home for many of my Hoosier constituents. While we do not yet know the full impact of the coronavirus pandemic on mental health, we do know it has forced Americans to isolate from their loved ones and other support systems, causing a troubling spike in mental health and substance abuse problems.

A Kaiser Family Foundation poll found that 45 percent of adults say that the outbreak has affected their mental health, almost half of adults. Among adults in Indiana who reported experiencing symptoms of anxiety or depressive disorder, almost 20 percent, one out of five, reported needing counseling or therapy but not receiving it, in the past 4 weeks.

I have a few questions related to this directed towards Dr. Durham. Dr. Durham, access has long been a barrier to adequate behavioral health care. The public health emergency is only exacerbating the existing challenges and increasing the need for providers and treatment.

How are providers responding to this increased need?

Dr. DURHAM. Thank you for the question. I think that you are absolutely correct that we have seen a lot of people, and a lot of uptake in services because of what we have all, I think, noted today, which is that there has been an increase in flexibility when we have added audio and video telehealth capability to all of our clinics throughout the country.

And like most have said previously, I do not think we should change that moving forward. We need to meet people where they are and whenever they can access the technology without having to necessarily come and drive in to appointments, or if you are in a rural community where you may not have access in your community to a mental health provider.

So, what has happened is that our clinics are full. We are seeing people back to back with telemedicine and our audio appointments. And what it leads to is that, you know, we have a workforce issue. And we need to figure out ways that we can expand on who is able to provide care, as Ms. Jett mentioned earlier. There are certain insurers that do not allow for certain services to be provided. And so, we need to look at that more deeply, the issue of who can provide services and be reimbursed for the services.

I am a firm believer that whatever you trained for and went to school for, you should be able to practice and get reimbursed appropriately for it. So, I think that telehealth has expanded so much for our communities, and I think there is more research to be done as well about which patient populations it works for and how we need to pivot in some other ways to make sure it is accessible for them too, due to other digital inequities, and maybe a lack of digital literacy as well. But it has definitely aided that process of engaging and reducing stigma, I think, in mental health. Not having to physically come in to see a mental health provider, I think, has helped substantially.

Senator YOUNG. Well, I agree that these additional flexibilities, based on my consultation with providers back home, have just been essential. So, I think it is really important that we continue to maintain these flexibilities.

If time remains, I will briefly touch on social determinants of health. Because we know that these are the economic and social conditions in which people live and learn and work and play. And they also impact one's ability to access transportation and stable housing. And by extension, these factors can positively impact the health and well-being of the most vulnerable Americans.

So, Dr. Durham, once again, just briefly, how might we better leverage existing programs and address the barriers to coordination between mental health and some of these social service programs that I alluded to? Is there anything that comes to mind that you see as a real opportunity for us in Congress?

Dr. DURHAM. So, I can talk based on my experience, just as a clinician and as someone who works in outpatient child psychiatry. We have folks at Boston Medical Center with exactly what you mentioned. They are struggling with food insecurity, housing insecurity, transportation issues—all of the social determinants. But what is lacking, most times from a Medicaid perspective, is we are not necessarily reimbursed for that time that we take to coordinate the care. It is very difficult to get case management as a psychiatrist, or as a social worker in our clinic, or we have LMHCs in our clinic—the time dedicated to coordinate all of those services that family may need from a case management standpoint are not necessarily reimbursed.

And so that happens but is carved out at other times during the day when maybe we have a gap, if you will, in our schedules. And I wholeheartedly agree that a person's mental health is affected by all of those social determinants. And the more that we can think about how we provide care and get reimbursed so that we can talk about all the social determinants, get them the services they need and also, as a provider, focus on their mental health, I think the better, you are right, our families would be. And then the communities would be as well, ultimately.

So many times that mechanism is funded by grants, and grants go away. And then we are stuck with, how do we help our families with all of the needs that they need in order to focus on the mental health issue at hand?

Senator YOUNG. Thank you so much. Yes, sustainable reimbursement for transportation to a primary care provider, and in underserved populations, so that we do not end up paying, as taxpayers, for something that becomes far more costly in the longer term, and certainly costly to that person's health, reimbursement to replace an air conditioning unit—or a heater—so that somebody does not become incredibly ill. It is the whole ounce of prevention notion. And we have just got to get better at that.

So thank you so much.

Senator CRAPO. We will have to move on to the next Senator, which is Senator Casey, who I understand is on the web.

Senator CASEY. Thank you, Senator Crapo. Thanks very much. I just have one question, and I know this may be plowing ground that has been plowed during the hearing, but I want to reiterate some of it.

I will direct my question to Dr. Durham and Dr. Miller. We know that, even before the COVID–19 pandemic, children were facing both behavioral and mental health crises all across the country. This need obviously is much greater because of the pandemic. And now kids are waiting weeks to months to get mental health care, both in the evaluation and the treatment. So, it is highly unlikely to get markedly better even as the pandemic is receding.

We have heard a lot today about telemedicine and the benefit it provides. But used alone, it does not help us with the question of increasing the number of trained professionals who can help both children and teens access the mental and behavioral health care that they need.

Primary care docs and nurses are often the first point of contact for kids, and for teens and their families, whether they are struggling with anxiety or depression or substance use disorder issues. Yet too often, many of these primary care providers believe they are not prepared to respond appropriately.

So, there is not a lot in the way of incentives to provide to child health providers to either engage in or expand their provision of mental or behavioral health care. So, we know that that lack of incentives can contribute to both racial and ethnic healthcare disparities, both in terms of care and outcomes.

So, to both Doctors, Dr. Miller and Dr. Durham, how do we better support or incentivize healthcare providers, advanced practitioners, and other therapists to increase or enhance their ability to respond to these mental health needs?

Dr. MILLER. Thank you for the question, Senator Casey. And I will just begin by briefly saying that I think you have your finger right at the center of this issue, which is that people, families, children, have to work too hard to get access to care. So how do we incentivize the places where the kids show up to make sure that they are providing adequate onsite mental health care?

And I think it begins with the flexibility of funding. One of the most profound barriers as to why people do not adopt integrated mental health care is because of the up-front startup costs. If they had flexible funding, what they could do is be a little more creative with how they were able to onboard a clinician to make sure that they were there in that pediatric setting to help that family and that child.

The second thing is that we have to provide some level of technical assistance. Integrating care, as powerful and potent as it is, can be difficult. And so an added incentive beyond just the flexible funding is helping practices make that change, make that transformation. Without that, sometimes we see people start and stop because of the difficulty of it.

Senator CASEY. Thanks. Dr. Durham?

Dr. DURHAM. Yes, thank you for the question. I will echo everything Dr. Miller said, and I will just add to it in that our TEAM UP for Children model, which is at FQHCs in Boston, the greater Boston area, did exactly that. You have to have some funding in order for those health centers to start doing some of that work. And so that is what some of the grant initiatives did.

But then on top of that, I would say that what we have also added to that care team—and make sure that it is a true team— is that the pediatrician or the pediatric primary care provider does not feel alone, that there is a behavioral health clinician and community health worker as a part of that model to get at kids that have the most needs—these are kids on our State Medicaid—to make sure, as the previous Senator mentioned, that we are tucking away housing, and food insecurity, and all of those other things so that we are not continuing to cost the system, but helping with that as well.

But I do think that that team effort, so that the pediatric primary care doc does not go at it alone, we have also integrated training within that, so they learn more about mental health conditions at the primary care level, which has been instrumental. And then also clinical work flows, because it is different, when we decide to start shifting from just physical health to both mental and physical health, that they have to shift their practice in some way. So, the technical assistance aspect, I think, is also very key.

Senator CASEY. Thanks very much. Thanks, Senator Crapo.

Senator CRAPO. Thank you.

And I understand Senator Warner is now with us. Senator Warner?

Senator WARNER. Thank you, Senator Crapo. And I thank the panel and the chairman for holding this hearing.

I know we have been talking about a variety of mental health issues. I want to talk about one that is quite close to home with me in terms of my own family, and that is some of the challenges around eating disorders.

We have seen from the Journal of Eating Disorders that about 62 percent of the individuals with eating disorders have seen an increase in stress due to COVID–19. We have seen a dramatic increase in binge eating as well.

I have seen around Virginia—again both on a personal basis and on a more global basis—how this disease can really challenge not only the afflicted, but whole families. As a matter of fact, eating disorders have the highest incidence of mortality of any mental health issue.

Dr. Durham, given your experiences as a physician specializing in pediatric and adult psychiatry, what do you think, both COVID- related and non-COVID-related, we can do to get ahead of this issue around eating disorders, from anorexia to bulimia to a host of other kinds of manifestations of this challenge?

Dr. DURHAM. Thank you for the question. This is not necessarily my area of expertise, but what I will say is that I understand, and can understand how eating disorders, among many other disorders that we treat during the pandemic, are on the rise. I think what happens when you are in a position of high stress, social isolation, lots of loss, is that you do not have all those reserves, those emotional reserves, that you had prior to the pandemic, and lack all the social connectedness that we all want and strive for.

And so, I think that is why we have seen rates rising in depression, anxiety, and folks maybe going back to some restrictive or binge-eating behavior. And we have also seen that for folks with substance use disorders, who had a period of sobriety for maybe years and now unfortunately have relapsed during this time because it has been stressful for everyone, and you sort of fall back to maybe things that felt more comfortable, or that were habit- forming at some point.

And so now, we have talked a lot too today about thinking about this critical time. But I do not think we have seen—you know, we need that year or two to see the devastating consequences of this pandemic, because I think it is going to take time for people to get back to their normal level of functioning, if you will, and to their own baseline.

And so, whatever we can do to extend services for telehealth and other services, and increase that flexibility, I think will be key moving forward.

Senator WARNER. I agree with you. I do think it is going to take us that time. What is the new baseline going to be? I mean, Dr. Miller, in your testimony you noted the need to integrate mental health within the primary care field and to modernize the workforce. The National Center of Excellence for Eating Disorders trained primary care practitioners on screening, brief intervention, and referral to treatment called SBIRT.

Do you view these cyber-trainings for primary care practitioners as helpful in addressing some of these workforce issues around mental health; not just eating disorders but more broadly?

Dr. MILLER. Yes. Thank you for the question, Senator Warner. And I think any time we do not ask, we do not know. So, we have to be able to screen to detect if there are issues that are under the surface that our patients and families are not necessarily raising on their own.

So, I think it is a positive thing to screen. However, I have to point out that screening alone without treatment is insufficient. We need to be providing incentives, as we have discussed today, to onboard experts, clinicians who can help when those individuals do come forward with a positive screening, if it is an eating disorder, if it is anxiety, and if it is depression. This is a very positive thing for us. It not only normalizes how people begin to talk about issues like eating disorders, but it also creates a team-based environment so that we can provide the most comprehensive care necessary for that patient.

Senator WARNER. Well, this is an area—I wish, Mr. Chairman, I was not as much of an expert as I have become over the last 12 or 14 years, but I appreciate the comments.

I want to go to Dr. Durham again. You know, when we are talking about practitioners, we had an enormous tragedy with Dr. Lorna Breen in Charlottesville, VA, who was a solo practitioner. In many ways the stress and overwhelming nature of COVID–19 unfortunately led her to, with the level of depression—she took her own life. Along with Senator Kaine and others in Congress, we introduced the Lorna Breen Health Care Provider Protection Act that would address professionals in terms of trying to make sure that we train folks on how to deal with these high-stress circumstances. Dr. Durham, I know we are down to the last couple of seconds.

Do you want to comment on how we make sure that we take care of patients, but also our providers?

Dr. DURHAM. Yes, in the last couple of seconds, I appreciate that. And I appreciate that that is happening, because we do need to take care of all of our providers. It has been an equally stressful time for all of us, no matter if you are a physician or a social worker, an LMHC, nurses; we have been working really hard. And I think that at a place like BMC, a lot of things have happened where they were even just doing wellness check-ins for all of our staff, from people that deliver food to patient rooms, to physicians, to the nurses. And I think that that is important.

And any time we can integrate more initiatives for the workforce, I think the better. We are going through this equally, as all of our patients are.

Senator WARNER. Thank you, Mr. Chairman. Thank you, Dr. Durham.

The CHAIRMAN. Thank you, Senator Warner.

Our next three are Senator Whitehouse, Senator Hassan, and Senator Warren.

Senator Whitehouse, are you out there?

Senator WHITEHOUSE. Thanks, Mr. Chairman. I am out here. I appreciate this hearing very much.

First, one of the things that I have gotten for feedback from my mental health community in Rhode Island is that the increase in telehealth during COVID had kind of a hidden benefit, very hard to quantify, but I heard it repeatedly, and that was the sense from practitioners that the qualitative input that they were getting through telehealth was actually better, more meaningful, than be- forehand when people had to find their way across town, wait in the waiting room, fill out the stupid clipboard, go into an unfamiliar room, and then have a chat with the practitioner. To be able to do it from a place of safety at home seemed to bring out better interaction, better substantive qualitative interaction.

And I am wondering if any of you have had that experience, or if you have seen any—I know it is hard to quantify, but has anybody tried to quantify it in any way?

Mr. BETLACH. Thank you for the question, Senator. The only thing I would add to that is that, in talking with providers, not only have they heard that from an impact, but also a lower notional rate. So, definitely——

Senator WHITEHOUSE. Yes, definitely a lower notional rate.

Mr. BETLACH. So, in addition to being able to have a better impact, you also have people showing up more for appointments. They have not had conflicts. They have not had transportation issues. So a number of those factors have been taken out of the equation, and as a result, more people have accessed services.

Senator WHITEHOUSE. So let me leave it at that. And if anybody else wants to expand on that for the record, please let me know. But I am going to take it as the agreement of the panel that there were those two improvements, both in showing up and in being engaged and getting better engagement as a result of telehealth.

The other topic I wanted to go into was the interface between law enforcement and mental health, which plays out first directly on the street with law enforcement and then, depending on how the individual engaged with law enforcement, maybe at the local police station or jail; and if not, then usually a ride over to the emergency room, where they get dropped on the unhappy ER docs to cope with.

So, Senator Cornyn and I are working on a bill to improve the engagement of law enforcement in this space so that there is an accredited curriculum and training programs for people so that they know they are getting the real deal in terms of training to improve crisis intervention teams and their engagement with law enforcement, to figure out how to improve the referrals to community- based mental and behavioral health service folks, and to improve de-escalation tactics. All of this, I think, is pretty important.

And I just wanted to get your sense—anybody who would care to respond—on the extent to which law enforcement today is the entry point for people who are in need of and have not received adequate mental health and behavioral health services and the extent to which it is a successful entry point.

Mr. BETLACH. Senator, thank you for the comments. In terms of the interaction between the mental health delivery system and law enforcement, I guess I would invite you to come out to Arizona and see what is going on with regards to the crisis system in our State in which, not only do we have robust mobile response teams but also crisis stabilization facilities to be able to work with law enforcement. There are thousands of drop-offs that occur annually within a 5-minute time span oftentimes.

There is also a lot of training in terms of the CIT model that you mentioned. So clearly there is a role, from my perspective, that Medicaid should be playing in helping to support the interaction and support of law enforcement, mental health providers, through a stabilization crisis infrastructure. And really, there has been a lot of discussion and a lot of new resources for States to be able to establish more robust systems.

There is also going to be an expectation from individuals as they dial 988 in the future in terms of what types of infrastructure will be available for individuals.

Senator WHITEHOUSE. Thanks. And I think my time is running out. So, if anybody else has best practices or really good local examples that you would like to share with us, if you could please get that information into the committee, both Senator Cornyn and I would be very grateful.

Thanks, all, for your terrific work and for helping get us through the COVID situation.

The CHAIRMAN. Thank you, Senator Whitehouse. Senator Hassan, and then Senator Warren.

Senator HASSAN. Well, thank you, Chair Wyden and Ranking Member Crapo, for this hearing. And to all of our witnesses, thank you so much for taking the time to be with us today.

Dr. Miller, I want to start with a couple of questions to you, and then I will move on to the other panelists. The demand for mental health and substance use disorder treatment and services skyrocketed during the COVID–19 pandemic, as millions of Americans grappled with grief, isolation, and economic uncertainty. We have helped meet that demand by providing new means to access mental and behavioral services such as telehealth, and there has been a lot of discussion about that this morning. Unfortunately, even as we move to make it easier to access some services, the stigma still associated with substance misuse prevents too many people from getting the behavioral health services they need.

Dr. Miller, how does the stigmatization of substance use disorder impact access to treatment and services, and what steps can Congress take to better integrate substance use disorder treatment into primary care settings?

Dr. MILLER. Well, thank you for your question, Senator, and thank you for your ongoing passion and views in this space.

You know, to your point on stigma, we know that only about 10 percent of individuals with substance use disorders receive care. And that tells me a lot about stigma. It says both socially that we do not talk about it as much as we should but, more importantly however, structurally we have these fragmented ways of individuals being able to get access to care.

One of the views that I think you are very familiar with, and that we have discussed today, is that we need to make it easier for individuals who are identified with a substance use disorder to be able to get access to care. That means bringing that care to where people are.

We have to train up our providers to identify it, and we have to train up our clinicians to treat it, and we have to recognize that undergirding all of the substance use disorders is also mental health. The reasons that we provide gold standard treatment for things like substance use disorders is because we need to provide counseling at the same time. This is how we begin to destigmatize substance use disorders and, hopefully, encourage more people to seek care.

Senator HASSAN. Thank you. I am also continuing to work on trying to change the X-waiver requirement as we move forward, because I think that stigmatizes the provision of treatment for some healthcare providers too.

Dr. Miller, I want to turn to another devastating public health crisis that we have to work on, which is the issue of suicides. A report published yesterday—and Senator Wyden mentioned it earlier—by the CDC found that, earlier this year, emergency department visits for suicide attempts by adolescent girls increased 51 percent on average when compared to 2019.

And I have heard directly from New Hampshire students about the mental health concerns that they have. That is why I have introduced the bipartisan STANDUP Act with my colleague, Senator Ernst, that is going to encourage the implementation of evidence- based policies and training in schools and communities across the country that will help to prevent suicide.

Dr. Miller, can you speak to the importance of providing kids and teenagers with the tools that they need to recognize if they, or someone they know, is at increased risk of suicide?

Dr. MILLER. Thank you again for the question, Senator. As the father of two children, I can tell you this is the one that I really want to make sure that we get right. We teach our youth, our kids, all about aspects of physical health. We even teach them things like how to drive a car, and even how to save someone's life with CPR. And so, yes, we have to be able to equip our youth and our schools, frankly, where our youth are basically a lot, with the ways to identify issues related to suicide.

In fact, there was one survey that came out from Mental Health America that showed how youth are talking more to each other around the issues of mental health, which includes suicide, rather than their parents.

So, because our youth are the front lines, we need to equip them with those skills necessary to know how to be there for one another. This could be the way to augment the workforce that we have discussed today. If we simply depend on our clinical workforce to address the demand, especially with our youth, we will fail.

We have to be more creative, more thoughtful, and most importantly, we have to have the youth at the table and with us as we design the solution to work with them on ways that they can better help each other.

Senator HASSAN. Thank you.

Mr. Betlach, I want to move on with a question for you. We increased Federal funding for home and community-based Medicaid services under the American Rescue Plan. This funding helps ensure that older adults and individuals with disabilities, including those with mental health conditions such as bipolar disorder and schizophrenia, can access mental health services outside of institutional settings.

Can you, from your experiences as Director at the Arizona Medicaid program, speak to the important role that home and community-based mental health professionals play in delivering care for individuals who experience severe mental health disabilities? And what can we do in Congress to expand access to home and community-based care for those struggling with mental health conditions?

Mr. BETLACH. Senator, the investment that you have made is really a once-in-a-generation investment in terms of where States are at in the ability to leverage that 10-percent home and community-based bump. And it is really broader, I think, than a lot of people appreciate. It is also on behavioral health services that States deliver through the rehab option as well. And those are incredibly important.

So, States are right now developing their plans. I am working with a number of States, and they are generating their options that they want to invest in. So, it is an exciting time for States. But States are feeling like there is a very significant time crunch here in terms of being able to establish this investment and do it in the right way.

So, I think those plans will be evolving. But there is clearly a unique opportunity, and these services are so important to be able to deliver services in the communities that serve these populations. So, it is an exciting time for States to have these resources to be looking at workforce issues, to be looking at being able to deliver more services in the community.

Senator HASSAN. Thank you. And thank you, Mr. Chair.

The CHAIRMAN. I thank my colleague. Senator Warren?

Senator WARREN. Thank you, Mr. Chairman.

COVID–19 is the worst public health crisis that our Nation has tackled in over a century, but it does not exist in a vacuum. The pandemic has exacerbated every preexisting public health problem facing our Nation. And that is especially true for substance use disorder, which often co-occurs with other mental health conditions.

Dr. Durham, I am sure that you are familiar with the data. Did substance use disorder and drug overdoses increase or decrease during the pandemic?

Dr. DURHAM. Thank you, Senator Warren. They definitely increased during the pandemic. I think DPH in Massachusetts reported, for black Americans in particular, a 69-percent increase over the pandemic——

Senator WARREN. Sixty-nine percent increase?

Dr. DURHAM. Yes, in Massachusetts, specifically. That could have been from various, you know—this is usually fentanyl-laced substances. Many times, cocaine use disorder is pretty prevalent in some of the black patients that we see, specifically at BMC. And so, we can think of lots of things that happened during this period. What happened to everyone happened also to the folks we see with substance use disorders: job loss, economic insecurity, housing insecurity, the loss of social supports. You know, substance use disorders are a remitting and relapsing disease. People sort of think of one moment in time you are sober, and then that's it. But it is not. And so, it is a chronic medical condition, and we should treat it as such.

Senator WARREN. So let me just push on this a little bit and let that sink in a little bit, that we saw a 69-percent increase in opioid deaths in Massachusetts.

You know, we were already, Nationwide, losing tens of thousands of Americans to drug overdoses. And the problem has only gotten worse. And I think this is where you were headed. It has gotten worse—differently in different communities.

So, you were serving on the front lines of this pandemic at Boston Medical Center, which serves many low-income patients and communities of color. As the coronavirus spread through Massachusetts and substance use disorder worsened, what patterns did you see in terms of the types of patients you saw at BMC, the types of communities that were affected? Can you just say a little more about that? I think that is where you were headed.

Dr. DURHAM. Yes, sure. Well, we predominantly serve about 70 percent black and Latinx at BMC, people who identify as black and Latinx, and about 30 percent do not speak English as their first language.

Just like many, I think many people were scared to come into the hospital at the beginning of the pandemic. And so I think what happened, though, is that we got high acuity as we hit December and January, where people were coming in with severe—whether that be mental illness, but also severe relapse on whatever substance that they may have been previously using and maybe had stopped. I think poverty and job loss, like I mentioned earlier—you know, health, access to health care in general, there was a change in that. We have talked a lot about telehealth, but it does not work for everybody.

And so, this is the particular population where I do not think it worked well. You needed to be on a Zoom link with your recovery coach. Did you have access to a computer and to get the Zoom link, and then have a smartphone? So, I will pause there.

Senator WARREN. That is very helpful. So, you have told us about the scope of the problem. You have told us about how it hits different communities differently. Let's talk a little bit about the solution.

In recent years, Congress has taken some steps, like passing the SUPPORT Act, to expand access to addiction treatment services. But it is clear that more resources are needed.

So let me ask you. Boston Medical Center is a national leader in addiction and substance use disorder treatment, research, and training. Would a significant Federal investment in substance use disorder prevention help lower overall deaths, reduce these disparities, and help support providers like BMC?

Dr. DURHAM. Absolutely. I think that we need parity in mental health and substance use treatment. I think we also silo substance use disorders from mental health disorders from physical health. The more we can combine all of that, because it is one person that presents, the better we will all be.

I do think that we need to start early with community outreach and more investment in the community. I think when we speak about black and Latinx communities in particular, we need more research that allows us to partner with community-based services to do some of that research, because we are not targeting that population well, and we need to invest dollars to do that.

Senator WARREN. Well, I really appreciate it. You know, we have an opportunity here not just to build back to where we were before the pandemic, but to drastically improve our public health infrastructure.

I was very happy to see President Biden's commitment back as a candidate to invest $125 billion over 10 years in substance use disorder and the opioid crisis. And that is why, in the coming weeks, I will be reintroducing my Comprehensive Addiction Resources Emergency Act, or the CARE Act. This legislation would provide State and local governments the resources to combat substance use; to invest in biomedical research, public health surveillance, and professional training; and to expand access to naloxone. I am looking forward to working with my colleagues to get this done. I appreciate all the work that all of you are doing. I hope you can get better support from Washington to continue to do it. Thank you, Mr. Chairman.

The CHAIRMAN. Thank you, Senator Warren. And I believe what you and Dr. Durham have just done in terms of laying out the 69- percent increase in substance abuse in your State really conveys the urgency of what this committee has to do. So, I thank you very much, and I thank you, Dr. Durham, because that is what this is all about.

Senator Warren and I talk about this all the time. The committee has a lot of stuff we have to deal with. We have all kinds of issues. But when you hear about a 69-percent increase in substance abuse, you say, ''This is something that cannot wait.'' So, I really thank you, Senator Warren.

And I am just going to wrap up with a couple of comments. I want to thank our witnesses. You all have been terrific. And I think you have seen from the Senators the very strong feelings about how important it is that we work on this, and we do it coming together in a very polarized political environment.

I do not know if any of you are aware of the Wyden story. My father wrote a book called ''Conquering Schizophrenia.'' It was about my late brother. And for years and years on end, my brother had schizophrenia and would be out on the streets in California, and the Wyden family went to bed at night worried that he was going to hurt himself or somebody else. And I think that is pretty typical of what families are facing when they are dealing with mental illness. And you all have described how many people fall between the cracks—the incredible stigma of this.

Chantay, thank you so much for describing what you are trying to do in rural Oregon, the part of the State I love so much, to try to reduce the stigma. And you all have laid out a lot of solutions here. You have laid out a lot of solutions, and I have been talking with Senator Crapo. We think that this is an issue where the committee can come together and do better.

We have currently reviewed the committee records. This is the second-ever hearing of the Senate Finance Committee on the issue of mental health care in our over 100-year history. Senator Stabe-now and Senator Daines are doing good work in the subcommittee, and I think now both Democrats and Republicans understand that we have to bring a greater sense of urgency and commitment and resources into this issue so that mental health is really in line with physical health, which of course was the dream of Senators Wellstone and Domenici. And I think I touched on it. I remember opening up the paper the next day, and I said to myself, ''Hallelujah; there is hope for Jeff Wyden and all the families who have suffered.'' And as you said very eloquently, Dr. Durham, in a lot of instances, the commitment to parity is honored more in the breach than in the observance.

So, I thank you all very much for your excellent testimony. It is a great kickoff to the committee's work in this area. I think you have heard from my Republican colleagues—they were raising important issues. I looked at the comments made by my Republican colleagues and my Democratic colleagues, and there was not an offbase idea in the house today. You can literally go up and down both sides of the dais and see Senators with great sincerity offering concrete ideas.

So we are going to wrap up for today. But for all of you and your colleagues who are out there on the web, we are wrapping up for today, but make no mistake about it: we are going to be consulting with you. This is a ''to be continued'' discussion.

Members know that questions have to be produced, what we call QFRs, within a week. And I want to thank our witnesses again.

And with that, the Senate Finance Committee is adjourned. [Whereupon, at 12:30 p.m., the hearing was concluded.]

Appendix: Additional Material Submitted for the Record

Prepared Statement of Thomas Betlach, MPA, Partner, Speire Healthcare Strategies

Chairman Wyden, Ranking Member Crapo, and members of the Senate Finance Committee, thank you for the opportunity to testify today on policy solutions for addressing mental health. I had the privilege of serving as the Arizona Medicaid Director for almost a decade and for a portion of the time, as the Mental Health Commissioner.

Medicaid serves over 70 million members, offering comprehensive mental health benefits to some of our country's most complex populations. In 2020, the Medicaid and CHIP Payment and Access Commission (MACPAC) published mental health statistics that showed, for non-institutionalized adults, 27.6 percent of the Medicaid population had an indicator of mental illness compared to 18.7 percent of the commercially insured population. And for individuals with Serious Mental Illness, the numbers were 8.2 percent for Medicaid, and 4.3 percent for commercial populations.[1]

[1] Behavioral Health in Medicaid Presentation, MACPAC, September 2020.

As you formulate health policy options, State Medicaid programs should be a critical component of the discussion. Understanding the system and the forces prevailing on it should be at the core of discussion.

The last year brought to light the extreme fragmentation of our healthcare delivery system at all levels. Our policy and program structures are in silos. Funding streams to support these populations follow those siloed program and policy structures. Providers gravitate towards these funding streams creating more complexity at the point of care. The very beneficiary the system is designed to serve is forced navigate the maze we created.

Fragmentation is often discussed, so I would like to explain how that fragmentation manifests in our system. When I became Medicaid director, individuals with serious mental illness had up to four different payers to navigate. Forty percent of that population were Medicaid and Medicare dual-eligible members. An individual had a Medicaid plan for physical health, a Medicaid plan for behavioral health, traditional Medicare and a Part D plan or a Medicare Advantage plan. Unfortunately, this level of fragmentation is common. The result is misaligned incentives and the bureaucracies of Medicare and Medicaid spending considerable time and resources creating payment rules and refereeing rather than focusing on improving care for our populations.

Now, in addition to fragmentation, Medicaid leaders are contending with the impact that the pandemic has had on an individual's mental health. It has been well documented that the pandemic has had a more negative impact on individuals with less means, both in terms of health and financial stress.

This last year has brought important issues such as social justice and health equity to the surface and at the same time there was rapid innovation. For example, the use of telehealth and the deployment of the 988 crisis hotline. Both will require much work ahead to ensure long-term success.

Today's environment has challenges. But States and Medicaid programs now have access to considerable investment resources to address these challenges and advance the delivery of mental health services.

1) Congress has authorized a 5-percent set-aside funding from the Mental Health Block Grant to be used for Crisis Systems.
2) Congress has authorized an 85-percent enhanced match in Medicaid for community mobile response teams.
3) Additional resources are now available for States that use the rehabilitation option to cover behavioral health services, which was

included in the 10- percent increased Federal funding for home and community-based services.

4) Finally, additional resources are available for expanding Certified Community Behavioral Health Clinics.

In February 2021, The National Association of Medicaid Directors (NAMD) published ‘‘Medicaid Forward: Behavioral Health,’’[1] outlining a series of strategies Medicaid programs are pursuing to advance mental health services for members. The strategies varied based on the unique populations served by Medicaid. This report highlighted initiatives such as, expanding access and improving timeliness to care, integrating physical health and behavioral health, and expanding access for the full continuum of care including crisis services.

Populations identified included children with complex needs, individuals experiencing homelessness, older adults, individuals with intellectual and developmental disabilities, and individuals involved in criminal justice.

The NAMD report provided proof that when implemented, the highlighted strategies make a difference.

Further, a March 2021 Bipartisan Policy Council report concluded that ‘‘integrating primary and behavioral health care is necessary and would ensure that individuals with behavioral health conditions and comorbid physical health problems receive high-quality access to care. Comorbid behavioral and physical health diagnoses are common. Addressing them together through integration can provide a patient-centered approach that can be cost-effective for payers and providers, reduce health disparities, and improve patient outcomes.’’[2]

Arizona provides a strong example of this, in 2011, we pursued a strategy to better integrate services for individuals with serious mental illness. This strategy was focused on driving integration at three levels.

1) Policy integration—Arizona merged behavioral health policy expertise into the Medicaid program and reviewed all policies that limited integrated services.
2) Payer integration—Arizona braided multiple funding streams including Medicaid, SAMHSA block grants, and local dollars to support housing and other non-Medicaid compensable services.

---

[2] Tackling America’s Mental Health and Addiction Crisis Through Primary Care Integration. Bipartisan Policy Council, March 2021, page 8.

3) Provider integration—Arizona created new incentives and supported providers in developing more coordination and integration at a provider level. This included opening up new codes to support the collaborative care model. This model has been shown to improve clinical outcomes and reduce costs by further integrating care at the primary care provider.

In 2018, Mercer consulting conducted an analysis of the integration efforts. Their final report for individuals with serious mental illness found that all measures of ambulatory care, preventive care, and chronic disease management demonstrated improvement. For example, Medication management for people with asthma (75- percent compliance) increased 35 percent. Just as important, all indicators of patient experience improved, with five of the 11 measures exhibiting double-digit increases. For example, shared decision-making improved 61 percent.[3]

Another opportunity highlighted by NAMD is to strengthen crisis systems. This issue is front and center with the implementation of 988. SAMHSA provided extensive thought leadership with the development of the Crisis Now model and the publication of the National Guidelines for Behavioral Health Crisis Care Best PracticeToolkit. This document provides the details on how to establish a system to serve anyone, anywhere at any time.

The Crisis Now model is based on three critical components.

1) Call center capability.
2) Twenty-four by seven Community Mobile Response Teams.
3) Twenty-three hour crisis receiving and stabilization units.

In Arizona, this system was developed over 20 years and serves all Arizonans. The call centers answer thousands of calls every month, meeting the State's expectations of three rings or less. Mobile response teams located throughout the State serve individuals in the community. Stabilization facilities provide services for individuals experiencing severe crisis episodes and offer continuous support for law enforcement to drop off individuals and to return to the field within 5 minutes. The financing for this system comes from creatively braiding multiple funding streams while leveraging Medicaid for support.

---

[3] Independent Evaluation of Arizona's Medicaid Integration Efforts, Mercer, 2018.

While we have seen improvement, there is clearly much more to do. We stand today at a unique moment with the power to address complex issues and continue the momentum of innovation by making strategic policy changes. To that end:

1) Congress and the executive branch need to develop and implement strategies holistically by ensuring Medicaid and behavioral health collaborate and partner in a meaningful manner. On several occasions Congress has leveraged the mental health expertise that lives at the Substance Abuse and Mental Health Services Administration (SAMHSA) to advance policy initiatives. This includes set-aside funding for first episode psychosis and crisis system planning. However, there does not appear to be sufficient expectations established by Congress that these important planning and investment dollars are to be linked to the Medicaid program. Unfortunately, the dollars often get siloed and the opportunity is suboptimal. SAMHSA traditionally works directly with its network of mental health commissioners, and Medicaid programs sometimes lack the expertise or bandwidth to leverage these opportunities. At the end of the day, Medicaid beneficiaries may or may not benefit from these forward-looking investments.
2) Congress should provide more flexibility with block grant funds for States to address social determinants of health as States look at ways to support these investments. As coverage has expanded, there may be opportunities for States to leverage block grants to support select social determinants for specific populations and improve outcomes.
3) Congress needs to legislate to establish payment parity between Medicare and Medicaid. Where Medicaid has led the way in developing paraprofessional staff such as peer support services and systems to support broader populations like Crisis, Medicare should follow. To achieve parity, Congress must act to have Medicare cover these and similar services.
4) Congress should continue to provide financial incentives for States to modernize the mental health infrastructure. Programs like Money Follows the Person worked well for home and community-based services. I am excited to see Congress using similar approaches for behavioral health services like community mobile response teams and CCBHCs. Congress should consider lending financial support

towards models that improve care and access. This approach should also be expanded to dual eligible members as well.

5) Congress should continue to evaluate the impact of the IMD 16-bed limits. While there have been efforts made to allow for some payments in select instances, some States have not been able to avail themselves of these opportunities. A good place to start the policy discussion is looking at select settings like crisis stabilization.
6) Congress should rectify the fact that behavioral health providers were excluded from the electronic health records incentive program provided through the HITECH Act. Data aggregation and analytics are an important component of improved care coordination. This is an investment that should be made to advance integration.
7) Finally, Congress should evaluate how graduate medical education financing policies negatively impact the ability to attract specialists, such as child psychiatrists, to meet the needs of the Medicaid population. Many States, like Arizona, are punished as a result of the Medicare formulas that are locked in at 1996 allocations.

We are at a critical moment in time to advance the delivery of mental health services, not only within Medicaid but for our entire country. Thank you for your time and interest in these topics.

Questions Submitted for the Record to Thomas Betlach, MPA
Questions Submitted by Hon. Catherine Cortez Masto

Question. Arizona has been a leader in behavioral health crisis services as the State's crisis now model has been incredibly successful in supporting individuals experiencing crisis, and creating a safety net for folks who have slipped through the cracks of our mental health system for far too long. Senator Cornyn and I have introduced legislation that seeks to empower communities across the country to build crisis services. The crux of our bill is insurance coverage—these are services that should be covered, no matter where people get their insurance.

What kind of difference would insurance coverage make as States look to build crisis services similar to the Arizona model?

Answer. Having all insurers provide coverage for crisis services would greatly benefit States. True parity would enable additional resources to be made available to support important crisis infrastructure. If all plans (e.g., commercial insurers and Medicare) covered a broad continuum of behavioral health services, it would reduce stigma, educate consumers on the importance, and improve access to behavioral health resources.

Question. What else can Congress do to facilitate the delivery of crisis services across the country?

Answer. Congress can continue to provide financial incentives like the block grant set-aside funding for crisis services and the additional funding for mobile response teams. Additionally, Congress can work closely with the administration to ensure appropriate coordination is occurring at the Federal level to maximize collaboration between agencies, including SAMHSA and Medicaid.

Question. In your testimony you also highlighted a recent report from the Bipartisan Policy Center on behavioral health integration.

What does that look like in practice and how easy or difficult would it be to implement this kind of integration into risk-based payment models such as Accountable Care Organizations, Medicaid Managed Care Organizations, and Medicare Advantage?

Answer. It is challenging to implement integration well with managed care. States should be thoughtful purchasers and make sure that appropriate contracts and policies are in place to support payer and provider integration. However, as more States have adopted integrated purchasing models, lessons learned and best practices are available to other States to enable them to successfully design and implement structures. State experience tells us that while it is challenging, if done correctly there are positive impacts associated with payer integration.

Question. What difference would that make in boosting access to services?

Answer. The Arizona experience shows that for individuals with serious mental illness there has been an increase in access when measured based on HEDIS scores. When done appropriately, integration results in additional providers being able to deliver behavioral health services.

Questions Submitted by Hon. John Barasso

Question. The healthcare professionals, along with all front-line workers, deserve our gratitude and appreciation. Their dedication to our communities during this pandemic is something we must recognize and never forget.

A top concern of Wyoming mental health facilities is making sure there are enough staff to care for their patients. It is especially challenging to attract and keep healthcare providers in rural communities. Can you discuss solutions related cilities to attract and maintain staff in rural areas?

Answer. Medicaid has done some excellent work expanding the behavioral health workforce through the use of peer supports. By leveraging individuals with lived experience, Medicaid has been able to expand access and better engage patients. Medicaid (and other payers) need to continue to expand the use of peer and family supports for behavioral health. In addition, the significant growth of telehealth, in response to COVID, expanded access and should continue to improve workforce capacity particularly in rural areas.

Question. Can you specifically discuss changes to GME policy you believe would improve the pipeline of mental health physicians?

Answer. There are a range of policy changes that Congress should consider with regards to GME. Three GME policy changes that would have a strong positive impact and improve capacity are:

- Change the Medicare formula to recognize the growth that has occurred especially in States like Arizona that are at an extreme disadvantage based on the Medicare formula being frozen for the past 25 years.
- Provide incentives for GME programs that specialize in behavioral health training.
- Increase expectations and create incentives so that more training can be done in outpatient clinics and in rural settings.

Question. As a doctor, I strongly support increasing access to mental health services, especially in rural communities. Senator Stabenow and I have previously introduced legislation for many years that would allow mental health counselors and marriage and family therapists to receive reimbursement from Medicare.

Can you discuss how the Department of Health and Human Services can improve access for mental health services, especially for those on Medicare?

Answer. Access will be improved when Medicare improves the overall benefits for behavioral health by expanding who can deliver services and where those services may be delivered.

Question. In particular, can you comment on the merits of allowing licensed professional counselors and marriage and family therapists to receive reimbursements from Medicare?

Answer. Some State Medicaid programs have determined that covering these codes are valuable in increasing access for members. Given the limited benefits within Medicare today for behavioral health services, especially in comparison to the robust Medicaid benefits, this is an important area for Congress to evaluate.

Questions Submitted by Hon. Tim Scott

Question. The toll that union-sponsored excuses for ''virtual learning'' has taken on actual kids is extraordinarily sad, especially for our Nation's most vulnerable children. In October 2020, a survey conducted by the Jed Foundation showed that 31 percent of parents said their child's mental or emotional health was worse than before the pandemic. Private insurance data also shows that while all health care claims for adolescents ages 13–18 were down in 2020 compared to 2019, mental health-related claims for this age group increased sharply. Additionally, the Centers for Disease Control and Prevention (CDC) reports 25 percent of parents whose children attended school virtually were more likely to report an overall worsened mental or emotional health compared to only 16 percent of parents of children attending school in-person.

What strategies and collaboration efforts would you recommend to encourage the infrastructural changes and technical assistance necessary to promote school safety and proactive approaches to mental health challenges?

Answer. We need to continue our efforts to train and support parents, teachers, staff, and students about the importance of behavioral health. Programs like mental health first aid have shown benefits towards reducing stigma and providing individuals with important tools on how to have challenging conversations.

Question. What programs within the Department of Health and Human Services' (HHS) purview are best poised to support children and schools as they return to complete in-person learning?

Answer. See above.

Question. How can we integrate more telehealth opportunities to expand access to mental health services in schools?

Answer. Medicaid and other purchasers should work with insurers and schools to leverage telehealth and other mobile technologies to engage students. These opportunities extend beyond just K–12 into higher education. Some States are evaluating policies that will expand the capacity to use schools as sites for delivering telehealth services.

Question. Telehealth has expanded rapidly as a result of the COVID–19 pandemic. Numerous studies have demonstrated the effectiveness of telehealth for behavioral health services. As telehealth becomes more common among healthcare providers, what can Congress do to ensure that patients do not suffer from unnecessary bureaucratic delays?

Answer. States with support from the Federal Government greatly expanded access to telehealth services for programs like Medicaid. Post-COVID, States will need to monitor access to ensure that inappropriate barriers are not being placed on the delivery of services. Access to care and the quality of the services being delivered are ultimately what Congress may want to consider evaluating as the telehealth evolution moves forward.

Question. There is a well-researched connection between unemployment and mental health. As recently as April 2021, despite billions of dollars of COVID–19 stimulus, aggregate employment remained 7.9 million jobs below its pre-recession level.

What impact will this failure to get people back to work have on mental health?

Answer. Recent surveys and studies indicated that individual stress levels are higher today than pre-COVID. There are many factors in place that have resulted in increased stress, including employment status. There will need to be continued efforts to provide education to individuals and families on the importance of mental health along with information on how individuals may access care in a timely matter.

Question. Last November, an article published in the Journal of the American Medical Association noted that multiple studies indicated that older adults may be less negatively affected by certain mental health outcomes than other age groups. Are these study outcomes consistent with your own professional experiences working with older adults?

Answer. This in not my area of expertise, and I do not feel comfortable commenting on this.

Question. Current network adequacy standards often allow networks of specialists who aren't taking new patients or who have long waiting lists. That means that many people needing treatment must go out of network to get care, and only those who can afford the high cost get it. One of the biggest challenges to access to behavioral health care services is that many behavioral health specialists don't participate in health plan networks.

Why is that, and how can we change that?

Answer. Market dynamics often drive provider utilization. It is clear that the country needs more specialists and a broader workforce to meet the increased demand. Congress should evaluate the impact of Graduate Medical Education funding and how that has resulted in constraints in behavioral health specialists. Medicaid has overcome some of the constraints by establishing a para-professional workforce of Peer supports.

Question. Outside of the public health emergency, telehealth services are restricted to certain geographic and clinical settings. Beneficiaries must live in a rural area and have an initial face-to-face visit with the distant-site provider. Once a relationship has been established, periodic in-person visits are also required. With few exceptions, patients must be located in a clinical setting and may not receive care from their homes. In addition, the distant-site provider cannot be located in a rural health clinic or FQHC.

Telehealth has been used broadly during the pandemic to expand healthcare access to individuals throughout the country. During the pandemic, Medicare significantly expanded the coverage of telehealth services. A recent Bipartisan Policy Center poll suggests that people receiving mental health and substance use services want a combination of in-person, video, and telephone services even after the pandemic has passed.

What telehealth expansions should remain after the pandemic?

Answer. I believe that consumers will expect all telehealth expansions to remain in place after the pandemic and purchasers and payers will need to ensure appropriate oversight is in place to drive the level of quality required from this platform.

Questions Submitted by Hon. John Cornyn

Question. Could you please explain why utilizing the primary care physician as the coordinator for a patient's mental health will result in better access to care and, ultimately, better patient outcomes?

Answer. Primary care physicians in many instances can serve as an initial access point for individuals with behavioral health needs. Like other acute or chronic issues, more serious cases may require a referral to specialists. However, a primary care provider may in fact be well-positioned to deal with the behavioral health needs of the patient in that moment. For many patients, the relationship with the primary care provider is already established and there will be more interactions. There also may be an ability to deal with stigma and educational issues around behavioral health diagnosis. Like many other cases that are more complex, primary care providers may not ultimately be the only provider involved with a patient but we need to do more to leverage and incentivize our primary care providers to meet the behavioral health needs of patients.

Question. Do you foresee any differences in integrating care with pediatricians and perhaps geriatricians as well?

Answer. Yes. Integration will look different for subsets of populations. Pediatricians need support for certain diagnosis and subpopulations. For example, children with more severe cases of autism may need to be referred to other providers for specialty services. More complex cases like children involved with the foster care system may require additional behavioral health supports. Populations served by geriatricians may require more robust specialty home and community-based services. Coordination between providers, patients and families are critical and pediatricians and geriatricians should be able to lean on insurers and managed care organizations to support and enhance service coordination.

Question. As COVID–19 closed down our society, healthcare providers still cared for patients. And with the pandemic came increased isolation, loneliness, anxiety, and depression.

Sadly, nearly 40 percent of American adults reported struggling with mental health or substance use. Anxiety and depression rose by 31 percent and serious suicidal ideation increased by 11 percent.

Points of access for those in crisis is a high priority for me. Last Congress I, alongside my colleague Senator Bennet, introduced the Suicide and Crisis Outreach Prevention Enhancement Act. This bill would reauthorize the National Suicide Prevention Lifeline for 5 years and collect more data on outcomes, providing a feedback loop of perfecting best practices. We think this legislation could save lives and help breakdown the stigma of seeking mental health care.

Can you describe the impact that you see this pandemic having on the need for access to mental and behavioral health services?

Answer. The pandemic has resulted in an increased need for behavioral health services. It has also increased expectations that these services be delivered through a full continuum of platforms including in-person, telehealth, and the ability to have individuals receive services in-home.

Question. What gaps do you continue to see in access to mental and behavioral health care?

Answer. Consistent with my testimony, we need to continue to support integration so that more patients can access behavioral health services in more settings. We need to continue to create incentives for a full continuum of services. The Lifeline program is a great start, but there is significant work to be done to enable success.

With the advent of 988, we need to make sure States are creating the infrastructure to respond to the expected increased demand. We also need a full continuum of crisis services. While Lifeline call center capacity is critical so are community services like mobile response teams and stabilization centers who handle more complex cases that cannot be resolved by call center teams. We need to create alternatives to emergency department boarding and short-term incarceration for those in crisis. We need to have Medicare and commercial carriers provide more financial support for behavioral health services and follow the lead Medicaid has established with broader services and provider access. We need to incentivize GME programs to create more specialists to support the behavioral health needs of patients.

Question. You mention in your testimony the National Association of Medicaid Director's recommendation of Crisis Systems. These are teams that are mobile, in the community and respond to individuals who may be experiencing a mental health crisis.

I am honored to work with my colleague from Nevada, Senator Cortez Masto, on the Behavioral Health Crisis Services Expansion Act. This bill would help communities establish a continuum of care for those undergoing a mental health crisis and support first responders and care providers by making such services reimbursable under Medicare and Medicaid.

This model would transform the way communities care for individuals in crisis and, in turn, it would help those who are most in need. I know you outlined the Crisis Now model in your testimony, but could you reemphasize the potential impact of such a crisis care system?

Answer. In Arizona, the Crisis Now model has been a critical part of the behavioral health continuum. It has provided robust call center teams that support individuals experiencing behavioral health crisis. Consistently, Arizona has one of the highest answer rates of any State for calls made to the Lifeline that originate from Arizona area codes. These call centers are able to support those in crisis by activating robust mobile response teams that serve all Arizonans (not just Medicaid members) in both urban and rural parts of the State. For the most complex cases, individuals may be served by short-term stabilization units. These stabilization units have also supported tens of thousands of law enforcement drop-offs that often occur in under 5 minutes. A robust crisis system can serve anyone anywhere at any time. Unfortunately, Arizona is somewhat unique in having this level of infrastructure. The overall impact is that people experiencing a behavioral health crisis are served in their time of need by individuals trained to deal with those in need. Crisis Now offers an appropriate array of vital services as an alternative to how people were treated previously through Emergency Department bed holds and incarceration.

Question. Do you see these teams as part of a larger strategy for addressing mental health?

Answer. Yes. The Crisis Now model serves individuals experiencing a crisis. We need to continue to expand access to prevent individuals from moving into crisis. We need to expand educational efforts around the importance of behavioral health and reduce stigma. We need to look at creative ways to deliver engaging behavioral health services through various platforms. We need to continue to improve culturally appropriate services and expand behavioral health access to address health equity issues. Crisis is an important step for improving behavioral health services but it is not the only policy focus that needs to be addressed to meet the needs of our country.

Submitted by Hon. Bill Cassidy, a U.S. Senator From Louisiana

American Telemedicine Association

901 N. Glebe Road, Suite 850
Arlington, VA 22203
T 703–373–9600
June 15, 2021

The Honorable Ron Wyden Chair
U.S. Senate Committee on Finance
Washington, DC 20510

The Honorable Mike Crapo Ranking Member
U.S. Senate Committee on Finance

Washington, DC 20510

Dear Chairman Wyden and Ranking Member Crapo:

On behalf of the American Telemedicine Association (ATA), I commend you for holding an important and timely hearing entitled, ''Mental Health Care in America: Addressing Root Causes and Identifying Policy Solutions.'' This hearing presents an excellent opportunity for members of your committee to thoughtfully consider the future of mental health care and how Congress can act to expand access to quality care for patients across the country. One such way you can accomplish this goal is to support the Telemental Health Care Access Act of 2021, bipartisan legislation championed by Senators Cassidy (R–LA), Smith (D–MN), Cardin (D–MD), and Thune (R–SD). The ATA enthusiastically endorses this important legislation and asks that you give it every possible consideration as you work together to identify policy solutions to improve mental health services.

As the only organization exclusively dedicated to expanding access to care through telehealth, the ATA appreciates and commends your committee's continued work to thoughtfully consider sound health care policies, including those impacting Medicare beneficiaries' access to telehealth services. Telehealth allows patients to receive safe, affordable, and quality care where and when they need it and has been a lifeline for millions of Americans during the COVID–19 pandemic. Before COVID–19, 65% of patients felt hesitant about telehealth, but now 87% want to continue using telehealth services post-pandemic.[4] Behavioral health services lend themselves particularly well to remote care, both because physical presence is not always clinically necessary for care and because of the great need for more access to mental health services.

We appreciate Congress's acting swiftly at the beginning of the COVID–19 Public Health Emergency (PHE) to ensure patients could safely access health care services from their homes. As you know, should Congress fail to act before the end of the current PHE, millions of Medicare beneficiaries will lose the choice to use these telehealth services. We look forward to continuing to work with you and your dedicated staff on policies that ensure these beneficiaries are not pushed off the telehealth cliff. Further, we commend you for already recognizing this looming cliff by including in the Consolidated

[4] How Americans Feel About Telehealth: One Year Later, SYKES' 2021 Telehealth Survey Report, April 9, 2021.

Appropriations Act, 2021, Pub. L. 116–260, a provision to ensure Medicare beneficiaries can access telemental services moving forward. However, one well-intentioned part of this policy provision, the in-person requirement, could have unintended negative consequences on Medicare beneficiaries.

In-Person Requirements for Telehealth Are Clinically Inappropriate

There is no clinical evidence for an arbitrary in-person requirement before a patient can access telehealth services. In fact, evidence has demonstrated that telemental services like telepsychology are just as effective as in-person visits.[5] Further, there is clear consensus that a provider can establish a relationship with a patient via a telehealth visit. The association of state regulators who oversee standards of medical care, the Federation of State Medical Boards, states that ". . . the relationship is clearly established when the physician agrees to undertake diagnosis and treatment of the patient, and the patient agrees to be treated, whether or not there has been an encounter in person between the physician (or other appropriately supervised health care practitioner) and patient."

In-Person Requirements Exacerbate Provider Shortages

The United States has a deficit of 6,000 mental health providers, and this shortage is expected to grow to a quarter of a million by 2030.[6] As we saw in 2020 and 2021, telehealth increases the capacity of the providers we do have to see more patients by removing geographic and other physical barriers. We must work together to increase the number of mental health providers to ensure all Americans get the care they need. However, explicitly denying a patient's access to mental health services based on his or her inability to find a scarce mental health provider is simply unreasonable.

---

[5] How well is telepsychology working? American Psychological Association, July 1, 2020.
[6] Triple-Tree: A New Era of Virtual Health Q2, 2021.

In-Person Requirements Increase Barriers and Worsen Health Inequities

The ATA strongly opposes statutory in-person requirements as they create arbitrary and clinically unsupported barriers to accessing affordable, quality health care. Requirements such as these could negatively impact those in underserved communities who may not be able to have an in-person exam due to provider shortages, work, lack of childcare, and/or other resources. Recent CDC data demonstrate that 23% of American adults do not have an existing relationship with a health care provider, and that statistic is alarmingly high in minority populations.[7] We cannot ignore the importance of providing all Americans, regardless of whether they have an established relationship with a medical provider, the opportunity to access life-saving health care.

Federal in-Person Requirements Unnecessarily Preempt State Laws

The in-person requirement for telehealth services is at odds with the direction telehealth policy has moved over the last decade. It disrupts Medicare's historical approach, which is to remain deferential to state laws on professional practice requirements and clinical standards of care. Today, no state practice of medicine law in the U.S. requires a prior in-person visit. The ATA urges Congress to ensure telemental health services continue post-pandemic but to recognize federal laws restricting these services are inappropriate. Instead, Congress should defer to states and individual payers to determine telehealth prerequisites. For the Medicare program, instead of codifying service-specific restrictions in statute, Congress should work with HHS to ensure the Secretary has the authority at the regulatory level to implement any appropriate health care requirements. By explicitly limiting care in statute, legislators will unnecessarily stifle innovation and tie the hands of regulators, providers, and patients.

For each of the reasons listed above, the ATA is proud to strongly support the Telemental Health Care Access Act and applauds the leadership of Senators Cassidy, Smith, Thune, and Cardin in introducing this essential legislation. We ask that you, too, consider the importance of this legislation and how we can work together to identify commonsense policies to not only

---

[7] Adults Who Report Not Having a Personal Doctor/Health Care Provider by Race/Ethnicity, KFF, Accessed June 8, 2021.

expand access to care but also ensure beneficiaries and federal taxpayers are protected. Thank you for your consideration, and please feel free to contact the ATA policy director Kyle Zebley should you have any questions about our support for thislegislation or ATA's broader federal policies.

Kind regards,
Ann Mond Johnson CEO
American Telemedicine Association

CC: The Honorable Bill Cassidy
the Honorable Tina Smith
The Honorable John Thune
The Honorable Ben Cardin

Health Innovation Alliance et al

June 22, 2021

Senator Bill Cassidy
520 Hart Senate Office Building
Washington, DC 20510

Senator Tina Smith
720 Hart Senate Office Building
Washington, DC 20510

Senator Ben Cardin
509 Hart Senate Office Building
Washington, DC

Senator John Thune
511 Dirksen 20510 Senate Office Building
Washington, DC 20510

Dear Senators Cassidy, Smith, Cardin, and Thune:

We write to thank you for your support of patients and providers in the mental health community by introducing the Telemental Health Care Access Act. We endorse your bill and applaud your efforts to ensure consistent coverage of mental health services furnished through telehealth.

Congress and the Administration have done much to utilize telehealth in response to COVID–19, and the results have been impressive. Prior to the pandemic just one percent of primary care visits were delivered via telehealth. Immediately after COVID–19 came ashore, primary care visits were delivered via telehealth more than 40 percent of the time. Telehealth improved access to care without generating cost increases for many, and at the exact time it was needed to help safeguard patients and prevent additional infections. It is a solid investment.

We were glad to see language pass through the Consolidated Appropriations Act of 2021 to remove Medicare restrictions on the mental health services delivered through virtual means, but we believe the inclusion of the in-person requirement every six months was unnecessary and a step in the wrong direction. Your legislation seeks to rectify that issue and we appreciate your leadership. Over the past 10 years, all 50 states and the District of Columbia have removed in-person requirements as a prerequisite to treatment through telehealth. In-person requirements on telehealth services create unnecessary barriers to care and can be especially harmful for those seeking mental and behavioral health services. The Health Resources and Services Administration reports a shortage of over 6,500 providers in the mental and behavioral health specialty. The scarcity of providers, particularly in rural and underserved areas makes lifting the in-person requirement even more critical. Those seeking care should not, and in many instances cannot, travel for hours to see an in-person provider.

By removing the automatic application of an in-person requirement for telemental health services in Medicare, Congress can improve health and lower costs while increasing access and utilization. This is where health care must head to become consumer-focused and responsive in the 21st century. We strongly urge Congress to pass the Telemental Health Care Access Act and continue increasing patient access to convenient at-home telehealth services. Thank you for considering our comments and for your leadership on this important issue.

Sincerely,

Health Innovation Alliance American Telemedicine Association STCHealth

CoverMyMeds HIMSS

PCHAlliance

National Council for Mental Wellbeing athenahealth

Alliance for Connected Care eHealth Initiative

Doctor On Demand Hims & Hers

Association for Behavioral Health and Wellness GO2 Foundation for Lung Cancer

Partnership to Advance Virtual Care Teladoc Health

Centerstone

American Psychiatric Association 3M Health Information Systems

American Foundation for Suicide Prevention American Psychological Association

The Michael J. Fox Foundation for Parkinson's Research American Medical Association

College of Healthcare Information Management Executives Connected Health Initiative

American College of Physicians Federation of American Hospitals American Heart Association Greenway Health

Marshfield Clinic Health System Association of American Medical Colleges American Medical Group Association Vanderbilt University Medical Center

Prepared Statement of Hon. Mike Crapo, a U.S. Senator from Idaho

Thank you, Mr. Chairman. Ensuring access to high-quality mental health services has been—and must continue to be—a priority.

Far too often, individuals with mental health, addiction, or substance use disorders find themselves isolated from their communities and separated from their providers. While Congress has taken decisive steps to address addiction, bolster behavioral health care, and curb substance use disorders, challenges remain. This committee has the ability to turn the tide.

We can begin by empowering States to craft innovative, targeted solutions. Medicaid functions most effectively when States have the flexibilities they need to address patients' unique care needs and adapt to unforeseen crises. As the Nation's largest payer of mental health and substance use disorder services, Medicaid must support, rather than subvert, State efforts to serve communities in need.

Unfortunately, the COVID–19 pandemic has highlighted—and exacerbated—the mental and behavioral health challenges we continue to confront. Loss of loved ones, increased isolation, and delayed treatment prompted a spike in anxiety, depression, and other debilitating conditions.

While many are returning to their pre-pandemic lives, we should not be content to allow our mental healthcare delivery system to revert to its preandemic ways. Whether for rural communities, urban areas, or tribes, telehealth has undoubtedly increased access to care. Through emergency flexibilities and permanent legislation authored by this committee late last year, we have taken crucial first steps toward modernizing telehealth coverage.

I look forward to working with you, Mr. Chairman, and with other members of this committee to build on those efforts in the months ahead. Further, by partnering with State and local leaders, we can spur care coordination, strengthen the mental health workforce, and drive value through delivery system reforms.

While there is no silver bullet here, I am confident we can tackle all of these challenges while upholding core principles of fiscal responsibility and program integrity.

Before concluding, it bares emphasizing that we must continue to make progress in improving understanding of mental health so that people in need are not afraid or ashamed to seek treatment. We cannot discount the impact of stigma on preventing those in need of treatment from receiving care. I look forward to hearing our witness testimony today to learn more about the solutions they have identified.

Prepared Statement of Michelle P. Durham, M.D., MPH, FAPA, DFAACAP, Assistant Professor of Psychiatry, Boston University School of Medicine; and Vice Chair of Education, and Psychiatry Residency Training Director, Department of Psychiatry, Boston Medical Center

Thank you, Chairman Wyden, Ranking Member Crapo, and distinguished members of the Senate Committee on Finance, for holding this hearing and providing me with the opportunity to speak today about the state of the mental healthcare system in America—where it's working, where it falls short, and how the Federal Government can play a role in helping to fill the gaps.

My name is Dr. Michelle Durham. I am a pediatric and adult psychiatrist at Boston Medical Center, and vice chair of education in the Department of Psychiatry, where I also trained for my residency, and now have the distinct honor of serving as the psychiatry residency training director. I hold a joint appointment at the Boston University School of Medicine as an assistant professor of psychiatry. Boston Medical Center (BMC) is an academic medical center and the largest safety-net hospital in New England. The patients we serve are predominantly low-income, with approximately half of our patients covered by Medicaid or the Children's Health Insurance Program (CHIP)—the highest percentage of any acute care hospital in Massachusetts.

The BMC emergency department, which includes 8 adult psychiatric emergency beds, is among the top ten busiest in the country. Mental illnesses are all too common among the patients BMC treats in our emergency department and across our continuum of mental health care services, which include outpatient integrated mental health care within our pediatric and adult primary care clinics and at local community health center partners, a mental health urgent care clinic, a crisis stabiliza tion unit, and our Boston Emergency Services Team (BEST) provides community-based evaluations and a jail diversion program. At present, BMC does not own or operate a locked inpatient psychiatric unit.

To give you a sense of who BMC serves, 70 percent of our patients identify as black or Latinx, approximately one in three (32 percent) speak a language other than English as their primary language, and over half live at or below the Federal poverty level. The patients we see at BMC who present with mental illness frequently have co-occurring substance use disorders, homelessness, malnutrition, and other health-related social needs linked to poverty. The current COVID–19 pandemic, structural racism, and economic crisis has further exacerbated the mental illness and trauma experienced by our patients. In my 10 years at BMC, I have never seen our mental healthcare services stretched so far beyond their capacity as they are now. Just the other day, we had 25 patients in our psychiatric emergency department—more than triple its capacity—presenting with a much higher level of acuity, some waiting for evaluation and others boarding awaiting placement in an inpatient psychiatric unit.

A severe lack of capacity in our country's mental healthcare system existed long before the COVID–19 pandemic. The reasons for this are multifactorial; however, for the sake of my remarks today I will broadly categorize them into issues related to the mental healthcare workforce and patient access to care.

It is widely understood and well-documented that America has a dearth of licensed mental health professionals, in general, and that particular areas of the country—largely rural and outside of the Northeast—are disproporionately impacted.[8] Even where I practice in Boston, which has one of the highest

---

[8] U.S. Health Resources and Services Administration. Health Professional Shortage Areas Data Dashboard. Last Updated: June 10, 2021. *https://data.hrsa.gov/topics/health-workforce/ shortage-areas.*

number of child and adolescent psychiatrists per capita in the country, the capacity is insufficient to meet the mental health needs of the community.[9]

Increased Medicare graduate medical education (GME) funding for psychiatry residency slots can help increase the physician workforce. Increased funding for loan forgiveness programs for those who work in underserved areas can help alleviate the $250,000 of debt that the average medical student has accumulated by the time their residency education is completed. The need to pay off medical school loan burden is also likely to cause physicians to pursue practice in more affluent areas, adversely impacting access to care for lower-income populations.[10]

Beyond the shortage of providers, the mental health workforce is not diverse—for instance, only 2 percent of psychiatrists identify as black—and not representative or reflective of the U.S. population.[11,12] In order to address this, we must understand that the issue at its root is a pipeline issue that requires holistic solutions. Just as we say in medicine, that a person's ZIP code is more influential than their genetic code in determining life trajectory and long-term health, where a person lives, the color of their skin, and language they speak is highly determinative of the quality of education and resources available, the level of exposure to the mental health field, and stigma associated with mental illness.

In terms of access to mental health services, COVID–19 led to an accelerated adoption of telemedicine. At peak, over 90 percent of our outpatient psychiatric visits were conducted via telehealth, which enabled BMC to maintain and exceed our pre-pandemic volume of service. That said, while telehealth is an important tool for ensuring patient access to mental health care, it does not work for everyone due to digital inequities that exist related to Internet access and digital literacy, especially among low-income communities.

Additional barriers to care exist as a result of disparate insurance coverage, lack of mental health parity, and insufficient insurance uptake by

---

[9] American Academy of Child and Adolescent Psychiatry. Practicing Child and Adolescent Psychiatrists Workforce Maps by State. Last Updated: March 2018. *https://aacap.org/AACAP/Advocacy/Federal_and_State_Initiatives/Workforce_Maps/Home.aspx.*

[10] Zimmerschied C. How med student loan burdens can deepen health disparities. American Medical Association. April 27, 2017. *https://ama-assn.org/education/medical-school-diversity/ how-med-student-loan-burdens-can-deepen-health-disparities.*

[11] Lin L, Stamm K, Christidis P. How diverse is the psychology workforce? American Psychological Association. 2018; 49(2). *https://apa.org/monitor/2018/02/datapoint.*

[12] American Hospital Association (2016). The State of the Behavioral Health Workforce: A Literature Review. *https://aha.org/system/files/hpoe/Reports-HPOE/2016/aha/Behavioral/FINAL.pdf.*

licensed mental health providers (especially for Medicaid). The social determinants of mental health and structural vulnerabilities inherently involved with treating low-income patients require more dedicated time with patients to provide appropriate care. Insufficient Medicaid reimbursement acts as a deterrent for providers to see Medicaid patients, producing a cascade effect in which the more oppressed, marginalized populations have limited to no access to mental health professionals.

I welcome the Senate Finance Committee's involvement in exploring ways for Federal policy to improve mental health care across various settings, as well as incentivize and seed the development and scaling up of innovative models of mental health care delivery in order to improve access. A few such examples include:

- Transforming and Expanding Access to Mental Health Care in Urban Pediatrics (TEAM UP) for Children, a pediatric integrated model in Federally Qualified Health Centers in Massachusetts, builds capacity of health centers to deliver high-quality, evidence-informed care to children and families. The model includes behavioral health clinicians and community health workers working with pediatric primary care providers to provide timely mental health treatment.
- The Massachusetts Child Psychiatry Access Program (MCPAP) improves access to treatment for children with behavioral health needs and their families by making child psychiatry services accessible to primary care providers across Massachusetts via remote consultation and education. This model has been expanded to other States such as Connecticut where I completed my fellowship.
- The Wellness and Recovery After Psychosis (WRAP) Program is tailored for people experiencing psychotic symptoms using a team-based approach and providing individual, group and family therapy, medication management, case management, and peer support.
- The Metro Boston Recovery Learning Community (MBRLC) offers peer-to-peer services for people in recovery from mental health and/or substance use issues through peer support, advocacy, and career coaching.

We are at a pivotal time in our country. Over a year into the COVID–19 pandemic, every person's mental well-being has been impacted in some way. The need for a more robust mental health care system has never been more clear or pronounced. Treatment for mental health issues should be accessible—no matter who you are, where you live or your ability to pay. Appropriate investment along the care continuum and for the mental health workforce can improve access to care and retention and recruitment of mental health professionals.

Mental health is health and should not be thought of or managed separate or apart from physical health in the ways it historically has been. The time is now to invest in a 21st-century mental healthcare system in America.

Thank you for your time. I look forward to the discussion.

Questions Submitted for the Record to Michelle P. Durham, M.D., MPH, FAPA, DFAACAP

Questions Submitted by Hon. Elizabeth Warren

Question. During your testimony and conversations with my staff, you mentioned that telehealth flexibilities were not enough to fully capture people with substance use disorder that encountered BMC providers (for example, it was harder to connect individuals that entered the emergency room with SUD services that were online, as opposed to available in person and in the moment). Congress should take steps to expand telehealth flexibilities beyond the pandemic, but it should also identify and seek to mitigate gaps that emerge when telehealth is the default.

What additional barriers, if any, did virtual telehealth services pose to patients in need of SUD services, and what specific steps should Congress take to address those barriers in advance of future pandemics?

Answer. Telehealth video was difficult for patients who didn't have reliable access to the needed technology (phones with video, computers, Internet, etc.) and a confidential place to have an appointment. Patients who need certain medications still were required to come into the clinic (e.g., methadone and injections for naltrexone or extended-release buprenorphine). Reimbursement for audio-only appointments al lowed clinicians to connect with folks who did not have access to technology with video capabilities and should be continued beyond the pandemic. Expanding mobile services for methadone and injectable medications would also help to reduce barriers to treatment. The infrastructure proposals before Congress that seek to expand broadband access would also be beneficial to enable more of the population to reliably access telehealth services. In addition, the Federal Government could work with local communities to establish centralized locations in the community where people can attend telehealth appointments.

Question. During your testimony, you raised the alarming statistic that black men in Massachusetts saw a 69-percent increase in overdoses and overdose deaths during the pandemic.

As Congress seeks to develop future legislation that responds to overdoses and overdose deaths through a health equity lens, what types of questions should members ask to ensure they are identifying challenges facing communities of color in SUD policy development?

Answer. I really appreciate this question. I think it's important for members of Congress to ask, ''Who is not at the table?'' It is important to include people with lived experience with addiction, including persons of color, in the conversation as they are so often left out, and ask them directly, ''What are the challenges you personally faced in getting the care you needed to get better?'' In addition, using a health equity lens, Congress could ask, ''How does SUD treatment offered to white patients differ from what is offered to persons of color, in terms of where services are offered, how they are advertised, and what specific treatment are offered to individuals? Data suggest that racial disparities exist in each of these arenas.

It is also important to acknowledge that stigma related to addiction and mental health is very real and differs by community and culture. Stigma is a challenge for ensuring access to care and stigma is a challenge for policymaking. Members of Congress can help reduce stigma by validating the experiences of persons of color with substance use disorders by inviting them to have a seat at the table in the development of SUD policy. Congress could seek to learn more about why stigma exists against seeking help, including the particular stigma associated with receiving medications for addiction, and what added stigma exists for persons of color who use drugs.

The Federal response to addiction should not focus on a specific class of substances like opioids at the exclusion of others as use patterns oftentimes cuts across racial/ethnic lines. In addition, use of more than one substance (or polysubstance use) is common and government policies and funding would do better to reflect that reality. As members of Congress are likely well aware, fentanyl is increasingly being mixed into other substances like cocaine, which users may ingest unknowingly, and may influence overdose and overdose death rates. The Congress could inquire, ''How does the availability of drugs and presence of fentanyl in the drug supply create further disparities in overdoses and overdose deaths for persons of color?''

There are numerous historical policies related to drug use that have resulted in the systematic exclusion of people of color from addiction treatment services. Reviewing past policies through a health equity lens can help to correct past inequities in order to create a more equitable and accessible SUD treatment system for persons of color. In particular, decriminalizing drug possession can help individuals get the treatment they need and avoid incarceration where comprehensive addiction services, including medications for addiction treatment, are rarely available. Additionally, a health equity lens should be applied to examining racial disparities in access to different medications for opioid use disorder, like methadone, which is more commonly prescribed to persons of color, and buprenorphine, which is more commonly prescribed to white patients, as well as the disparate regulations pertinent to these treatments. Research is necessary to better characterize the needs of people of color and to design addiction treatment programs that may be more responsive to their goals and expectations—the Federal Government can play a role in catalyzing and seeding this research. Additionally, Congress can create sustainable funding and additional incentives for integrated mental health and primary care services, which especially for low-income populations, like those served at BMC, should incorporate the capacity to address social determinants of health.

Question. In your experience as a provider, how do you see these communities left out of SUD conversations, and what preemptive steps should policymakers take to center these communities in policy discussions?

Answer. The one-size-fits-all approach of the American health care system does not work for all communities—i.e., expecting patients to show up to clinic to get care, instead of bringing care to places and people that communities trust. For example, care provided in houses of worship, community centers or home visits. In general, there's not a lot of focus on prevention and promotion in our addiction and mental healthcare system. Greater investment in community-based organizations and support services, such as case management focused on psychosocial needs, would help reach more people that the current system fails to catch. It also could help to create a seat at the table in SUD policy discussions for community health workers (CHWs) and recovery coaches.

Questions Submitted by Hon. Catherine Cortez Masto

Question. In your testimony you touched on the continuum of crisis services that are provided by Boston Medical Center.

If you were to be able to expand the capacity of programs like the behavioral health urgent care clinic or the crisis stabilization unit, would you expect to see changes in ER volume or even hospital readmissions?

Answer. Expanding the continuum of crisis services at Boston Medical Center (BMC) would probably not realistically impact the volume of patients we see presenting with behavioral health issues in the emergency room (ER) or inpatient setting. A regional approach to expand the full continuum of care services, not just crisis services, including an emphasis on prevention and moving upstream to address health-related social needs, behavioral health integration in primary care settings, and other means of enabling individuals to access outpatient mental health services when they need it, would be more likely to reduce reliance on ER and inpatient mental health services. Timely response is key and can potentially avoid requiring ER or inpatient-level care.

Question. You spoke about the workforce challenges that we're seeing across the country, and the lack of diversity among providers that seems to exacerbate access issues among LGBT populations, communities of color and underserved communities.

Do you think expanding the types of clinicians who can practice behavioral health services would help to build the pipelines of providers who can meet the needs of diverse communities?

Answer. Increased use of behavioral integration in primary care and allowing mental health professionals to work to the full extent of their license within scope of practice could help address workforce shortages and improve access to behavioral health care. Including CHWs and peer support in care models, and reimbursing them for their time is crucial to better serving the needs of diverse communities.

Question. How else can Congress develop a provider workforce that is able to serve diverse communities most effectively?

Answer. As I mentioned in my testimony, I see the provider workforce shortage as a pipeline issue. Additional education and training opportunities writ large and for communities of color in particular would go a long way. Increased resources should be targeted to historically disinvested communities. Barriers to education and training can be addressed with additional funding for scholarships for people of color and individuals from low-income communities to complete their primary education and higher education, as well as loan repayment programs to reduce the financial burden/barriers to getting people into the field. Addressing stigma in the community—what it means to work in the mental health profession, and what it means to get mental health care—is imperative as well. In terms of legislation before Congress, the Pursuing Equity in Mental Health Act (S. 1795)—which you've cosponsored and has passed the House as H.R. 1475—if passed by the Senate would help provide additional resources to recruit and sustain a diverse mental health workforce. BMC is very much in support of S. 1795/H.R. 1475.

Questions Submitted by Hon. John Barasso

Question. The healthcare professionals, along with all front-line workers, deserve our gratitude and appreciation. Their dedication to our communities during this pandemic is something we must recognize and never forget.

A top concern of Wyoming mental health facilities is making sure there are enough staff to care for their patients. It is especially challenging to attract and keep healthcare providers in rural communities.

Can you discuss solutions related to workforce development you believe will improve the ability of mental health facilities to attract and maintain staff in rural areas?

Answer. The mental health burden in some communities, rural, urban, and suburban, is tremendous, and requires significantly more resources to adequately support the mental health workforce and address the need. Overtaxing the limited mental health resources that exist in high need areas contributes to high churn among mental health professionals. A model like the Massachusetts Child Psychiatry Access Program (MCPAP), which I referenced in my testimony, is one way to stretch existing resources and increase access to psychiatric consults for primary care providers in rural areas.

Question. Can you specifically discuss changes to GME policy you believe would improve the pipeline of mental health physicians?

Answer. Increased funding for GME slots in general, as proposed in the Resident Physician Shortage Reduction Act (S. 834/H.R. 2256), and targeted to a particular specialty, such as addiction medicine and addiction psychiatry, as proposed in the Opioid/SUD Workforce Act (S. 1438/H.R. 3441), would help significantly improve the pipeline of mental health physicians.

Question. As a doctor, I strongly support increasing access to mental health services, especially in rural communities. Senator Stabenow and I have previously introduced legislation for many years that would allow mental health counselors and marriage and family therapists to receive reimbursement from Medicare.

Can you discuss how the Department of Health and Human Services can improve access for mental health services, especially for those on Medicare?

Answer. One way HHS could help improve access to mental health services is by removing the Medicare cap on the number of inpatient psychiatric days a beneficiary can have in their lifetime—this is a lack of parity with physical health care. People under age 65 who are chronically or severely mentally ill and on Medicare, who need inpatient mental health care, end up stuck in the hospital emergency department because of this restriction.

Question. In particular, can you comment on the merits of allowing licensed professional counselors and marriage and family therapists to receive reimbursements from Medicare?

Answer. People should get reimbursed for what is in their scope of practice, so I don't see any reason why licensed professional counselors (LPCs) or marriage and family therapists (MFTs) should not receive reimbursement from Medicare for the services they are trained to provide.

Questions Submitted by Hon. Tim Scott

Question. The toll that union-sponsored excuses for ''virtual learning'' has taken on actual kids is extraordinarily sad, especially for our Nation's most vulnerable children. In October 2020, a survey conducted by the Jed Foundation showed that 31 percent of parents said their child's mental or emotional health was worse than before the pandemic. Private insurance data also shows that while all health care claims for adolescents ages 13–18 were down in 2020 compared to 2019, mental health-related claims for this age group increased sharply. Additionally, the Centers for Disease Control and Prevention (CDC) reports 25 percent of parents whose children attended school virtually were more likely to report an overall worsened mental or emotional health compared to only 16 percent of parents of children attending school in-person.

What programs within the Department of Health and Human Services' (HHS) purview are best poised to support children and schools as they return to complete in-person learning?

Answer. I'm not sure of the particular programs within HHS that may best support children and schools as they return to in-person learning, but either way more therapists are needed in schools. Kids spend most of their waking hours in school so it is best to make mental health services and supports available to them there.

In addition, mental health support for school teachers, staff, administrators, and parents of school-aged children will be vitally important as kids look to adults for modeling especially during times of transition and uncertainty. The Federal Government can and should play a role in helping to facilitate connections to care within the community in instances when it is beyond the capacity of school (e.g., funding and supporting crisis management services in the community). All of this should be integrated into a prevention and promotion framework, which includes psychoeducation and group intervention, in order to help kids and adults connect the dots of what they have experienced and identify how trauma may manifest and when to ask for help.

Question. How can we integrate more telehealth opportunities to expand access to mental health services in schools?

Answer. I think it would be very impactful if students could access telehealth in schools. Schools or community health center partners should be outfitted with the technology to enable access for kids who may not have the necessary technology or private space at home, assuming the location of the child is no longer relevant for reimbursement. Parents will have to be involved to a certain extent with the care of minors, particularly with respect to prescribing medication, so it will be important for schools and communities to set up systems and processes to engage parents without creating additional barriers.

Question. Telehealth has expanded rapidly as a result of the COVID–19 pandemic. Numerous studies have demonstrated the effectiveness of telehealth for behavioral health services.

As telehealth becomes more common among health care providers, what can Congress do to ensure that patients do not suffer from unnecessary bureaucratic delays?

Answer. Congress can help to ensure parity for mental health services with physical health services. In my experience, prior authorization for behavioral health services is not level with physical health and should be addressed to reduce unnecessary barriers to care.

Question. There is a well-researched connection between unemployment and mental health. As recently as April 2021, despite billions of dollars of

COVID–19 stimulus, aggregate employment remained 7.9 million jobs below its pre-recession level.

What impact will this failure to get people back to work have on mental health?

Answer. Engaging people with meaningful work, financial security, and structure is helpful for maintaining and supporting mental health. In places where insurance is more closely tied to work, rising or stagnant unemployment could reduce access to health care for people facing unemployment.

Question. Last November, an article published in the Journal of the American Medical Association noted that multiple studies indicated that older adults may be less negatively affected by certain mental health outcomes than other age groups.

Are these study outcomes consistent with your own professional experiences working with older adults?

Answer. N/A.

Question. Current network adequacy standards often allow networks of specialists who aren't taking new patients or who have long waiting lists. That means that many people needing treatment must go out of network to get care, and only those who can afford the high cost get it. One of the biggest challenges to access to behavioral health care services is that many behavioral health specialists don't participate in health plan networks.

Why is that, and how can we change that?

Answer. Low reimbursement and administrative burden, including dealing with prior authorization, act as deterrents to providers accepting health insurance. Improving reimbursement and expanding team-based care models that support integration of behavioral health into primary care settings could help.

Question. Outside of the public health emergency, telehealth services are restricted to certain geographic and clinical settings. Beneficiaries must live in a rural area and have an initial face-to-face visit with the distant-site provider. Once a relationship has been established, periodic in-person visits are also required. With few exceptions, patients must be located in a clinical setting and may not receive care from their homes. In addition, the distant-site provider cannot be located in a rural health clinic or FQHC.

Telehealth has been used broadly during the pandemic to expand health care access to individuals throughout the country. During the pandemic, Medicare significantly expanded the coverage of telehealth services. A recent Bipartisan Policy Center poll suggests that people receiving mental health and substance use services want a combination of in-person, video, and telephone services even after the pandemic has passed.

What telehealth expansions should remain after the pandemic?

Answer. Particularly for the patients that I see at Boston Medical Center, a majority of whom are low-income, maintaining coverage and reimbursement for audio-only telehealth is essential. Insurers should also not require an in-person visit for mental health visits in order to permit continued telehealth use (e.g., requiring one in-person visit within 6 months of the first telehealth appointment). The decision of whether to see a patient in person or virtually should instead be up to the discretion of the clinician.

Questions Submitted by Hon. John Cornyn

Question. Your testimony outlines the collaborative care model and integrated care. I can appreciate the benefit of this collaboration between practitioners, and I too am concerned about the education and support our primary care physicians receive for addressing mental health.

The Massachusetts Child Psychiatry Access Program, as you claim, "improves access to treatment for children with behavioral health needs and their families . . . via remote consultation and education." Telehealth is a tool that delivered positive results during the pandemic and is largely here to stay. And I look forward to working with my colleagues on ensuring patients have access to care through telehealth, including mental health care.

What type of education regarding mental health is offered to primary care physicians in collaborative care models?

What about outside of those care models?

Do you have any recommendations for Congress to consider regarding disseminating mental health best practices or education items to primary care physicians?

Answer. Congress could play a role in funding a national technical assistance program for collaborative care models, including access to start-up capital to get behavioral health clinicians, managers, and systems in place. Training and education works best when built into clinicians' workflow/time. Additional research funding is needed in order to learn more about the best forms of integrated care for different patient populations.

Prepared Statement of Chantay Jett, MA, MFT, Executive Director, Wallowa Valley Center for Wellness

Introduction/Background

Good morning, Chairman Wyden, Ranking Member Crapo, and members of the Senate Finance Committee. Thank for you for the opportunity to appear before the committee to discuss policy solutions to address both the mental health and substance use crises impacting the United States and in particular the rural and frontier areas of our percent. My name is Chantay Jett, and I am executive director of Wallowa Valley Center for Wellness (WVCW), which provides community-based mental health and substance use treatment services in the most remote region of the great State of Oregon.

We represent a truly frontier area of our Nation where the cows outnumber the people and our closest major airport is in Boise, ID—nearly 4 hours away. We are literally at the end of the road where everybody knows everybody, which unfortunately contributes to both stigma and lack of access for people seeking treatment services. I am here to tell you that the Certified Community Behavioral Health Clinic (or CCBHC) model has truly made a difference in our frontier community. I hope every State in the near future has the opportunity to use the resources this model has made available to us to meet the specific needs of our wonderful community.

The State of Oregon participates in a 10-State demonstration of the Excellence in Mental Health and Addiction Treatment Act that this committee helped to establish in 2014 through the bipartisan leadership of Senators Stabenow and Blunt. The Center for Wellness is one of 12 CCBHCs that operate in our State. We provide high-quality, integrated, community-based mental health and substance use services to individuals, while also screening for possible co-morbid conditions like heart disease, diabetes, and HIV/AIDS. Among the most important services that CCBHCs provide—both in Oregon and nationwide—are immediate access to Medication Assisted Treatment (MAT) for substance use and 24-hour emergency psychiatric care.

Prevalence of Behavioral Health Conditions in Oregon/ Mental Health Professional Shortages

Please permit me to provide some very brief context of CCBHCs within rural and frontier counties in the State of Oregon. According to the Oregon Health Authority (OHA), our State reports higher rates of mental health conditions, including severe and persistent mental illness and suicidal ideation. The COVID–19 pandemic has only exacerbated an ongoing mental health and substance use crisis in rural Oregon.

OHA also details a lack of access to mental health and substance use care, especially in frontier communities which face greater distances for referral to outpatient and inpatient services. To give you a sense, there is no stoplight within a 76-mile radius of Wallowa County. The OHA reports average wait times of as much as 6 months Statewide due to a lack of providers. However, we are the lucky ones, because the CCBHC model helped created an internal reorganization of service delivery which resulted in same day access to care.

Wallowa Valley Center for Wellness: The Ccbhc Experience

Prior to becoming a CCBHC, The Center for Wellness was heavily reliant upon grants. Grant funding is crucially important, but it carries limitations. Grants typically end every 2 to 3 years; they all have different reporting requirements and different program specifications, which unfortunately results in more time spent filling out paperwork, rather than treating our patients.

By contrast, the CCBHC prospective payment system permits us to do three big things. First, The Center for Wellness is able to contract with more skilled clinicians—including psychiatrists and medical professionals to prescribe Medication Assisted Treatment for patients with opioid use disorder. This directly results in decreased wait times and reduced emergency department utilization.

Secondly, the CCBHC program is designed to expand access to underserved populations. In our case, becoming a CCBHC really opened the door for mental health care to veterans as it requires the staffing of services specifically for veterans. According to the Veterans Service Organizations (VSO) in our county, there are at least 1,000 community members who have donned the uniform out of 7,000 residents. One of our CCBHC funded clinicians has been invited to the weekly PTSD groups at the Veterans of Foreign Wars (VFW) for veterans and their families. Becoming a CCBHC has allowed us to increase our services to 23 veterans in our community. This may not seem significant to you, but it's an increase of 300 percent— a big deal for us here in rural Oregon.

Thirdly, consistent CCBHC resources are a fundamental driver of integrated care. In Oregon, the CCBHC demonstration financing has made it possible to integrate with a local Federally Qualified Health Center (FQHC) allowing primary care, specialty medical services, and behavioral health services to be accessible under the same roof. We also share a single Electronic Health Record with our partner FQHC and local critical access hospital to permit immediate care coordination. Patients tell me that it is such a relief to not have to retell their story with every multidisciplinary provider they see. I will add that if there is no open acute psychiatric bed in our hospital or an acute bed is too distant in time traveled, we are lucky to have a great neighbor and partner across the State line in Idaho to access acute care psychiatric hospitalization. This component of care coordination and partnership with primary care and hospitals even across State lines is imperative because patients with severe mental illness and substance use challenges have shockingly high rates of chronic conditions, encompassing everything from cirrhosis to emphysema to heart disease. The CCBHC model allows us to have these partnerships and get patients the services they deserve in a timely manner.

In closing, I strongly believe that this model represents the future of community-based mental health care and substance use treatment in the United States. This is why I am asking you to make this model available to every State nationwide. As a percent, we can do better than first treating mental health and substance use in hospital emergency departments, homeless shelters, and the county jails. Investing in CCBHC's is streamlining services in efficient ways that drive costs down over the entire continuum of care. Despite being from a tiny frontier community at the end of the road in northeastern Oregon, I hope you see that CCBHCs make an enormous impact.

Again, thank you for the opportunity to testify, I am happy to answer any questions you may have.

Questions Submitted for the Record to Chantay Jett, MA, MFT Question Submitted by Hon. Ron Wyden

Question. I understand you employ a range of physician and non-physician providers.

Can you tell the committee more about the clinical staff you employ who can and cannot receive Medicare reimbursement? In rural and frontier counties it is very difficult to find licensed providers in this workforce shortage landscape.

Answer. Many of the service providers, such as peer support, case management, skills training, Supported Employment, Early Assessment Support Alliance (EASA), Assertive Community Treatment Team (ACT), med management, and Substance Use Providers (SUD) are not compensated at all by Medicare. The Licensed Clinical Social Workers we employ along with psychiatrists are compensated less than the value of the service they provide.

Question. In a typical year, about how much does Medicare's provider policy cost your clinic?

Answer. Wallowa Valley Center for Wellness writes off more than $500,000 per year in uncovered Medicare services.

Questions Submitted by Hon. John Barasso

Question. The healthcare professionals, along with all front-line workers, deserve our gratitude and appreciation. Their dedication to our communities during this pandemic is something we must recognize and never forget.

A top concern of Wyoming mental health facilities is making sure there are enough staff to care for their patients. It is especially challenging to attract and keep healthcare providers in rural communities.

Can you discuss solutions related to workforce development you believe will improve the ability of mental health facilities to attract and maintain staff in rural areas?

Answer. Attracting and retaining a highly qualified workforce requires easier loan repayment programs and equalizing the requirements for school BH, primary care BH and community BH. We currently see the other sectors being able to pay more for less requirements and we cannot compete with this. The solution is to create an environment of equal parity in base salary for behavioral health workers as well as parity with the paperwork administrative burden placed only on the community mental health programs, as well as primary care providers sharing the risk for acute care hospital placements. I believe these three practices would remove a significant barrier to workforce development and the inability to offer competitive employment for a spouse/partner of a master's level clinician.

Question. Can you specifically discuss changes to GME policy you believe would improve the pipeline of mental health physicians?

Answer. As a community mental health program, we do not deal specifically with the guidelines and policies related to GME programs on the primary healthcare side. I do not feel like I could offer an educated answer to your question.

Question. As a doctor, I strongly support increasing access to mental health services, especially in rural communities. Senator Stabenow and I have previously intro duced legislation for many years that would allow mental health counselors and marriage and family therapists to receive reimbursement from Medicare.

Can you discuss how the Department of Health and Human Services can improve access for mental health services, especially for those on Medicare?

Answer. Medicare reimbursement for Licensed Professional Counselors (LPCs) and Licensed Marriage and Family Therapists (LMFTs) would vastly improve access to care. Currently, a consumer has to either wait for an available (and scarce) LCSW or pay full fee for services, both of which are unacceptable. The ability to conduct telephonic and video sessions has addressed some barriers to care and these services must continue to be reimbursed/billable regardless of the status of COVID.

Question. LMFTs and LPCs are as qualified or more to serve our community members, and the alliance between Medicare and LCSWs is purely an outcome of effective lobbying not good practice. In particular, can you comment on the merits of allowing licensed professional counselors and marriage and family therapists to receive reimbursements from Medicare?

Answer. Please see above.

Questions Submitted by Hon. Tim Scott

Question. The toll that union-sponsored excuses for ''virtual learning'' has taken on actual kids is extraordinarily sad, especially for our Nation's most vulnerable children. In October 2020, a survey conducted by the Jed

Foundation showed that 31 percent of parents said their child's mental or emotional health was worse than before the pandemic. Private insurance data also shows that while all health care claims for adolescents ages 13–18 were down in 2020 compared to 2019, mental health-related claims for this age group increased sharply. Additionally, the Centers for Disease Control and Prevention (CDC) reports 25 percent of parents whose children attended school virtually were more likely to report an overall worsened mental or emotional health compared to only 16 percent of parents of children attending school in-person.

What programs within the Department of Health and Human Services' (HHS) purview are best poised to support children and schools as they return to complete in-person learning?

Answer. Regardless of the location of the instruction, a global event like COVID impacts the mental health of students. DOE and HHS need to partner on grasping the impact of collective trauma. Educators and school-based counselors need to recognize and support the lasting effects that COVID has had on our Nation and world and help students gain an understanding and normalize the emotional response to a life changing event.

Question. How can we integrate more telehealth opportunities to expand access to mental health services in schools?

Answer. A barrier to tele-health BH services is ensuring IT systems have the necessary permissions to ''talk'' to teach other. Our experience is that the school's Internet blocks our access.

Question. Telehealth has expanded rapidly as a result of the COVID–19 pandemic. Numerous studies have demonstrated the effectiveness of telehealth for behavioral health services.

As telehealth becomes more common among health care providers, what can Congress do to ensure that patients do not suffer from unnecessary bureaucratic delays?

Answer. Unnecessary bureaucratic delays are often due to the payment structure and how Medicare and private insurance will not pay for less expensive evidence-based services such as IPS-supported employment, case management, skills training, etc.

Question. There is a well-researched connection between unemployment and mental health. As recently as April 2021, despite billions of dollars of COVID–19 stimulus, aggregate employment remained 7.9 million jobs below its pre-recession level.

What impact will this failure to get people back to work have on mental health?

Answer. Like students, the entire Nation has experienced collective trauma, and employers need to recognize that status quo employment practices and some of the barriers to things like affordable housing and child care have a ripple effect across the employment rate.

Question. Last November, an article published in the *Journal of the American Medical Association* noted that multiple studies indicated that older adults may be less negatively affected by certain mental health outcomes than other age groups.

Are these study outcomes consistent with your own professional experiences working with older adults?

Answer. Actually, older adults identify ''not needing'' MH support but that does not correlate with overall health outcomes and behaviors (such as obesity, smoking, gambling, alcohol abuse, and suicide). Our older community members cite stigma and rugged individualism as factors in avoiding MH services. This is also relevant to accessing/pursuing preventative medical care. ''I'm not sick, so why should I see a doctor?''

Question. Current network adequacy standards often allow networks of specialists who aren't taking new patients or who have long waiting lists. That means that many people needing treatment must go out of network to get care, and only those who can afford the high cost get it. One of the biggest challenges to access to behavioral health care services is that many behavioral health specialists don't participate in health plan networks.

Why is that, and how can we change that?

Answer. In my opinion, this problem is specific to the failure of health plan networks. The most common feedback I hear is that ''the network is full and not accepting any new providers.'' This is something providers in private practice face; this is not generally an issue in a community mental health program which employs a wide range of behavioral health specialists within their own programs.

Question. Outside of the public health emergency, telehealth services are restricted to certain geographic and clinical settings. Beneficiaries must live in a rural area and have an initial face-to-face visit with the distant-site provider. Once a relationship has been established, periodic in-person visits are also required. With few exceptions, patients must be located in a clinical setting and may not receive care from their homes. In addition, the distant-site provider cannot be located in a rural health clinic or FQHC.

Telehealth has been used broadly during the pandemic to expand health care access to individuals throughout the country. During the pandemic, Medicare significantly expanded the coverage of telehealth services. A recent

Bipartisan Policy Center poll suggests that people receiving mental health and substance use services want a combination of in-person, video, and telephone services even after the pandemic has passed.

What telehealth expansions should remain after the pandemic?

Answer. All of them! We are finding greater engagement to care by being offering an array of access points for folks. Even in the pandemic our yearly hours of service only fluctuated by about 60 hours from the previous year. However, the number of visits nearly doubled due to shorter encounters made possible through a variety of video, telephonic and in-person visits.

Prepared Statement of Benjamin F. Miller, PSY.D., Chief Strategy Officer, Well Being Trust

Chairman Wyden, Ranking Member Crapo, and members of the committee, my name is Dr. Benjamin F. Miller, and I am the chief strategy officer for Well Being Trust, a national foundation started in 2016 through a gift by the Providence Health System that is focused on advancing the mental, social, and spiritual health of the Nation.

I am a clinical psychologist by training and have spent most of my adult life pursuing strategies that can advance mental health to a place of priority within our society. This goal has guided much of my work during my time as the founding director of the University of Colorado's Farley Health Policy Center and continuing today in my capacity as an adjunct professor at Stanford School of Medicine and at Well Being Trust.

It is an honor to be able to speak to you today about an issue that every American is experiencing—an issue that we need to aggressively pursue, and which COVID–19 has all but exacerbated especially among communities of color and other marginalized people: our mental health. Several government reports highlight how broken our mental health system is. The 2020 DoD Inspector General report that found over 50 percent of service members and their families who needed mental health care did not receive it.[13] SAMHSA found that over 56 percent of adults with mental illness did not receive any treatment in the past year, nor did 35 percent of those with serious mental

[13] https://www.dodig.mil/reports.html/Article/2309785/evaluation-of-access-to-mental-health-care-in-the-department-of-defense-dodig-2/.

illness.[14] And a recent GAO report highlighted a multitude of issues at multiple levels for mental health, including ongoing challenges with health insurance, enforcing laws like mental health parity, and finding the right clinician who can help.[15] In one survey, almost 30 percent of people reported not seeking care because they did not know where to go.[16]

The need to solve for these and other existing problems is real and immediate. Clear pathways do not exist for people seeking mental health care—there are not obvious doors to enter, and we have no system that routinely is able to identify and treat people in a timely manner. This is perhaps our greatest challenge as we emerge from the devastating COVID–19 pandemic.

With broad majorities in both parties now understanding the importance of addressing mental health, I believe it is the time to enact immediate fixes for people in need, as well as begin to lay the foundation for a reimagined mental health system—a mental health system that is grounded in community and an integral part of our broader healthcare infrastructure.

There are three key priorities I believe this committee should consider as it pursues both short- and long-term reforms for mental health.

First and foremost, we need to bring mental health care to where people are. This includes schools, and even our workplaces, but to most immediately meet this moment, the best place to start is in primary care, the largest platform of healthcare delivery. In one poll, 70 percent of adults agreed that it would be more convenient if their mental health and substance use services were integrated into their primary care doctor's office.[17]

To do this, we must create more global and flexible funding mechanisms for primary care practices who are working to integrate mental health. Our payment mechanisms often reinforce a siloed delivery model, and this must change.

By first using existing payment structures like those found in Medicaid Managed Care Organizations, Medicare Accountable Care Organizations, and Medicare Advantage plans to expand mental health integration work, primary

---

[14] https://www.samhsa.gov/data/sites/default/files/cbhsq-reports/NSDUHDetailedTabs2018 R2/NSDUHDetTabsSect10pe2018.htm.

[15] https://www.gao.gov/products/gao-21-437r.

[16] https://www.thenationalcouncil.org/press-releases/new-study-reveals-lack-of-access-as-root-cause-for-mental-health-crisis-in-america/.

[17] https://bipartisanpolicy.org/download/?file=/wp-content/uploads/2021/03/BPC-MC- FINAL-Slide-deck-on-Mental-Health-Analysis-Poll.pdf.

care practices would have the flexible financial resources to onboard mental health clinicians as a part of their integrated care team.

Second, we must reconsider the design and capabilities of our workforce. Demand for care has far outpaced the supply of mental health clinicians, and it is inconceivable to rely upon clinician recruitment strategies alone to meet our ever-growing need. There are two things we can do simultaneously to address this workforce issue.

First, we can map out mental health utilization and gaps to better determine where services are needed and for whom.[18] Without this we run the risk of widening disparities or putting money into places or programs people are not using for their mental health.

Second, we invest in our community workforce—those like peer support specialists, community health workers, or more broadly, lay people in our communities. We train them in mental health skills to help become the first line of mental health support, complementing our clinical enterprise and enhancing the overall capacity for communities to address mental health needs.[19]

Finally, we must modernize and connect our Federal programs and systems to collaboratively solve for common mental health problems. I realize it is hard to ask committees to work across jurisdictional boundaries, but so many aspects of our mental health need to be understood together and implemented together—at the State and community level. Because there are multiple agencies, funding streams, and programs that support mental health, performing a landscape analysis can create a strategy for synergistic efficiencies by breaking down silos across Federal agencies and departments and allow for a more cohesive plan for mental health.

In closing, I thank the committee again for holding a hearing on mental health. This is our moment to be bold in what we can do to boost our Nation's well-being, and ultimately save lives.

Context

In 2019, 156,242 Americans were lost to alcohol, drugs, or suicide—one person every 31⁄2 minutes. 39,043 of those deaths were tied to alcohol

---

[18] https://www.thelancet.com/journals/lanpsy/article/PIIS2215-0366(21)00073-0/fulltext.

[19] https://onlinelibrary.wiley.com/doi/abs/10.1111/jrh.12229.

misuse—a 4-percent increase over 2018—and drug-induced deaths in 2019 increased by 5 percent to account for 74,511 of the totals.[20]

Annual Deaths from Alcohol, Drugs, and Suicide in the United States, 1999–2019

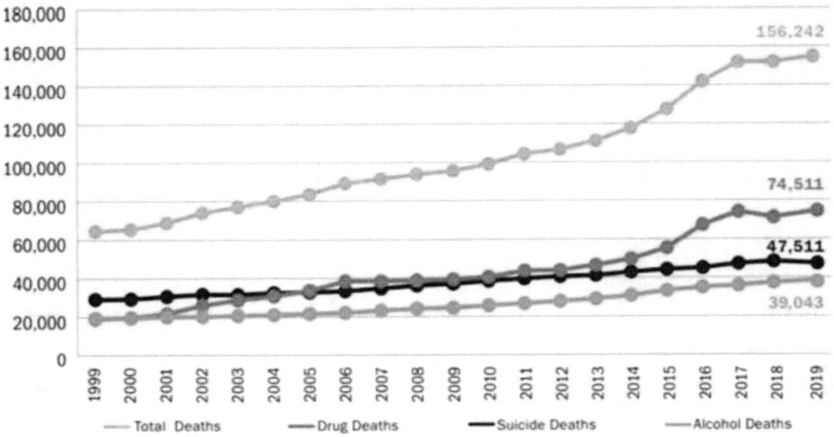

Source: TFAH and WBT analysis of National Center for Health Statistics data

A few things to note. First, this data represents societal behaviors before COVID–19. While we do not have all the data from 2020 yet, preliminary CDC data suggests a 27-percent increase over 2019 in drug overdose deaths offering a glimpse into how much worse it could be.[21] In addition, between 2003 and 2018, the age-adjusted suicide rate reported by the CDC increased by more than 30 percent—and early data indicates that this number will continue to grow in the face of COVID–19.[22]

Second, the data highlight our ongoing problems with health disparities. In these data, we saw a 2-percent increase in drug overdose deaths in whites but a 15- percent increase in blacks and Latinos, an 11-percent increase in American Indians, and a 10-percent increase in people of Asian descent. These are statistically significant differences that highlight how even dominant legislative responses to major issues like our opioid crisis can work well with some populations but not all. These ongoing disparities require a level of

---

[20] https://wellbeingtrust.org/news/pain-in-the-nation-annual-deaths-due-to-alcohol-drugs-or-suicide-exceeded-156000/.

[21] https://www.cdc.gov/media/releases/2020/p1218-overdose-deaths-covid-19.html.

[22] https://stacks.cdc.gov/view/cdc/100479.

attention in system design that is currently missing. Simply decreasing the supply of opioids overall without addressing the demand and its underlying causes leaves us in a place where unintended consequences are likely to occur, such as increases in deaths from synthetic opioids or some sub populations failing to sufficiently benefit from even the most well-intentioned reforms.

Finally, it's important to see these data points for what they are—a macro trend line going in the wrong direction. While the calculations are ongoing, the projections informed by the CDC data and others suggest that our problems are only getting worse and are overwhelming communities. We must stop trying to see substance us disorder and mental, physical and behavioral health as separate issues—they are all interconnected. Assessing and addressing all is essential to achieve the outcomes and well-being we want for individuals and society as a whole. But in order for us to do this, and do this well, we need a system that can take care of all aspects of our health and not just the pieces. In fact, COVID–19 has given our Nation an opportunity to see mental health for what it is—a foundation to our overall health and well-being

As seen below, Kaiser Family Foundation has tracked the mental health impact of COVID–19 throughout the pandemic. This is truly an issue that impacts us all.

In early 2020, the number of adults who said worry and stress related to the coronavirus was having a negative impact on their mental health increased from about one-third (32 percent) in March 2020 to roughly half (53 percent) in July 2020.[23] While the impact appears to have normalized, data from March 2021 finds thatalmost half of adults report negative mental health impacts due to COVID–19.

In another survey conducted in the fall of 2020, almost 80 percent of surveyed registered voters described how COVID–19 had impacted their mental health. In the same survey, 9 out of 10 people believed that elected officials should be doing more for mental health.[24] And when compared to the rest of the world, the U.S. has a much higher mental health burden from COVID–19 than other high-income countries.[25]

---

23 https://www.kff.org/coronavirus-covid-19/poll-finding/mental-health-impact-of-the-covid-19-pandemic/.

24 https://wellbeingtrust.org/news/viacomcbs-well-being-trust-2020-mental-health-survey/.

25 https://www.commonwealthfund.org/publications/issue-briefs/2020/may/mental-health-conditions-substance-use-comparing-us-other-countries.

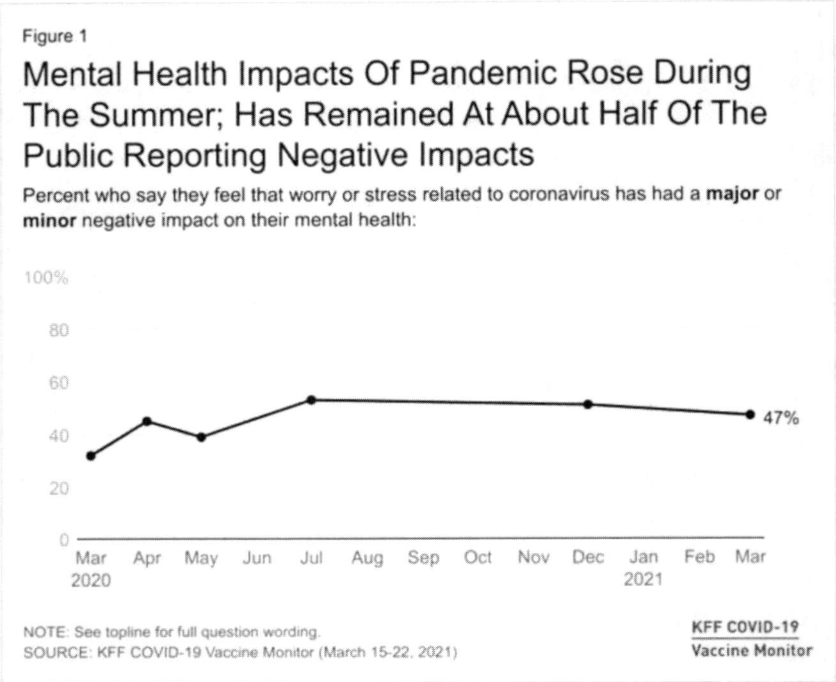

Perhaps most concerning is the impact that COVID–19 has had on our kids and younger adults. Thirty-one percent of 18–29-year-olds report stress has had a major impact on their mental health. Schools are overwhelmed by the mental health needs of students but must make difficult decisions on where to invest their limited resources.

Some of these issues are the expected result of a national health emergency; however, our Nation's fragmented approach to mental health and addiction impedes treatment and has exacerbated these problems. In addition, some facets of society, like our Nation's jails and prisons, are full of people with mental health and addiction needs. Many of these people had significant unmet need for mental health and addiction services before they were incarcerated. And too often, these needs unaddressed by the time they move back into community settings—further stressing the ability of local systems to adequately respond.[26] These national problems and others are a constant threat against the well-being of our communities until comprehensive reforms are embraced.

---

[26] https://www.mhanational.org/issues/access-mental-health-care-and-incarceration.

It should be no surprise that when people don't have any place to go, they show up in the emergency department—but these are often some of the worst places for people to go who are in a mental health crisis as they are often ill-equipped to manage acute psychiatric crises potentially exacerbating an already existing problem. Data from the CDC found that compared with 2019, the proportion of mental health-related visits to emergency departments for children aged 5–11 and 12–17 years old in 2020 increased approximately 24 percent and 31 percent, respectively.[27]

To make this crisis even more challenging, two commercial payers[28],[29] 16,17 have stated that they will retroactively review why a person went to the ED, and if they determine it wasn't warranted, they can restrict or deny these Americans coverage. Imagine showing up thinking you are having a heart attack only to be told it's a panic attack, and then have to pay out of pocket after the cause of the emergency was diagnosed. This could further discourage American families from seeking out help, and while one payer has temporarily walked back this policy,[30] it remains something that could reemerge.

In summary, unaddressed mental health and addiction needs will negatively impact the collective spirit and well-being of individuals, families, and communities. The 116th Congress passed landmark legislation establishing streamlined crisis hotlines (988 crisis hotlines), which could very well overwhelm an already fragile system without support. I am hopeful that this committee might take the opportunity afforded by this legislative effort to begin laying the foundation for a truly modern system of care that works to integrate mental health through delivery, financing, and policy.

Below I outline the three areas that I believe hold the most promise for mental health.

1. Reimagine Care Delivery

Mental health is local. We need to consider all the places that people show up with need and be prepared with a mental health response. From community settings like schools, and workplaces to health delivery settings like primary

---

[27] https://www.cdc.gov/mmwr/volumes/69/wr/mm6945a3.htm.

[28] https://www.uhcprovider.com/en/resource-library/news/2021-network-bulletin-featured-articles/0621-ed-facility-commercial-claims.html.

[29] http://file.anthem.com.s3-website-us-east-1.amazonaws.com/04591CAEENABC.pdf.

[30] https://www.nytimes.com/2021/06/10/health/united-health-insurance-emergency-care.html.

care, one of the best ways we can begin to enhance access and more proactively address mental health needs is to integrate mental health.

What does this look like? At a high level it means that the location—whether it's a primary care office or a school—has the resources to have an onsite mental health professional who can help identify, treat, and coordinate. This approach helps us begin to better distribute mental health services throughout the community in an effort to better be responsive to needs. Below I outline a few specific policy ideas that can support this reimagined approach to mental health.

Primary Care

Care for those seeking mental health services is fragmented in many of today's local systems, leaving even the most connected of people waiting for help. The issues that contribute to the problems in our current care delivery systems include: (1) unnecessary care limitations restricting where and how a person can get access to care; (2) referrals being the dominant intervention for mental health in most healthcare settings; and (3) care approaches remain fragmented with team-based interventions remaining an aspirational goal in most settings. Integrating mental health into primary care addresses all three of these issues head on.

The Bipartisan Policy Center's report on mental health and primary care integration offers several key recommendations for this committee to consider.[31] And rather than list all of those recommendations here, I would encourage the committee and staff to look into the report at the three major areas the report covers: transforming payment and delivery to advance value-based integrated care, expanding and training the integrated workforce, and promoting technology and telehealth to support integrated care.

Additional integration recommendations include:

- *Creating a definition for mental health and primary care integration.* The definition should allow for local adaptation and flexibility in how practices implement an integrated model of care. There are operational definitions that have been created, which may prove

---

[31] https://bipartisanpolicy.org/download/?file=/wp-content/uploads/2021/03/BPC_Behavioral-Health-Integration-report_R02.pdf.

useful in this process.[32] The evidence for integration is that patients like it, clinicians like it, it saves money from total costs, the costs are currently borne by practices and are unsustainable.[33,34] The National Academies' report on Implementing High Quality Primary Care published last month with support from four Federal health agencies, points to mental health integration in primary are as the team-based intervention most supported by evidence.

- *Fixing the financing of integrated mental health in primary care because practices typically bear the cost, one size will not fit all, and flexible financing options will allow for practices to create a model of care that works best for their community. I have offered an example below from Colorado.*

Western Colorado's Rocky Mountain Health Plans (RMHP) has pursued a comprehensive approach to mental health integration and found the model necessary to meet the needs of their members, wherever they choose to access care. Specifically, they have implemented enhanced, non-volume-based payment models to promote and sustain integrated mental health clinicians in advanced primary care sites. Their payment models sustain services that are often not recognized in conventional private payer or State programs, such as health and behavioral encounters or care coordination services. These embedded mental health clinicians provide immediate support for the emotional well-being of patients and families and improve the overall capacity of scarce primary care providers to serve the population.

Additionally, when extended or specialty therapy is necessary, primary carebased providers receive reimbursement for care alongside other provider options in the inclusive network. They admit all willing and qualified providers promptly to their mental health provider network, credentialing over 90 percent of all complete applications within 45 days, often a major rate limiting factor in expanding our workforce.

Patrick Gordon, RMHP's CEO, attributes the positive performance of their health plans to comprehensive primary care and integrated mental health. They routinely exceed quality benchmarks

[32] https://integrationacademy.ahrq.gov/products/lexicon.
[33] https://www.ncbi.nlm.nih.gov/pmc/articles/PMC5698230/.
[34] https://jamanetwork.com/journals/jama/fullarticle/2545685.

set by the State of Colorado in their year-to-year agreements and have achieved Commendable accreditation distinction from the National Committee for Quality Assurance, as well as statutory and contractual financial performance requirements that require an annual return of 2 percent savings to taxpayers.

The key? They have embraced a new model of care that pays for mental health differently in primary care settings. This model begins to take us away from traditional fee-for-service codes and embraces the power of what can happen when we push for flexibility in our financing that supports the concept of a team working in concert to improve health. A recent report from the National Academies reinforces this by recommending paying for primary care teams to care for people, not doctors to deliver services.[35] A forceful charge to move away from volume-driven payment mechanisms that may reinforce a siloed approach to mental health.

Future Accountable Care Organization efforts and primary care value-based payment models should include specific incentives to promote mental health integration.

In addition, as States move away from carved-out financial models for mental health, new arrangements emerge that better support integrating care. Each decision of how mental health is financed can have an impact on how care is delivered on the ground.[36] We should continue to promote payment models that reinforce the concept of a team and facilitate easier access for mental health services in primary care.

- Assuring that our mental health workforce is trained and prepared to work in integrated settings.

Most mental health clinicians are trained to work in specialty mental health settings. While some training programs have recognized the importance of training their mental health clinicians to work in places like primary care, without proper training, many mental health clinicians may not adapt to a primary care culture, making it difficult to sustain integrated efforts.

To this end, the Federal Government could consider:

---

[35] https://www.nationalacademies.org/our-work/implementing-high-quality-primary-care.

[36] https://www.ohsu.edu/sites/default/files/2021-05/McConnell%20et%20al.%20Financial% 20 Integration%20of%20Behavioral%20Health%20in%20Medicaid.pdf.

- ✓ Expanding financial support for continuing education programs that prepare providers to work in integrated settings;
- ✓ Increasing financial support for programs that recruit diverse students into primary care and mental health professions and improve access to and affordability of healthcare education;
- ✓ Creating learning collaboratives for integrated programs and increasing preference for integration as a quality improvement activity under programs like MIPS; and
- ✓ Funding the incubation of new models of integrated training for primary care and mental health professionals in medical schools/other training institutions.

- Providing technical assistance to primary care practices looking to integrate mental health.

Integrating care requires a change in workflow and overall practice culture. It becomes about the team and not just the individual clinician. Practices could benefit greatly from having some form of technical assistance to help them with this transformation. Recent evidence from the Agency for Healthcare Research and Quality demonstrates that this facilitation is key to enabling transformation and for speeding it up.[37,38] There are two immediate options to help here:

- Provide appropriate funding for the Primary Care Extension Program; and
- Establish grant funding for technical assistance for implementation and the ongoing delivery of integrated care.

Schools

Federal policies, initiatives, regulations, and guidance are important tools for the promotion and widespread adaption of comprehensive school mental health systems. In addition to Federal agencies with responsibility over the well-being of children and youth such as the Department of Education (DOE)

---

[37] https://www.ncbi.nlm.nih.gov/pmc/articles/PMC8118489/.
[38] https://www.ncbi.nlm.nih.gov/pmc/articles/PMC6827672/.

and the Department of Health and Human Services (HHS), congressional champions are increasingly leaning into their role in this space.

We have a patchwork of grants at SAMHSA, and elsewhere that either promote school climate or integrate mental health services, and ESSA allows flexibility, but we need an ambitious goal of making sure that our initiatives reach every school and that they're equipped to engage all of the school staff in promoting the mental well-being of the students and addressing the needs of those with mental health conditions.

Before the pandemic, clinicians were seeing alarming trends in adolescent mental health, with increased reporting of depression, anxiety, and suicidal ideation. Unfortunately, those trends were accelerated by the pandemic. Emergency room visits for mental health for adolescents 12–17 rose by 30 percent last year. To put it simply, America's children are in trouble.

The good news is that we know what can be done to help alleviate this mental health crisis in our youth. We want to see strong community and family supports, and importantly we know that one of the best chances we have to get children the mental health care they need is actually in the one place they all have to go every day, and that's in our school systems. The adoption of comprehensive mental health systems in our school systems will help make sure that every child has the opportunity to thrive, while also making sure we offer immediate help to those who might be falling through the cracks.

Congress has a significant role to play in promoting school mental health. Federal policies, initiatives, regulations, and guidance are important and necessary tools for the widespread adaption of comprehensive school mental health systems.

Congress can provide three major lanes of support to comprehensive school mental health programs: providing funding via appropriations, grants, and initiatives; setting up sustainable funding mechanisms and incentives such as increasing the Federal Medicaid matching rate for school-based health services and working with schools to support their ability to bill Medicaid; and scaling up technical assistance centers and programs to provide ongoing support for implementation at the district and school levels.

However, and important to note, promoting school-wide mental health is not a one-and-done program—it's a process of engaging staff, students, and parents to identify needs and continuously improve. And to accomplish this, schools need support.

Making concrete investments in school mental health won't just address the current crisis we find ourselves in, it will pay dividends for generations, giving all children the chance to thrive, and building a next generation resilient and prepared workforce.

2. Reconsider the Design and Capabilities of our Workforce

To make it easier for people to access and pay for mental health care, we need a different way of thinking about workforce—one that helps us respond to mental health needs in a timely manner and do so in a high quality and effective way. Solving these problems goes beyond simply adding more clinicians.

The existing mental health workforce access challenges within our communities are well understood. They result in the following statistics:

1) Thirty-three percent of those seeking care wait more than a week to access a mental health clinician;
2) Fifty percent drive more than one-hour round trip to mental health treatment locations;
3) Fifty percent of counties in the U.S. have no psychiatrist;
4) And only 16 percent of active psychologists are from minority populations despite comprising 40 percent of the U.S. population;[39] and
5) Only 10 percent of practicing psychiatrists are from underrepresented minorities.[40]

There are two immediate steps we can take to best begin to address our workforce shortage problem.

First, we can map out mental health utilization and gaps to better determine where services are needed and for whom.[41] We should look at where people are showing up for care and who is available to help. Without this important foundational step, we run the risk of widening disparities or putting money into places or programs people are not using.

---

[39] American Psychological Association. Demographics of the U.S. psychology workforce: Findings from the American Community Survey. Washington, DC, 2015.

[40] Wyse R., Hwang W.-T., Ahmed A.A., Richards E., Deville C. Diversity by Race, Ethnicity, and Sex Within the U.S. Psychiatry Physician Workforce. Acad Psychiatry. 2020;44(5):523–530.

[41] https://www.thelancet.com/journals/lanpsy/article/PIIS2215-0366(21)00073-0/fulltext.

Second, we need to invest in our community workforce—those like peer support specialists, community health workers, or more broadly, lay people in our communities with no formal role or title. We train them in mental health skills to help become the first line of mental health support, complementing our clinical enterprise and enhancing the overall capacity for communities to address mental health needs.[42] Frameworks have been proposed that offer guidance on how best to enhance our mental health workforce, and much of it begins with strengthening our unlicensed and community-based workforce.[43] Solutions for the mental health workforce can be broken down further into three distinct buckets of improving our current workforce, enhancing the pipeline for the future workforce, and creating a new community workforce.

Current Workforce

We should take the clinicians we have out there in the field and retrain or prepare them to work in new settings. For mental health clinicians, this might be primary care or schools. We should also look to our unlicensed workforce—peer support specialists and community health workers and seek ways to support, finance, and scale their work.

The education, training, and development of new generations of health professionals will be needed to address existing and expected unmet needs in areas such as crisis care and maternal and childhood mental health. The following steps should be taken in the short-term to address immediate areas of unmet medical need and prepare for expected increases in service requests once the 988 community crisis hotlines come online in the near future.

- Increase funding for Medicare residency slots. Without this, it's nearly impossible to increase the number of clinicians like psychiatrists. Of note, parity implementation and enforcement may also help here considering that some clinicians eligible to bill for services may be under-reimbursed making it less desirable to fill a residency slot.

---

[42] https://onlinelibrary.wiley.com/doi/abs/10.1111/jrh.12229.

[43] https://thinkbiggerdogood.org/enhancing-the-capacity-of-the-mental-health-and-addiction-workforce-a-framework/.

- Make permanent 1135 waiver allowing Medicaid providers in another State to provide Medicaid services (though State licensing laws still apply).
- Promote telehealth and other digital service options to expand the service reach of our existing medical professionals.
- Incentivize providers to take additional Continuing Medical Education (CME) classes on current mental health best practices.[1]
- Focus existing federally funded quality improvement organizations on mental health integration across diverse primary care practices and for serving diverse populations, and finance additional learning collaboratives as necessary.

Future Workforce

We should provide prospective healthcare professionals with the appropriate training by making mental health a core curricular component of medical school education. In addition, we should train our future clinicians to understand what it's like to work within a team-based, multidisciplinary setting and provide incentives to higher education institutions to offer training in integrated mental health care, through graduate medical education (GME), graduate nursing education (GNE), and other programs.

While increasing our future workforce is necessary, it alone cannot solve our workforce problem. The time and resources needed will always present limitations to the numbers of new mental health and medical professionals our Nation can train at any one time. Therefore, steps should be taken to expand workforce capabilities in new ways to address current and expected service needs.

Policymakers should consider the following reforms to help local systems begin to update their local workforce capabilities:

- Develop non-medical multi-discipline community workforces to help address service requests that do not require a medical license to satisfy. Offering up payment mechanisms like Medicare to support critical services like peer support specialists would go a long way in strengthening this approach.

- Promote the use of innovative technologies like automated testing and screening platforms to reduce the requirements on medical professionals.
- Develop innovating payment methods and coverage designs like global payments to promote additional testing services from non-medical and technology platforms to better identify and improve access to the right care at the right time.

Community Workforce

We should empower everyone to perform tasks that traditionally clinicians would. There's robust literature out there on it, and it seems to solve several problems at once.[44]

We must also recognize that there are never going to be enough clinicians to meet service demands. Even as we reform Medicare and Medicaid to help primary care better integrate mental health, we will still run into the issue of finding time to undergo trainings and recruit mental health professionals to join their practice in the short term. And in truth, many mental health needs people have are not going to be solved solely at a clinical level, e.g., housing, employment, etc. Of course, we will need people to be able to diagnose and prescribe, but we also need many more people to be able to teach important skills for navigating recovery or building a sense of community that supports people in times of crisis. Ideally, these skills would be spread out across many people and can mutually reinforce one another.

In the long term, we are likely to never have enough clinicians to meet the community's demand without additional effort to increase the pipeline. Like what we've seen successfully work in other countries, we need to tap into our unlicensed yet credentialed workforce—such as peer support specialists and community health workers—and also adopt models that empower everyone to take on mental health at a local level. Innovative technologies such as digital therapeutics and telehealth can open up new access opportunities to train communities as well as reach individuals in need.

Congress and this committee could consider grants or financing mechanism to States to help them sort out the regulatory and multipayer financing issues that often stymie creative and innovative ideas for mental health.

---

[44] https://pubmed.ncbi.nlm.nih.gov/29914185/.

- Modernize Federal Programming and Operations Strategies

We must modernize and connect our Federal programs and operational systems to collaboratively solve for common goals within communities, and to better bring mental health into the national mainstream. Like when corporations merge, we should do a landscape analysis and create a national strategy for synergistic efficiencies among the 55 or more payment systems and thousands of programs that support mental health care in our communities today. Such a step can also help identify redundancies and inefficiencies by allowing for modern programming strategies to break down these silos across all Federal departments and agencies to allow for a more cohesive system for the future. For example, modern Federal funding and programming strategies might allow families and individuals to access a host of different Federal health care, workforce and educational services from multiple different Federal agencies, departments and programs through community and health system access routes.

There are a host of additional steps we can take such as doing a better job of enforcing and expanding existing mental health parity laws that equate mental health and physical or improving care coordination for physical, mental, and behavioral care. In addition, public and private means of coverage.

Communities and local health systems are on the front lines of managing services critical to the mental health and well-being of all Americans. Traditionally, the Federal Government's role has been to provide funding and other resources to these communities to help them manage their service needs. There are dozens of programs, funding streams, and other Federal resources available to communities and local health systems to support the provision of mental health services. However, allowing local communities greater flexibility to plan, program, and allocate these resources would allow programs the opportunity to manage their service needs while investing in local system innovations.

Policymakers should consider reforms to key Federal financing authorities as a means of promoting greater local control over how resources are programmed. At the same time, policymakers can improve how the Federal Government plans for and allocates funds to communities to help maximize on these critical investments and better justify new expenditures that might be required in the future.

Policymakers should consider:

- Establishing a national strategy for how the Federal Government can establish ''smart'' or collaborative financing strategies to improve the efficiency of Federal spending, leverage new uses of existing funds, and create better budgetary certainty for local communities. The 21st Century Cures Act, which became law, contained provisions intended to establish such a strategy. Policymakers might consider steps already taken by the agency in response to the act to establish such a national strategy more quickly.
- In 2016, there was a Community Solutions Task Force that had a focus on solving major challenges facing communities.[45] Congress could use this as a model for mental health and ensure that in each policy it works on it specifically enables cross-agency and community-level collaboration.
- Repositioning the Family First Prevention Services Act (FFPSA) and Community Mental Health Services Block Grant (CMHSBG) to act as lead funding authorities for the various acts with overall responsibility for managing and verifying performance aspects related to Federal funds and other resource allocations meant to support the provision of mental health services within local communities.
- Requiring the Federal Government to regularly update the Committees of Jurisdiction in the House and Senate on the goals of the reformed financing process including progress against those goals.
- While the resources provided for by the Federal Government are substantial, overly prescriptive Federal requirements and lack of collaboration amongst the various Federal authorities in charge of overseeing these resource allocations impede the ability of communities to use these resources effectively.
- As example, the Community Mental Health Services Block Grant (CMHSBG) requires communities seeking funding to ''ensure that community mental health centers provide such services as screening, outpatient treatment, emergency mental health services, and day treatment programs.'' While community mental health centers play an important role, such requirements on local system performance unnecessarily tie the hands of officials struggling to manage growing

---

[45] https://obamawhitehouse.archives.gov/the-press-office/2016/11/16/fact-sheet-establishing-council-community-solutions-align-federal.

service needs—especially in areas where solutions would otherwise exist except for Federal regulation.

- Reviewing the Federal requirements under existing community mental health Federal funding streams and considering easing requirements that unnecessarily impede care.
- Including program sustainability measures with new sources of funding or other resources meant to support the operation and modernization activities of local systems.
- Modern Federal laws like 988 promote modern programming strategies such as program sustainability best practices combined with local autonomy measures to ensure that local officials have sufficient freedom to establish successful and predictable local systems for individuals in need. The ability of local systems to improve their own systems operations through use of information sharing that leads to evidence development and best-practice adoption can help pave the way for continuous system improvement. Such a ''system of learning'' can provide Federal policymakers and local officials greater ability to collaborate and plan for program modernization today and in the future.
- Developing information-sharing and best practice development processes to provide local communities and Federal policymakers insights into the need for and design of future reforms.

While the above areas are the three priorities I have chosen to focus on for today—reimagine care delivery, reconsider the design and capabilities of our workforce, and modernize Federal programming and operations strategies—outlined below are several other notable issues this committee should consider.

Other Issues and Recommendations to Consider
Mental Health Parity and Health Insurance Coverage

- The Finance Committee could take aggressive steps to ensure parity enforcement in Medicaid managed care and expansion populations, which is critical to both mental health equity and racial equity. There could now be an opportunity to engage consumers in setting key indicators of access and track progress with intensive oversight from CMS/CCIIO.

- The Finance Committee could ensure parity be applied to Medicare and Medicare Advantage. This will require eliminating discrimination against MH/ SUD that is baked into title XVIII of the Social Security Act, and ensuring the full continuum of services are covered, including all intermediately levels of care.[46]
- The Finance Committee could require Medicaid and Medicare Advantage plans to follow Generally Accepted Standards of Care and use level of care criteria from non-profit clinical specialty associations as outlined in the Federal case *Wit v. United Behavioral Health.*

988 And Crisis Response

- The Finance Committee could make the CAHOOTS enhanced match permanent and extend it to a comprehensive range of crisis services to create a continuum beyond response.
- The Finance Committee could make sure Medicare and commercial insurance plans cover crisis services and look to Medicaid crisis benefits as a model.

Questions Submitted for the Record to Benjamin F. Miller, PSY.D. Question Submitted by Hon. Catherine Cortez Masto

Question. In your testimony you noted that it is ''inconceivable to rely upon clinician recruitment strategies alone to meet our ever-growing need.'' Stakeholders across the behavioral health spectrum—including policymakers—are looking at overwhelming workforce challenges.

You mentioned peer support services as one solution. Can you elaborate on how peers help to address unmet need?

Answer. Bringing a workforce that has experience, both firsthand and through additional training, into clinical and community settings can be a powerful tool in enhancing the capacity of our systems and our frontline

---

46 https://www.realclearpolicy.com/articles/2020/12/30/medicare/must/cover/mental/health /654797.html.

licensed workforce. And the evidence is clear that peer support services (PSS) work.1 In fact, in 2007 CMS lifted up PSS as an evidence-based practice, and—while Medicare still does not pay for these services—many State Medicaid programs have adopted the model.

There are three characteristics that stand out about PSS.

First, as the name implies, they are peers to those they are serving meaning they have some form of personal or lived experience. In the mental health and addiction field, having a person that knows the challenges of what you are going through can be a powerful tool for healing unto itself.

Second, these peers are equipped with skills that not only allow them to be more than supportive, but also to intervene with evidence-based skills that can be further beneficial to the person they are trying to help. This allows peers to provide higher-touch care than the current workforce would allow, while also ensuring that other clinicians work at the top of their licensure.

Third, PSS can offset the load placed on clinicians and become an extension of clinical services and clinical settings. When we look at wait times for clinicians, it forces us to begin to look to more creative ways to help people in a more expeditious timeframe. PSS do just that—there is an endless supply of individuals with lived experience who can be trained as peers.

For PSS to scale, however, it could benefit from several policy changes. Medicare and most commercial health insurers do not cover PSS, as well as other mental health crisis services, Assertive Community Treatment, Coordinated Specialty Care (for early psychosis), and other team-based interventions. Allowing PSS services to be eligible for Medicare payment would go a long way in helping expand this service line.

In the immediate term, the committee could ensure that mental health and substance use peers could be offered as a supplemental benefit by Medicare Advantage plans, and that they can offer PSS services in the context of integrated mental health care already billable under Medicare, as the recently introduced PEERS Act of 2020 in the House would support. Peers also have a clear role in promoting value in Medicare Accountable Care Organizations (ACOs), and the committee could direct CMS to provide technical assistance to ACOs to better integrate PSS.

And while outside of the scope of PSS specifically, it is important to note that Medicare only covers certain licensed mental health clinicians (e.g., LCSW, psychologists) to bill for services, which leaves a major challenge in building and diversifying the clinical workforce. Medicare has not updated its mental health provider licensure standards since 1989 and is still unaccountable to the Mental Health Parity and Addiction Equity Act. This presents major gaps in coverage for Medicare beneficiaries and can further interrupt continuity of care—leaving families to pay out of pocket or forego essential care entirely. It seems time to modernize Medicare policies for mental health in general and address PSS as we do so.

Questions Submitted by Hon. John Barrasso

Question. The healthcare professionals, along with all front-line workers, deserve our gratitude and appreciation.

Their dedication to our communities during this pandemic is something we must recognize and never forget.

A top concern of Wyoming mental health facilities is making sure there are enough staff to care for their patients. It is especially challenging to attract and keep healthcare providers in rural communities.

Can you discuss solutions related to workforce development you believe will improve the ability of mental health facilities to attract and maintain staff in rural areas?

Answer. Mental health workforce recruitment and retention is a major need, especially in rural communities. And while I will address this issue, I think it's critical that we think beyond simply finding more clinicians and opening up the pipeline. As I have written about in my testimony, only choosing to focus on these pipeline issues, including attracting the right kinds of clinicians to the settings they are most needed, does not provide immediate relief nor does it enhance a mental health clinic or systems capacity to see more people. If our focus can become on better creating new pathways to allow for individuals to be identified and treated, it's inevitable that new solutions emerge beyond just a clinical workforce.

I believe that Congress and this committee should pursue options like Community Initiated Care (CIC), a concept based on a rich evidence-based often called ''task-sharing'' or ''task-shifting.'' This is a model of intervention that is not dependent on licensed clinicians and has shown to be highly effective by allowing non-specialized, trained workers, and even ''lay'' members of the community to learn mental health skills.[47]

Community initiated care is a broadly inclusive concept that democratizes knowledge and empowers individuals to learn how to respond to mental health

---

47 https://www.commonwealthfund.org/publications/2021/feb/making-it-easy-get-mental-health-care-examples-abroad.

and addiction issues. Effective components include training and supporting community members to ensure that they acquire the knowledge, skills, and competencies necessary to deliver high quality evidence-informed programs for prevention and early intervention of mental health concerns.

Bringing more mental health skills into the community can help solve several issues at once—it can make the workforce more readily available because we are creating capacity for communities to intervene on issue of mental health and addiction.

To this end, Congress and this committee could consider grants or financing mechanism to States to help them sort out the regulatory and multi-payer financing issues that often stymie creative and innovative ideas for mental health like the community initiated care model described above. Offering up payment mechanisms like Medicare to support critical services like peer support specialists or a community workforce could go a long way in strengthening this approach and making it more viable. SAMHSA could push out pilot programs with community health workers, community-based organizations, and other community-based non-professionals to deliver psychological interventions based on the learnings from global mental health. Currently, SAMHSA funds gatekeeper type programs through non-specialists as well as peer-specialists programs, but there has been less support for these community based models. A final option is to consider pilot programs with additional funds through block grants if States commit to exploring the community initiated care approach.

Question. Can you specifically discuss changes to GME policy you believe would improve the pipeline of mental health physicians?

Answer. The first step to growing our pipeline of mental health clinicians is to increase funding for Medicare residency slots. Without this, it will be nearly impossible to increase the number of clinicians like psychiatrists.

Parity implementation and enforcement may also help here, considering that some clinicians eligible to bill for services may be under-reimbursed. A lack of reimbursement makes mental health a less desirable residency slot.

So too would modifying primary care residency training programs. Primary care remains one of the largest platforms for mental health delivery in this country. However, not all residency programs train the future workforce much in mental health—family medicine training programs do train their residents in mental health and in most cases, expose them to onsite mental health clinicians who they can work and train beside. Internal medicine and pediatrics residents get much if any such training.

To change this, we should create mental health training requirements in all primary care residency programs modeled off of family medicines current requirements. In addition, residency programs should also require and support mental health integrated in primary care so that all trainees are acculturated to working in such models and can advocate for them later. If medical education had additional resources and incentives to bolster mental health and substance use training for more categories of clinicians, this would further extend the workforce.

In addition, I shared some ideas in my testimony that I feel could be additive to changes in GME policy. For example:

- Make permanent 1135 waiver allowing Medicaid providers in another State to provide Medicaid services (though, State licensing laws still apply).
- Promote telehealth and other digital service options to expand the service reach of our existing medical professionals.
- Incentivize providers to take additional Continuing Medical Education (CME) classes on current mental health best practices.
- Focus existing federally funded quality improvement organizations on mental health integration across diverse primary care practices and for serving diverse populations, and finance additional learning collaboratives as necessary.

Question. As a doctor, I strongly support increasing access to mental health services, especially in rural communities. Senator Stabenow and I have previously introduced legislation for many years that would allow mental health counselors and marriage and family therapists to receive reimbursement from Medicare.

Can you discuss how the Department of Health and Human Services can improve access for mental health services, especially for those on Medicare?

Answer. One of the best ways to improve access to mental health services is to first consider who is eligible to bill what, where, and for whom.

CMS can ensure that Medicare payments for mental health integration are properly valued and that primary care clinicians have the necessary support and technical assistance they need to implement integrated care. Implementing integrated care models requires time, effort, and practice expenses that may not be fully captured in the current valuation. Further, interested clinicians might not have access to resources they need to set up integrated care in their practice. CMS should work with clinicians to identify barriers for the adoption of integrated care in Medicare, including misvaluing of codes, to ensure that beneficiaries get access to effective care.

Recently, CMS launched the Community Health Access and Rural Transformation (CHART) model, which could be a promising approach to building the infrastructure for defragmentation and care transformation in rural America. One strategy that HHS could consider is building on the Community Transformation Track of the CHART model but with a specific focus on ensuring comprehensive access to mental health and substance use treatment, unlocking the full range of innovations from virtual care, peer support services, and integrated care models.

The committee could also work with CMMI to ensure that alternative payment models (APMs) currently in progress adequately incentivize implementation of integrated care for Medicare beneficiaries. Model evaluations indicate that past APMs have had little effect on mental health outcomes. However, as mental health has been subject to chronic underinvestment—especially in rural communities—it counts against the benchmark for shared savings when providers implement effective early intervention (such as integrated care models), unless it very rapidly reduces hospitalizations. To address this issue and incentivize investment in early intervention, CMMI could:

- ✓ Adjust risk adjustment in ACOs, CPC+, and others to accommodate expected costs from integrated care in mental health, and pair with appropriate quality measure recommendations to ensure accountability; or
- ✓ Temporarily waive costs from integrated care models from shared savings calculations.

Question. In particular, can you comment on the merits of allowing licensed professional counselors and marriage and family therapists to receive reimbursements from Medicare?

Answer. Allowing other mental health clinicians outside of psychologists and licensed clinical social workers the chance to bill Medicare could be a slight help in our never-ending numbers game for the clinical workforce—how to get more. There are several benefits to allowing LPC and LMFT to bill Medicare, but the top one is infusing thousands of new clinicians into the workforce.

Questions Submitted by Hon. Tim Scott

Question. The toll that union-sponsored excuses for ''virtual learning'' has taken on actual kids is extraordinarily sad, especially for our Nation's most vulnerable children. In October 2020, a survey conducted by the Jed Foundation showed that 31 percent of parents said their child's mental or emotional health was worse than before the pandemic. Private insurance data also shows that while all healthcare claims for adolescents ages 13–18 were down in 2020 compared to 2019, mental health-related claims for this age group increased sharply. Additionally, the Centers for Disease Control and Prevention (CDC) reports 25 percent of parents whose children attended school virtually were more likely to report an overall worsened mental or emotional health compared to only 16 percent of parents of children attending school in-person.

What programs within the Department of Health and Human Services' (HHS) purview are best poised to support children and schools as they return to complete in-person learning?

Answer. Each agency within HHS offers incredible programs to help support our Nation's children. This includes Project AWARE at SAMHSA, Healthy Schools at CDC, school-based billing under Medicaid, support for school-based health centers at HRSA, and support for families' social and economic needs via the Administration on Children, Youth, and Families (ACYF).

The biggest problem with these programs is scale—these programs benefit the grantees, but don't help most of the children who need them.

To meet this moment, interagency collaboration is needed to coordinate and leverage all available resources to support States and local school systems to provide effective mental health supports for their students. CMS also needs to work with States to help them streamline appropriate billing for mental health services in schools under Medicaid. Several advocacy organizations have also offered up the idea of creating a White House Office on Children and Youth, and/or a Federal Children's Cabinet to help specifically on many of these issues above.

Question. How can we integrate more telehealth opportunities to expand access to mental health services in schools?

Answer. Congress has already done incredible work promoting access to virtual mental health consults for children in primary care by funding HRSA's Pediatric Mental Health Care Access Program. Congress can integrate more telehealth opportunities in schools by expanding this program further initiating a similar program to support integration with schools as well. As part of this work, CMS can provide technical assistance to States for ensuring that their current approach to Medicaid billing supports telehealth for children's mental health in schools. With these investments in infrastructure and attention to sustainability, millions more children can gain access to virtual mental health services where they are—in schools.

We should also allow States to continue utilizing telehealth flexibilities put in place during the pandemic which facilitate schools both delivering mental health services and billing Medicaid for those services. For example, during the pandemic audio only was an allowable modality of telehealth services, both in terms of being able to deliver services and bill for services delivered using audio only. Other flexibilities include allowing school districts to access out of State providers for telehealth which helps address some of the workforce shortage issues and in general, just allowing school health provider types to bill Medicaid for services delivered.

Congress should also support States in expanding their school Medicaid programs. States that had expanded their school Medicaid programs to allow for billing for non-IEP (individualized education program) services were able to do significantly more Medicaid claiming for telemental health services.

And finally, there should be guidance issued to schools on how best to utilize telehealth to expand access to mental health services in schools. More guidance is needed to help States and school districts navigate Federal policies around telehealth, including reimbursement procedures.

Currently, there is no designated guidance on telehealth for schools, and it would be a perfect opportunity for cross-agency collaboration to develop a piece that supports school districts in expanding access to mental health services in schools via telehealth.[48]

Question. Telehealth has expanded rapidly as a result of the COVID–19 pandemic. Numerous studies have demonstrated the effectiveness of telehealth for behavioral health services.

As telehealth becomes more common among healthcare providers, what can Congress do to ensure that patients do not suffer from unnecessary bureaucratic delays?

Answer. It's going to take time for Congress to ensure that every American has access to broadband—this is needed so that everyone has access to telehealth and that existing disparities aren't made worse. However, in the

---

48 https://healthyschoolscampaign.org/dev/wp-content/uploads/2021/03/Providing-Health-Services-During-School-Closures-March-2021.pdf.

interim, to make sure the greatest number of American can most immediately access telehealth services, Congress should make permanent some of the policies they temporarily put in place during the pandemic. Congress should make audio-only telehealth services permanent, enact payment parity, and allow for telehealth to be available for all forms of outpatient care.

Question. There is a well-researched connection between unemployment and mental health. As recently as April 2021, despite billions of dollars of COVID–19 stimulus, aggregate employment remained 7.9 million jobs below its pre-recession level.

What impact will this failure to get people back to work have on mental health?

Answer. There is a well-researched connection between unemployment and mental health, but it just makes sense: financial insecurity can increase stress, and stress can exacerbate underlying mental health and addiction issues.[49]

Unfortunately, despite billions of dollars of COVID–19 stimulus funds, as recently as April 2021 aggregate employment remained 7.9 million jobs below its pre recession level. And the longer it takes use to close that gap, the great risk we run of seeing an increase in the number of lives lost to suicide and drug overdoses.

Question. Last November, an article published in the Journal of the American Medical Association noted that multiple studies indicated that older adults may be less negatively affected by certain mental health outcomes than other age groups.

Are these study outcomes consistent with your own professional experiences working with older adults?

Answer. That study found that older adults appeared to experience less mental health impacts during the early days of the COVID–19 pandemic that other age groups. The article also notes the following:

> The data from various studies contrast the numerous personal stories about how difficult the pandemic has been for the older population. This divergence likely represents the heterogeneity that is a hallmark of aging. Also, resilience captured at the population level may not translate to individuals in specific circumstances. Thus far, there is not a clear understanding of which risk factors and protective factors are the

---

[49] https://wellbeingtrust.org/wp-content/uploads/2020/05/WBT/Deaths-of-Despair-COVID-1 9-FINAL.pdf.

strongest determinants of mental health outcomes, although these may vary from person to person.

Many older adults do not have the resources required to deal with the stress of COVID–19. This may include material (*e.g.,* lack of access to smart technology), social (*e.g.,* few family members or friends), or cognitive or biological (e.g., inability to engage in physical exercise or participate in activities or routines) resources. Clinicians and caregivers must estimate resource availability and consider how the absence of resources can be mitigated for a given individual and family. Of particular importance is the role of technology, which has emerged as an important factor for maintaining social connection as well as accessing mental health services.[50]

In general, older adults are heavily impacted by mental health problems, although in different ways than their younger counterparts. For example, among men, suicide rates are the highest for those over 75 years of age.[51] Other recent studies find relatively consistent prevalence of depression across adulthood.[52] Although risk factors evolve with age, mental health remains a serious issue and older adults often do not have access to appropriate care that meets their particular needs. This is in part why any conversations on Medicare reform must begin to address the deficiencies in the program for mental health and substance use disorders.[53]

Question. Current network adequacy standards often allow networks of specialists who aren't taking new patients or who have long waiting lists. That means that many people needing treatment must go out of network to get care, and only those who can afford the high cost get it. One of the biggest challenges to access to behavioral healthcare services is that many behavioral health specialists don't participate in health plan networks.

Why is that, and how can we change that?

Answer. The consequences of inadequate networks can be devastating for American families. Inadequate networks are a major driver of enormous disparities in out-of-network utilization for mental health and substance use disorder (MH/SUD) treatment compared to physical health care. Patients are far too often forced to find out-of-network MH/SUD services because in-

---

[50] https://jamanetwork.com/journals/jama/fullarticle/2773479.

[51] https://pubmed.ncbi.nlm.nih.gov/32487287/.

[52] 6 https://www.cdc.gov/nchs/products/databriefs/db303.htm.

[53] 7 https://www.realclearpolicy.com/articles/2020/12/30/medicare_must_cover_mental_health_654797.html.

network services are not available, and are therefore exposed to much higher out-of-pocket costs, balance billing, and more aggressive insurer utilization controls. Data from Milliman shows out-of-network MH/SUD utilization for both inpatient and outpatient facilities is more than five times higher than out-of-network physical health utilization.[54]

Strong network adequacy standards are essential to ensuring access to MH/SUD care. Unfortunately, for many types of health plans, network adequacy standards are weak, if existent all, and often qualitative in nature. Weak standards effectively contribute to inadequate networks that result in Americans not receiving the MH/ SUD services they need, at enormous cost to individuals, families, and our society. For example, while Federal law requires Medicaid managed care and Affordable Care Act qualified health plans (QHP) to maintain adequate networks, Federal law simply defers to a hodgepodge of State regulatory standards, which often fail to establish concrete access standards that are plainly transparent to consumers, providers, and health plans alike. According to a recent report by the Legal Action Center, only seven States have created standards for State-regulated plans relating to the three most meaningful network adequacy measures: appointment wait times, provider/enrollee ratio, and distance standards.[55]9

Importantly, self-funded health plans subject to the Employee Retirement Income Security Act of 1974 (ERISA), which are exclusively regulated by the U.S. Department of Labor, are not subject to any legally imposed network adequacy standards at all. Given that the majority of Americans in ERISA plans are covered by self-funded plans, this significant gap in law leaves tens of millions of Americans without a right to adequate networks.

Strong, quantitative network adequacy requirements should be expanded to all types of health plans. These requirements should include provider/enrollee ratios that only measure providers who are active plan providers (measured by billings within the last 6 months to prevent ‘‘ghost’’ networks), as well as appointment wait times (i.e., timely access standards) and distance standards. Timely access and geographic standards directly

---

[54] Steve Melek, et al., Addiction and mental health vs. physical health: Widening disparities in network use and provider reimbursement, Milliman, November 19, 2019, https://assets.milliman.com/ektron/Addiction_and_mental_health_vs_physical_health_Widening_disparities_ in_network_use_and_provider_reimbursement.pdf.

[55] Ellen Weber, Spotlight on Network Adequacy Standards for Substance Use Disorder and Mental Health Services, Legal Action Center, May 2020, *https://www.lac.org/resource/spotlight-on-network-adequacy-standards-for-substance-use-disorder-and-mental-health-services.*

measure patient access to care and should be required together. After all, care that is theoretically available now but at a great distance or theoretically available nearby but not when needed is tantamount to no care at all. All health plans that cannot ensure suitable, timely and geographically accessible in-network care should be required to cover the cost of out-of-network treatment, without any additional cost-sharing for patients.

Standards should be set, measured and enforced separately for MH and SUD providers, with requirements that plans meet timely access, distance, and patient/ enrollee ratios for the full range of provider types and settings that are necessary to treat MH/SUD. While telehealth should be allowed to help plans meet network adequacy requirements in areas with few providers (e.g., rural areas), the availability of telehealth providers should not be allowed to replace patients' ability to access in-person care.

Placing the obligation of maintaining adequate networks on health plans—particularly by requiring health plans to pay for out-of-network care without additional cost-sharing by patients—is the only way to ensure that patients are not continuously victimized by insurers' phantom networks and inaccurate provider directories. Only when insurers must bear the financial risk of out-of-network coverage will they have sufficient incentive to maintain accurate provider directories and recruit sufficient providers into their networks.

Question. Outside of the public health emergency, telehealth services are restricted to certain geographic and clinical settings. Beneficiaries must live in a rural area and have an initial face-to-face visit with the distant-site provider. Once a relationship has been established, periodic in-person visits are also required. With few exceptions, patients must be located in a clinical setting and may not receive care from their homes. In addition, the distant-site provider cannot be located in a rural health clinic or FQHC.

Telehealth has been used broadly during the pandemic to expand healthcare access to individuals throughout the country. During the pandemic, Medicare significantly expanded the coverage of telehealth services. A recent Bipartisan Policy Center poll suggests that people receiving mental health and substance use services want a combination of in-person, video, and telephone services even after the pandemic has passed.

What telehealth expansions should remain after the pandemic?

Answer. Telehealth has been used broadly during the pandemic to expand healthcare access to individuals throughout the country, as Medicare significantly expanded the coverage of telehealth services.

Outside of the public health emergency, telehealth services are restricted to certain geographic and clinical settings. Beneficiaries must live in a rural area and have an initial face-to-face visit with the distant-site provider. Once a relationship has been established, periodic in-person visits are also required. With few exceptions, patients must be located in a clinical setting and may not receive care from their homes. In addition, the distant-site provider cannot be located in a rural health clinic or FQHC. These are all barriers that will emerge again if the emergency order provisions for telehealth expire—with consequences. For example, placing an in-person requirement back on the patient works against patients as it restricts access to telehealth for those individuals with transportation issues, those in provider shortage areas, or other access barriers. It also prevents the use of telehealth for new patients experiencing a crisis.

The uptick in telehealth utilization for mental health signals that people enjoy when care comes to them—and Americans should continue to have that choice post-pandemic. That's why Well Being Trust supported a Bipartisan Policy Center report earlier this year that highlighted the importance of removing site of service, geographic, and established patient restrictions for telehealth services.[56]10 In addition, it called for the elimination of the two-way video requirement, which will begin to help address the digital divide and access disparities for those without broadband or video technology.

Congress should make permanent audio-only telehealth services, enact payment parity, and allow for telehealth to be available for all forms of outpatient care. Congress therefore must also, as many have pointed out, make sure broadband is accessible and affordable as to not further disparities, and encourage that we ask clinicians using telehealth services to measure outcomes to show that they work for mental health.

Questions Submitted by Hon. John Cornyn

Question. Your testimony provides a piece to the puzzle of mental health policy that our Nation is currently lacking: strategy. I would like to follow up on this point with a few questions.

Your testimony included thoughts on how the Senate Finance Committee and U.S. Senate should pursue reforms for immediate problems strategically

[56] https://bipartisanpolicy.org/report/behavioral-health-2021/.

so that these efforts can also allow communities to begin modernizing local systems of mental and behavioral health.

Could you elaborate on those thoughts?

How should Congress pursue legislation to support these twin goals?

Answer. Good mental health is foundational to the health and well-being of every American. Our society, however, treats mental health all too often as a system of medical services for people experiencing a mental health crisis. It spends very little time investing thinking about how we can prevent some of these episodes from occurring in the first place or how to help young people develop strong foundations and self-care tools so that individuals might avoid a mental health crisis in the first place.

Immediate steps need to be taken by Congress to address unmet medical needs such as increasing the availability of the workforce to manage the expected increase in call volume from 988. S.B. 1902 holds great promise in helping address this issue by clearly laying out standards for what should be in a crisis continuum, assuring comprehensive coverage of these services, and finding sustainable funding mechanisms.

However, any legislative vehicle required to pass these reforms could also be used to lay the groundwork for a modern, more wholistic approach to solving our Nation's mental health needs. We need to get ahead of our problems if we are to solve many of them, and reforms at the local level are needed to get us there. We can achieve this by creating opportunities for Americans at all stages of life to participate in mental health and well-being.

First and foremost, we need to enhance the capabilities of local workforces and programs to increase service availability for local communities. Some of that can be addressed through medical professional workforce development but we cannot solve our need for services through them alone. The development of non-medical community workforces and use of digital therapeutics are two steps that Congress can undertake to broaden the response beyond the need to increase the numbers of local medical workforces. The benefits of the overall availability of services within local communities should have the added benefit of taking some of the burden off of health professionals thereby allowing them greater capacity to address the most severe cases.

Second, I believe the Federal Government needs to reimagine its approach to funding mental health and addiction services in local communities. There are numerous autonomous Federal funding streams and other resources that have been developed over the years but no comprehensive strategy for how they all work together to best support Federal interests. This lack of coordination and differing funding authorities needlessly places undue administrative burden and cost on communities which can lead to inefficient spending and diminished results. outdated approaches to addressing mental health and addiction issues are contributing to ineffective community approaches that don't do enough. Communities in this country need to go through the same type of process to reimagine local operations—a process to help them reform and hold them accountable for improved operations and programming could help improve the effectiveness of the Federal effort even further.

Third, establishing foundations for good mental health should begin early. Our formative years, from birth through the age of 18, are critical to an individual's overall mental health and well-being. Creating early opportunities for education and the development of self-help tools to help a person manage mental health throughout their lives can go a long way to preventing some medical issues before they arise, and help every American build the tools they will need to succeed. There is an immediate need to reinforce this approach right now in our schools, assuring that the staff, the students, and all those connected have access to mental health services and supports.

Lastly, there are concrete steps that Congress can take to improve local health system approaches to mental health care. Some of these ideas are already being advanced by members of the Senate. Others I am happy to provide.

Legislatively speaking, I believe that the Senate Finance Committee has unique statutory authority to lead the charge on larger reform. While a comprehensive solution will need to involve the Public Health Service Act as well, the Family First Prevention Services Act presents a unique model that if adapted could help initiate the type of system and generational reforms that are needed today. In the interest of helping support your efforts, I am in the process of developing a draft legislative outline for your consideration and should be delivering that to you in the next couple of weeks.

Taken together, these steps can begin to create opportunities for Americans at all stages of life to pursue and embrace mental health and well-being.

Question. Your testimony touched on a key concept—updating Federal approaches to funding care for local communities.

How can we more efficiently spend Federal funds already allocated today to local communities?

Also, in what ways can modern technologies improve community and Federal Government return-on-investments?

Answer. The Federal Government spends very inefficiently on mental health and addiction care. There are dozens of Federal programs and authorities created over the years by Congress with no overarching Federal strategy for how they are to work together. This fact contributes to duplicative and other wasteful spending practices.

In addition, some of the Federal rules governing these authorities—such as spending requirements that prevent long-term planning of awarded funds—encourages wasteful and inefficient spending by communities fearful of missing out on Federal dollars. The lack of an overarching strategy for how the Federal Government funds communities, combined with the time and cost of running separate regulatory channels, needlessly adds administrative burden on both communities and Federal officials as well.

As for communities, being more efficient with Federal funds need not only rely upon spending efficiencies alone. For instance, there are numerous programmatic improvements already vetted and proven to save money (under the Family First Prevention Services Act and other sources) that many local communities have failed to adopt. In addition, self-sustainability provisions and other mechanisms to ensure efficient programming and spending can be added to reform efforts to ensure they maintain fiscal integrity.

Digital technologies offer other options for improving access while improving spending efficiencies. Digital therapeutics (like cognitive behavioral therapy) offer communities alternative sources of medical service without the commiserate cost of training and employing medical professionals. Best practice and evidence development aided by modern digital technologies such as AI can help systems identify where future improvements can be made.

Digital therapeutics along with non-medical workforces also have the added benefit of freeing up medical professionals so that they can focus on the highest-acuity patients. Where local systems are able to recognize and use such alternative service providers, access to care can increase beyond what a traditional workforce can provide—at a lower cost.

Question. You write in your testimony that, ‘‘we need to bring mental health care to where people are.’’ This includes schools, workplaces, and primary care. As primary care is the largest delivery of health care this inclusion makes sense, but as you note, there are some barriers.

Can you expand on this thinking?

Answer. Bringing mental health care to where people are is a way of speaking to the need to engage individuals in all phases of their lives in ways most conducive to securing engagement. Fragmentation of mental health and addiction care has made it an ongoing challenge for people to get easy and timely access to services. By bringing care to where people are, we begin to offer more timely opportunities for engagement and lessen the likelihood that a person does not get much-needed care. Delaying care does not lead to improvement—we must be more responsive to our communities needs by assuring care is integrated into the settings they present. We need to pursue novel models that integrate care and support those models with the appropriate payment mechanisms.

Erasing the stigma and improving societies embrace of mental health can best be achieved by engaging people at all stages of life. The stigma of mental health and addiction in our society may be one of the biggest barriers our Nation faces. As a society, we are taught by example to avoid talking about or seeking help for mental illness and give little thought to building familiarity with the pursuit of well-being. Parents typically do not realize the extent to which their own behavior is held up as a model for children. Society does not typically teach children the basics of mental health or the importance of building self-care tools early on as a means of preparing for the years to come. As we grow older, there are many different things that can reinforce these avoidance lessons. The net result is a community approach that encourages people to ignore mental and behavioral issues until they manifest as healthcare issues. By then, our lack of familiarity with these areas makes treatment very difficult on people who may have a long course of treatment and recovery ahead of them.

If we are to achieve more positive outcomes in areas of mental health and addiction, we need to break this stigma for current and future generations. For those alive today, that means finding ways to engage people who might otherwise avoid these issues altogether. Each generation alive today can benefit from opportunities to engage in mental and behavioral well-being. If we are to succeed in breaking the stigma for them, we need to create opportunities that relate to where they are in their lives. For children, basic education on the ABCs of mental health can help establish familiarity and strong foundations upon which to deal with issues of mental and behavioral health later in life. For families of young children or those expecting, educational and medical services for mental health can be better integrated in the physical care model in a physician offices or other site of service. For adults and seniors, access to wellness, treatment, and referral services through community workforces or community access points like employers can help begin to break down barriers and make it easier for people interested in taking the next step to more easily find answers.

All policies should be scrutinized for how they limit a person getting access to mental health care—in some cases further fragmenting care—and how they may inadvertently reinforce stigma.

Prepared Statement of Hon. Ron Wyden, a U.S. Senator from Oregon

The Finance Committee meets this morning to discuss mental health care in America. This issue ought to bring Democrats and Republicans together, starting with a single, clear lodestar: every American must have mental health care when they need it.

The shameful reality is, the United States does not come close to meeting that bar today. Multiple Federal laws say that mental health care is supposed to be on a level playing field with physical health care. In practice, however, the system still reflects the dangerous, old stigma against recognizing and treating mental illness, and that's why millions of people are falling through the cracks.

For someone with a mental illness, it can be nearly impossible to find a provider who can meet your needs, or one who accepts insurance—particularly in rural areas or in communities of color. Insurance claims too often get denied or cut off too quickly. Particularly for those experiencing homelessness, the outcome of a mental health crisis is too often incarceration instead of treatment.

Prior to the pandemic, one in five Americans was living with a mental illness. All the evidence suggests the pandemic is adding to the crisis. The proportion of Americans reporting symptoms of anxiety or depression has nearly quadrupled. On Friday, the Centers for Disease Control and Prevention released a new report finding that over the last year, suicide attempts among teenage girls were up by more than 50 percent. Meanwhile, a study the Government Accountability Office conducted at my request found that many provider offices closed or cut staff during the pandemic, resulting in too many patients turned away.

There's a lot for this committee to work on. There are a few key challenges. First, the country needs a larger mental health workforce. There simply are not enough providers, whether it's psychiatrists or therapists or staff in inpatient facilities. For example, due to a major staffing shortage, the psychiatric hospital in Salem is currently being staffed in part by members of the Oregon National Guard. That's in a State capital, where there are people and resources focused on this issue. Other areas have it worse. More than one in three Americans lives in an area with a severe shortage of mental health professionals.

Second, insurance companies must not cut corners when it comes to mental health coverage. This issue comes up all the time during town hall meetings I hold in Oregon—people describing having their claims denied. In other cases, insurance only covers a portion of the treatment people need. Furthermore, it doesn't make any sense to leave somebody experiencing a true mental health crisis waiting for a green light from an insurance company before they can get treatment.

Third, this committee must address the racial inequities in mental health care. Black and Latino Americans are roughly half as likely as white Americans to receive treatment for a mental illness. Suicide rates are much higher among black children. There aren't enough black, Latino, and Native American mental health providers. This is a basic matter of healthcare equity, and there's a long way to go.

Finally, the Finance Committee ought to build on areas of recent progress. For example, early in the pandemic this committee led the fight to get Medicare to cover mental health services via telehealth. In December, the Congress made that permanent. This is going to be a game changer, particularly for seniors who live in rural areas. It would work outside of traditional Medicare too.

Senator Stabenow has long been a champion of mental health care. Today the committee will hear about the success of Certified Community Behavioral Health Clinics, a program she fought for and created. These clinics are up and running in 40 States, including Oregon. It's an approach that works, and it's meeting big needs. I believe the Congress ought to look at ways to build on its success.

In March, the Congress also passed a big down payment for a pioneering new approach on mental health services and law enforcement called the CAHOOTS program. It originally comes from Eugene, OR, and it has expanded in bigger cities and rural areas around the State. Under this approach, when there's a 911 call dealing with someone experiencing a mental health crisis, CAHOOTS sends trained health professionals as first responders instead of just police. Healthcare providers like it; law enforcement likes it. The American Rescue Plan included a billion-dollar down payment to help States build their own programs like CAHOOTS. Now the Congress needs to consider what comes next to build these programs successfully and make sure people are getting the help they need, even after the immediate crises end.

It's clear there's a lot of work to be done. Members on both sides have important ideas addressing these issues and more. I want to continue working with members in the weeks ahead, because I believe there's a big need and a big opportunity for legislation on mental health.

Communications

American Academy of Family Physicians
1133 Connecticut Ave,. NW, Suite 1100
Washington, DC 20036–4305
(800) 794–7481
(202) 232–9033

June 25, 2021

The Honorable Ron Wyden
Chairman
U.S. Senate
Committee on Finance
Washington, DC 20510

The Honorable Mike Crapo
Ranking Member
U.S. Senate
Committee on Finance
Washington, DC 20510

Dear Chairman Wyden and Ranking Member Crapo:

On behalf of the American Academy of Family Physicians (AAFP) and the 133,500 family physicians and medical students we represent, I applaud the committee for its consideration of the mental health challenges in the U.S. I write in response to the hearing: ''Mental Health Care in America: Addressing Root Causes and Identifying Policy Solutions'' to share the family physician perspective and the AAFP's policy recommendations for ensuring all patients who need mental health care are able to access it.

Mental illness is highly prevalent in the United States and is associated with an increased risk of morbidity and mortality. There are significant gaps in the provision of mental health care services in the U.S., especially related to vulnerable populations. While psychiatric and other mental health professionals can play an important role in the provision of high-quality mental health care services, primary care physicians are the main providers for the majority of patients. Most people with poor mental health will be diagnosed and treated in the primary care setting. Mental illness also complicates other medical conditions, making them more challenging and more expensive to manage. Together, this makes mental health an important issue for primary care physicians.

Screening for mental illness is not new to family medicine but has more recently been linked to quality metrics and payment. Screening for mental illness can be an important strategy for decreasing morbidity, as well as preventing adverse maternal and child health outcomes associated with perinatal depressive symptoms, postpartum depression, or maternal suicide.[57,58,59] While important, screening in a busy practice can seem overwhelming, but practices can leverage technology, empower staff, and utilize wellness visits to complete this screening.[60]

Integrating mental health into primary care settings, as well as the blending of primary and preventive medicine into traditional mental health settings, represents a more holistic approach to treatment than the traditional consultative and referral models. Integrating primary care and mental health services increases access for patients by making mental health services available in their regular primary care clinics. When integrated into primary care, mental health clinicians can impact the care of more patients than in the specialty mental health referral sector.[61] In the primary care setting, mental health clinicians take on a more consultative and team-based role and focus on helping primary care physicians treat mental health disorders. In this context, mental health clinicians typically reach more patients, and have short er and more problem-focused encounters than in the context of traditional specialty mental health.

The Collaborative Care Model, supported by various organizations including the AAFP and the American Psychiatric Association, is a model for

---

[57] LeFevre ML, U.S. Preventive Services Task Force. Screening for Suicide Risk in Adolescents, Adults, and Older Adults in Primary Care: U.S. Preventive Services Task Force Recommenda- tion Statement. *Ann Intern Med.* 2014;160(10):719.

[58] Kendig S, Keats JP, Hoffman MC, et al. Consensus bundle on maternal mental health: Perinatal depression and anxiety. *Obstet Gynecol.* 2017;129(3):422–430.

[59] Yonkers KA, Wisner KL, Stewart DE, et al. The management of depression during preg-nancy: A report from the American Psychiatric Association and the American College of Obste- tricians and Gynecologists. *Obstet Gynecol.* 2009;114(3):703–713.

[60] Savoy M, O'Gurek DT. Screening your adult patients for depression. *Fam Pract Manag.*2016;23(2):16–20.

[61] Collins C, Hewson DL, Munger R, Wade T. Evolving models of behavioral health integration in primary care. Milbank Memorial Fund. 2010. Accessed January 22, 2018.

the successful integration of primary care and behavioral and mental health.[62] At its core, the idea of collaborative care is anchored in team-based care, often in the context of a medical home, and steered by primary care physicians. It involves behavioral health specialists and consulting mental health professionals delivering evidence-based care that is patient-centered.

The collaborative care model at its core is: (1) team driven, (2) population focused, (3) measurement guided, and (4) evidence based. These four elements, when combined, can allow for a fifth guiding principal to emerge—accountability and quality improvement. Collaborative care is team-driven, led by a primary care clinician with support from a ''care manager'' and consultation from a psychiatrist who provides treatment recommendations for patients who are not achieving clinical goals. Other mental health professionals can contribute to the Collaborative Care Model. Collaborative care is population focused, using a registry to monitor treatment engagement and response to care. Collaborative care is measurement guided with a consistent dedication to patient-reported outcomes and it utilizes evidence-based approaches to achieve those outcomes. Care remains patient centered with proactive outreach to engage, activate, promote self-management and treatment adherence, and coordinate services.[63]

The AAFP urges Congress to support the adoption of the Collaborative Care Model by funding grant programs for primary care practices and encouraging Center for Medicare and Medicaid Innovation models for behavioral health integration.

Telemedicine for mental health is a growing interest in primary care and tele- health initiatives for mental health care are expanding rapidly. While the research is limited on this topic, there are a growing number of studies assessing the benefits, comparative effectiveness with face-to-face visits, and cost comparisons. From January to March 2020, at the beginning of the COVID–19 pandemic, telehealth visits increased by 135% compared to that time period in 2019, and 93% of those visits were for non-COVID concerns.[64] In addition, mental health concerns increased rapidly during the pandemic. Four in ten adults reported symptoms of anxiety, an increase from one in ten the year prior, and more than half of all young adults ages 18–24 reported

---

[62] American Psychiatric Association Academy of Psychosomatic Medicine. Dissemination of integrated care within adult primary care settings. Accessed January 22, 2018.

[63] Ibid.

[64] Koonin LM. Trends in the Use of Telehealth During the Emergence of the COVID–19 Pandemic—United States, January–March 2020. MMWR Morb Mortal Wkly Rep. 2020;69. doi:10.15585/mmwr.mm6943a3.

symptoms of anxiety and depression and were more likely than other age groups to report substance use and suicidal thoughts.[65] Other trends should a disproportionate effect on mental health for communities of color, mothers, and essential workers.[66] The AAFP is supportive of efforts to expand access to mental health services via telehealth and encourage Congress to address the legislative barriers outlined in our previous testimony and Joint Principles for Telehealth Policy. In particular, the AAFP strongly believes that the permanent expansion of telehealth services should be done in a way that advances care continuity and the patient-physician relationship. Telehealth for mental health can help address the shortage of over 6,000 mental health professionals in the U.S., particularly for rural and underserved areas that face a disproportionate impact of the shortage.[67]

Trauma-informed care, an approach to engaging individuals with a history of trauma that recognizes their traumatic experiences, and how it affects their lives, is a promising practice that may facilitate healing and help prevent the consequences of exposure to trauma.[68,69] An estimated 60% of adults in the U.S. have experienced a traumatic event at least once in their lives.[70] Exposure to trauma, such as intimate partner violence, sexual abuse, rape, neglect, terrorism, war, natural disasters, and street violence predisposes those affected to poor physical and mental health outcomes.[71] The principles of trauma-informed care include: realizing that there is a high prevalence of trauma and it has serious effects; recognizing the signs and symptoms of trauma; responding to the high prevalence by integrating knowledge about trauma into

---

[65] Panchal N, Kamal R, 2021. The Implications of COVID–19 for Mental Health and Substance Use. KFF. Published February 10, 2021. Accessed June 17, 2021. https://www.kff.org/coronavirus-covid-19/issue-brief/the-implications-of-covid-19-for-mental-health-and-substance-use/.

[66] Ibid.

[67] Mental Health Care Health Professional Shortage Areas (HPSAs). KFF. Published November 5, 2020. Accessed June 17, 2021. *https://www.kff.org/other/state-indicator/mental-health- care-health-professional-shortage-areas-hpsas/.*

[68] Oral R, Ramirez M, Coohey C, et al. Adverse childhood experiences and trauma informed care: The future of health care. *Pediatr Res.* 2016;79(1–2):227–233.

[69] Decker MR, Flessa S, Pillai R V., et al. Implementing trauma-informed partner violence assessment in family planning clinics. *J Women's Heal.* April 2017:jwh.2016.6093.

[70] National Council for Behavioral Health. Trauma-informed approaches learning communities. Accessed January 22, 2018.

[71] Agency for Healthcare Research and Quality. Trauma-informed care *(https://www.ahrq.gov/ncepcr/tools/healthier-pregnancy/fact-sheets/trauma.html).* Accessed January 22, 2018.

practices, procedures, and policies; and avoiding retraumatizing individuals by using best-practices in screening and history taking.[72]

Disparities are pervasive in all aspects of health, including mental health conditions. While mental health conditions can affect everyone, regardless of culture, race, ethnicity, gender or sexual orientation, some populations experience those conditions at a higher rate.

- American Indian and Alaska Natives (28.3%) experience higher rates of mental illness than white (19.3%), black (18.6%), Hispanic (16.3%), or Asian (13.9%) adults.[73]
- Individuals from the lesbian, gay, bisexual, transgender, and questioning (LGBTQ) community are two or more times as likely as heterosexual individuals to have a mental health condition, and LGBTQ youth are two to three times more likely to attempt suicide than heterosexual youth.[74]
- Nearly one-fifth (18.5%) of the veterans who returned from serving in either Iraq or Afghanistan suffer from either major depression or post-traumatic stress disorder.[75]
- The prevalence of mental illness is similar for individuals living in either rural or metropolitan areas, but the mental health care needs are more often unmet in rural communities due to inadequate services.[76]

Disparities in mental health illness and mental health care are related to coverage and availability of care, quality of care, rates of health insurance, stigma, cultural insensitivity, racism, bias, homophobia, discrimination in treatment settings, and language barriers.[77]

---

[72] *Ibid.*

[73] National Alliance on Mental Illness. Mental health by the numbers *(https://www.nami.org/mhstats)*. Accessed January 22, 2018.

[74] *Ibid.*

[75] Tanielian T, Jaycox LH, Schell T, et al. Invisible wounds. Mental health and cognitive care needs of America's returning veterans. RAND Corporation. 2008. Accessed January 22, 2018.

[76] Substance Abuse and Mental Health Services Administration. Results from the 2015 National Survey on Drug Use and Health: Detailed Tables *(https://www.samhsa.gov/data/sites/default/files/NSDUH-DetTabs-2015/NSDUH-DetTabs-2015/NSDUH-DetTabs-2015.pdf)*. Preva- lence estimates, standard errors, P values, and sample sizes. 2016. Accessed January 22, 2018.

[77] National Alliance on Mental Illness. Mental health by the numbers *(https://www.nami.org/mhstats)*. Accessed January 22, 2018.

College students face unique mental health concerns, such as non-suicidal self-injury and serious suicidal ideation.[78] There are approximately 20 million students enrolled in U.S. colleges and universities, and the rates of serious mental health concerns is rising in this population.[79,80] According to the Center for Collegiate Mental Health's 2017 Annual Report, 52.7% of students attended counseling for mental health concerns; 34.2% took a medication for mental health concerns; 9.8% were hospitalized for a mental health concern; 27% purposely injured themselves without suicidal intent; and 34.2% seriously considered attempting suicide, with 10% making a suicide attempt.[81] In fact, some data suggest that suicide may be the most common cause of death in college students.[82]

Attention-deficit/hyperactivity disorder (ADHD) is another prevalent disorder in college students that family physicians may encounter. ADHD's prevalence is estimated to be between 2–8% among college students, and this condition is frequently associated with other psychiatric comorbidities and increases individuals' risk of psychosocial and substance-use problems.[83]

Tobacco use is prominent among individuals living with mental illness. Thirty-six percent of adults with any mental illness use tobacco products, compared with 25.3% for adults without a mental illness.[84] In addition, people who have any mental illness are only half as likely to quit smoking compared to individuals without a mental illness.[85] One study found that nearly half of all deaths were tobacco-related for persons who received substance abuse

---

[78] Center for Collegiate Mental Health. 2017 Annual Report *(https://sites.psu.edu/ccmh/files/2018/01/2017_CCMH_Report-1r3iri4.pdf)*. Accessed January 22, 2018.

[79] Ibid.

[80] National Center for Education Statistics. Fast facts. Back to school statistics (https://nces.ed.gov/fastfacts/display.asp?id=372). Accessed January 22, 2018.

[81] Center for Collegiate Mental Health. 2017 Annual Report *(https://sites.psu.edu/ccmh/files/2018/01/2017_CCMH_Report-1r3iri4.pdf)*. Accessed January 22, 2018.

[82] Turner JC, Keller A. Leading causes of mortality among American college students at 4-year institutions. Conference Paper: American Public Health Association 139th Annual Meeting and Exposition. Washington, DC 2011. Accessed January 22, 2018.

[83] Unwin BK, Goodie J, Reamy BV, Quinlan J. Care of the college student. *Am Fam Physician.* 2013;88(9):596–604.

[84] Centers for Disease Control and Prevention. Tobacco use among adults with mental illness and substance use disorders *(https://www.cdc.gov/tobacco/disparities/mental-illness-substance-use/index.htm)*. Accessed January 22, 2018.

[85] Centers for Disease Control and Prevention. Vital signs: Current cigarette smoking among adults aged ≥ 18 years with mental illness—United States, 2009–2011. *MMWR.* 2013;62(05):81– 87.

services, or who received both substance abuse and mental health services.[86] Therefore, addressing tobacco addiction among individuals living with mental illness is an important strategy for decreasing preventable mortality and morbidity among individuals living with a mental illness.

The AAFP has position papers that detail substance use disorders and addiction and tobacco prevention and cessation.

Payment for primary care physicians has historically been inadequate for office visits for mental health diagnoses. This limitation in reimbursement interfered with the family physician's ability to offer comprehensive care and management of mental health conditions, as well as the ability to integrate, from a business perspective, with behavioral health services. However, new coverage policies adopted by the Centers for Medicare and Medicaid Services (CMS) are more promising and may incentivize primary care physicians to provide treatment for mental and behavioral health conditions.[87] These policies, effective January 1, 2017, emphasize collaborative care, where primary care physicians are expected to work in partnership with a behavioral health care manager, and consult with mental health specialists. While targeting populations with Medicare, these policies may also encourage private insurers to offer similar options and may incentivize more family physicians to offer behavioral and mental health care to other populations.

Health care for all people with mental illness should be "affordable, nondiscriminatory, and includes coverage for the most effective and appropriate treatment."[88] Coverage for mental illness should be equal in scope to coverage for other illnesses and all clinically-effective treatments appropriate to the needs of individuals with mental illness should be covered.

Thank you for the opportunity to provide testimony on this important issue. For further questions, please contact Erica Cischke, Senior Manager, Legislative and Regulatory Affairs at ecischke@aafp.org.

Sincerely,
Gary L. LeRoy, M.D., FAAFP

---

[86] Bandiera FC, Anteneh B, Le T, Delucchi K, Guydish J. Tobacco-related mortality among persons with mental health and substance abuse problems. PLoS One. 2015;10(3):e0120581.

[87] Press MJ, Howe R, Schoenbaum M, et al. Medicare payment for behavioral health integration. *N Engl J Med.* 2017;376(5):405–407.

[88] National Alliance on Mental Illness. Public policy platform of the National Alliance on Mental Illness*(https://www.nami.org/getattachment/learn.more/mental-health-public-policy/public-policy-platform-december.2016(1).pdf).* Twelfth Edition. 2016. Accessed January 22, 2018.

Board Chair
End notes

https://www.aafp.org/dam/AAFP/documents/advocacy/health/it/telehealth/TS- SenateFinanceCmte-DavisTelehealth-051921.pdf.
https://www.aafp.org/dam/AAFP/documents/advocacy/health/it/telehealth/LT- Congress-TelehealthHELP-070120.pdf.
https://www.aafp.org/about/policies/all/substance-use-disorders.html.
https://www.aafp.org/about/policies/all/tobacco-preventingtreating html#:~:text=The%20AAFP%20opposes%20all%20forms,of%20tobacco%20products%20to%20chil dren.

American Hospital Association

800 10th Street, NW Two CityCenter, Suite 400
Washington, DC 20001–4956
(202) 638–1100

On behalf of our nearly 5,000 member hospitals, health systems and other health care organizations, our clinician partners—including more than 270,000 affiliated physicians, 2 million nurses and other caregivers—and the 43,000 health care leaders who belong to our professional membership groups, the American Hospital Association (AHA) appreciates the opportunity to submit this statement for the record.

America's hospitals and health systems play a central role in delivering behavioral health care and are uniquely positioned to help patients navigate the behavioral health resources that are available in communities. Psychiatric and community hospitals are a vital source of care for behavioral health patients, providing treatment for a full range of psychiatric and substance use disorders (SUD) by stabilizing patients, establishing and providing quality treatment regimens, and transitioning patients to outpatient and community-based services. The AHA strongly supports efforts to increase access to, and improve the quality of, behavioral health care.

Even before the COVID–19 pandemic, one in five American adults was estimated to have a behavioral health condition, and nearly 60% of adults with behavioral health disorders reported not receiving services for their conditions. But the nation's level of unmet behavioral health needs has been exacerbated by the COVID–19 pandemic. As of June 14, the Centers for Disease Control and Prevention (CDC) reports that more than 33 million Americans have been infected with COVID–19, and, of those, more than 597,000 have died.

The effects of high unemployment, anxiety over the risk of contracting COVID–19, grief over the death of loved ones, isolation from neighbors and friends, and an increase in domestic violence and child abuse are all increasing the incidence and prevalence of mental health conditions and substance use disorder. For example, one in three adults reported symptoms of an anxiety disorder in 2020, compared with one in 12 in 2019.

In addition, the inability to access in-person group therapy and medication-assisted treatment (MAT), in part because of social distancing requirements, has led many with substance use disorders to relapse. According to the CDC, overdose deaths spiked after the start of the pandemic, driven by synthetic opioids such as fentanyl.

Further, the behavioral health effects of COVID–19 are manifesting at a time when the nation's behavioral health care system is ill-prepared to meet the nation's needs. According to the Substance Abuse and Mental Health Services Administration (SAMHSA), only 43% of U.S. adults with mental illness received treatment in 2018, and a JAMA study found that 50.6% of U.S. youth aged 6–17 with a mental health disorder received treatment in 2016.

Unfortunately, due to financial pressures, hospitals' capacity to care for behavioral health patients has been significantly diminished, exacerbating a trend that began decades ago. The number of state-funded psychiatric beds per capita decreased by97% between 1955 and 2016, with the per capita psychiatric inpatient bed count approximately 70% lower than the average among developed nations, as noted by a March 2019 National Association for Behavioral Healthcare report. Lack of access to psychiatric inpatient services and resources will exacerbate existing sever shortages in psychiatric beds nationally. This trend, combined with new closures, will result in more preventable deaths from psychiatric and substance use disorders and more cases of emergency room boarding. As the number of psychiatric beds has declined, the demand for inpatient services has continued to increase, and correspondingly, wait times for those beds has increased dramatically as well.

To address the urgent need for greater access to behavioral health services, the AHA offers the following recommendations to the Committee on Finance.

Address Physician Shortages

At the core of our health care system is a well-trained, diverse workforce. But critical physician shortages deprive many communities of access to needed care. The Association of American Medical Colleges estimates that the United States faces a shortage of between 54,100 and 139,000 physicians by 2033.

In the 1997 Balanced Budget Act, Congress froze the number of Medicare-funded residency slots at 1996 levels, based on projections that the nation would soon have a surplus of physicians. Over the past 24 years, millions more Americans have attained health insurance, the nation's population has grown and aged, and more physicians are retiring—leading to a crisis in physician access. The shortage is even more acute for substance use disorder providers. A recent report from the National Academies of Sciences, Engineering and Medicine highlighted the dearth of clinicians with specialized training in MAT, and SAMHSA has estimated that only 10% of the 22 million Americans with an SUD receive treatment.

Last December, Congress lifted the cap on Medicare-funded residency positions, allowing growth for the first time since 1997. That provision, in the Consolidated Appropriations Act, 2021, created 1,000 new slots that will begin to be distributed in fiscal year (FY) 2023. Increasing the number of Medicare-funded slots would help ease current shortages, and bolster the foundation of our health care system.

The AHA supports the Opioid Workforce Act of 2021, introduced by Senators Margaret Wood Hassan and Susan Collins, which would help abate the national shortage of opioid treatment providers by increasing the number of resident physician slots in hospitals with programs focused on SUD treatment. Existing shortages of SUD treatment providers have led to lengthy waiting periods for treatment and increased mortality from opioid misuse and addiction. The Opioid Workforce Act would help address existing shortages by adding 1,000 Medicare-funded training positions in approved residency programs in addiction medicine, addiction psychiatry or pain medicine. These new slots would constitute a major step toward increasing access to SUD treatment for communities in need. We look forward to working with you to ensure passage of this important legislation.

Repeal the IMD Exclusion

Since 1965, the Institutions for Mental Diseases (IMD) exclusion has prohibited federal payments to states for services for adult Medicaid beneficiaries between the ages of 21 and 64 who are treated in facilities that have more than 16 beds, and that provide inpatient or residential behavioral health treatment. The discriminatory IMD policy was established at a time when behavioral health conditions were not considered medical conditions on the same level as physical health conditions, state-operated psychiatric facilities were a primary setting for behavioral health care, and patients were admitted for longer-term stays.

We know that successful treatment requires access to the full continuum of care— namely, inpatient care, partial hospitalization, residential treatment and outpatient services. Different types of patients require different clinical services from across the care continuum. Investing only in outpatient care and failing to provide states with relief from the IMD exclusion would continue to deny many of these patients access to the most clinically appropriate care. Additionally, advances in behavioral health care have allowed for shorter inpatient stays and more outpatient treatment options, while funding challenges have led to a decline in the number of inpatient psychiatric beds. Repealing the IMD exclusion would help reverse this decline.

Eliminate Medicare's 190-Day Limit on Inpatient Psychiatric Treatment

Medicare covers only 190 days of inpatient care in a psychiatric hospital in a beneficiary's lifetime. This discriminatory limit erects a barrier to accessing care for indi viduals who have gone beyond their 190-day limit, particularly those with a chronic mental condition.

As the nation looks to recover from COVID–19 pandemic, an even greater mental health crisis awaits. Medicare beneficiaries who did not seek inpatient care during the pandemic because they hesitated to leave their homes or because they have conditions that were exacerbated by the pandemic will need inpatient services. Further, as the nation's elderly population continues to grow and life expectancy continues to rise, the 190-day limit will severely affect access to needed care. To effectively address the needs of America's seniors, Congress should repeal Medicare's 190-day limit on inpatient psychiatric care.

Make Telehealth Flexibilities Permanent

Telehealth services, including for mental health and SUD treatment, have improved access to care. The increased use of telehealth since the start of the public health emergency (PHE) is producing high-quality outcomes for patients, enhancing patient experience, and protecting access for individuals susceptible to infection. With the appropriate statutory and regulatory framework, this beneficial shift in care delivery could continue to improve patient experiences and outcomes and deliver health system efficiencies beyond the pandemic. The AHA urges the Committee to consider making these flexibilities permanent.

Additionally, telehealth policies should work together to maintain access for patients by connecting them to vital health care services and their personal providers through videoconferencing, remote monitoring, electronic consults and wireless communications. We support the following: elimination of the 1834(m) geographic and originating site restriction; coverage and reimbursement for audio-only services; an expanded list of providers and facilities eligible to deliver and bill for telehealth services, including rural health clinics and federally qualified health centers; a national approach to licensure so that providers can safely provide virtual care across state lines; and, adequate reimbursement for the substantial costs of establishing and maintaining a telehealth infrastructure, among others.

Promote Integration of Physical and Behavioral Health

The use of electronic health records (EHR) can promote the integration of physical and behavioral health care. Yet, significant barriers remain for the adoption of EHRs by behavioral health providers. The 2009 HITECH Act incentivized EHR adoption with payments for providers who participate in the Medicare and Medicaid Promoting Interoperability Programs; however, psychiatric hospitals are ineligible for these programs. In addition to this financial pressure, the nature of behavioral health records—that is, that they are often narrative or follow a different structure than physical health records—as well as conflicting regulatory requirements regarding information sharing has led to far lower adoption of EHRs in psychiatric hospitals compared to general acute care hospitals. We urge the Committee to create opportunities for behavioral health providers to acquire interoperable electronic health records that enable improved information sharing among providers and with public health and other government agencies.

Conclusion

The AHA is encouraged that the Committee is examining ways to improve Americans' access to mental health and substance use disorder treatment. We stand ready to work with the Committee as you consider legislation to expand vital behavioral health services to patients and families.

American Psychological Association

750 First Street, NE Washington, DC 20002–4242
202–336–5800
202–336–6123 TDD
https://www.apa.org/

Statement Submitted by Katherine B. McGuire, Chief Advocacy Officer

The American Psychological Association (APA) thanks the Committee for the opportunity to offer solutions to strengthen the nation's mental health system, which even prior to the COVID–19 pandemic could not meet the needs of people in need of care. APA is the nation's largest scientific and professional nonprofit organization representing the discipline and profession of psychology. APA has more than 122,000 members and affiliates who are clinicians, researchers, educators, consultants, and students in psychological science.

As the U.S. Government Accountability Office (GAO) recently found, ''longstanding unmet needs for behavioral health services'' continue to persist and were in fact ''worsened by new challenges associated with the COVID–19 pandemic'' (GAO, March 31, 2021). Over the past year, the pandemic created ''a cascade of societal challenges, including illness and death, prolonged social isolation, job loss, and reliance on remote work and online education'' while also ''cast[ing] a bright light on the destructive effects of health, educational, employment, legal, and criminal justice disparities and inequities'' (American Psychological Association, August 2020). The results of APA's ''Stress in America'' survey series during this time tell a compelling story about the mental health impact of the pandemic on everyday Americans, particularly on communities of color and other underserved communities (American Psychological Association, 2021). This impact manifests in a highly individualized manner, which includes but is not limited to higher rates of emotions associated with prolonged stress, such as anxiety, stress and anger; unexpected fluctuations in weight; disruptions in sleep; and increased consumption of alcohol and dangerous substances.

Innovative solutions are urgently required if we are ever to meet the challenge of addressing the long-term mental health impact of this pandemic while remedying preexisting barriers to accessing these services. However, there is no single solution to addressing this crisis, and the Committee and its members will need to improve policies in multiple areas, including the following:

- *Preserve Recent Expansions in Medicare Coverage of Mental and Behavioral Health Services Furnished by Telehealth.* Congress's and CMS's decision to expand Medicare coverage of mental and behavioral services via telehealth—including those furnished via audio-only communication—prompted a long-overdue expansion of mental health services to many communities that traditionally lacked access to such services. Audio-only services in particular are a critical (and often the only) link to mental and behavioral health services for many individuals and communities that are less likely to have reliable access to technological training or broadband technology, such as older adults, individuals with disabilities, people in rural and frontier areas, lower-income families, and communities of color.

  We remain concerned, however, that this access expansion will abruptly end once the current public health emergency ends, and we hope this Committee will help avoid this ''access cliff '' and permanently authorize Medicare to cover audio-only telehealth for mental, behavioral, and substance use disorder services. Specifically, we urge the Committee to approve legislation such as the bipartisan bill H.R. 3447, introduced by Reps. Jason Smith and Josh Gottheimer. This bill would permanently establish Medicare coverage of mental, behavioral, and substance use disorder services furnished via audio-only telehealth, provided that the patient has at least one in-person or audio-video telehealth visit within the past 3 years.

Additionally, while APA supported Congress's decision to eliminate certain site- of-service requirements on Medicare tele-mental health coverage in the year- end budget and COVID package (Pub. L. 116–260), we are concerned that the new six-month in-person service requirement will inequitably limit access to services. Accordingly, APA asks the Committee to take up and pass the bipartisan Telemental Health Care Access Act (S. 2061) sponsored by Senators Cas- sidy, Smith, Thune, and Cardin, which removes this arbitrary and unnecessary barrier to coverage of tele-mental health services. AP A also hopes that members of this Committee will consider introducing a Senate counterpart to Representative Matsui's Telemental Health Care Access Act (H.R. 4058), which in addition to removing this in-person service requirement, will also eliminate the aforementioned site-of-service requirements for behavioral health services.

Finally, we hope this Committee will support a bipartisan bill co-sponsored by Senator Stabenow, the Tele-Mental Health Improvement Act (S. 660), which will—both during and shortly after the pandemic—place coverage and reimbursement for mental health and substance use disorder services on the same footing as services provided in-person. We hope members of this Committee will also consider long-term measures to address the inequities in reimbursement between care furnished in person and care furnished via telehealth.

- *Support Innovative Approaches to Combating the Resurgent Opioid and Substance Use Disorder Crisis.* Despite Congress' commendable efforts to combat the opioid epidemic, the COVID–19 pandemic worsened rates of opioid and substance use. According to CDC data, over 88,000 individuals died due to a drug overdose between August 2019 and August 2020, an astounding 26.8% increase over the previous year (Ahmad, et al. 2021). CDC data also shows that while opioids, and especially fentanyl, continue to account for the bulk of overdose deaths, the use of psychostimulants such as methamphetamine increased by 46% over the previous year (Volkow, 2021). The drug overdose crisis demands a strong public health response which meets individuals with substance use disorders where they are. The CAHOOTS Act (S. 764) introduced by Chairman

Wyden embodies this approach, and we urge both its enactment and the adoption of mobile crisis intervention services by Medicaid programs nation- wide.

- We urge the Committee to advance similarly innovative approaches to this crisis, such as those outlined in: (1) the bipartisan Medicaid Reentry Act (S. 285), co-sponsored by Senator Whitehouse, which allows inmates within 30 days of release to enroll in Medicaid to reduce the risk of relapse upon release; (2) Sen. Hassan's Mainstreaming Addiction Treatment Act (S. 445), which eliminates the unnecessary and counterproductive requirement that prescribing providers obtain a waiver from the Drug Enforcement Agency (DEA) before prescribing buprenorphine for the treatment of substance use disorders; (3) S. 854, legislation introduced by Sen. Grassley to designate methamphetamine as an emerging drug threat; and (4) S. 1457, the STOP Fentanyl Act of 2021—introduced by Senators Warren, Whitehouse, Baldwin, and Booker—that, among other provisions, would remove barriers to the establishment of contingency management programs, an evidence-based form of behavioral treatment developed by psychologists for treatment of methamphetamine, cocaine, and other substance use disorders (De Crescenzo, et al., 2018).
- *Allow Clinical Psychologists to Practice Independently in All Medicare Treatment Settings.* Current law requires physician supervision of psychologists' treatment of Medicare patients in certain settings, such as partial hospitalization programs, surgical centers, and community mental health centers. Medicare is the last health insurer that requires physician supervision of psychologists. Unlike Medicare, *all* other health insurers and state licensure laws allow psychologists to practice independently in *all* treatment settings.
- Most older Americans with mental disorders do not receive mental health treatment from a mental health specialist, and older Americans are much more likely to be prescribed psychoactive drugs—even without an established diagnosis for a mental disorder-than to receive psychotherapy or other behavioral health services, despite the ongoing opioid epidemic and concerns about overmedication in nursing homes and other facilities. Allowing clinical psychologists to practice independently in all treatment settings, as they can do

through other health insurance programs, would contribute to reversing this trend. Medicare patients would benefit from improved access to psychologists' services, including psychological and neuropsychological assessments, psychotherapy, and health and behavior assessments and interventions.

- *Incentivize Adoption of a Broad Array of Integrated Care Models.* APA appreciates the Committee's discussions around the integration of primary care and mental health services. Integrated care is an innovative way of improving patient outcomes and satisfaction with care, as well as reducing overall treatment costs, but it requires significant changes to primary care practices' physical offices, information technology systems, management procedures, clinical staffing and policies, health records and data tracking practices, and provider education and training. With these challenges and given differences in patient populations and the goals of the integration effort, there is no ''one size fits all'' approach to effective integrated primary care. As stated in a recent review, ''[t]here are several models and differing levels of integration described in the literature, suggesting that approaches to integration should be responsive to the needs and context of the community'' (Vogel et al., 2017, p. 81).

  We urge the Committee to provide support for the implementation of integrated care programs by primary care providers that gives them the flexibility to blend services, models, and interventions in a way that best meets the needs of their patient populations and reflects the healthcare workforce in their community. Support should be made available for all evidence-based integrated care programs meeting the following four criteria:

  ✓ A multi-professional approach to patient care;
  ✓ A structured management plan;
  ✓ Scheduled patient follow-ups; and
  ✓ Enhanced inter-professional communication.

- *Support Programs that Strengthen Access to School-Based Mental Health Services.* The pandemic continues to have an outsized impact on children and youth, with nearly a third of parents reporting that their child experienced some degree of harm to their emotional or mental health during the pandemic (Gallup, 2020). This population is of concern not only due to their higher overall vulnerability to stress, but also because of the increased risk they will experience adverse childhood experiences (ACEs) such as various forms of abuse, neglect, and household dysfunction. As schools are a key provider of mental and behavioral health services to children, the pandemic often cut off access to mental health services for many children (Nuamah, et al., 2020).

- To aid the nation's school-age children in recovering from the mental, social, and educational impact of the COVID–19, we ask that members of the Committee support the following pieces of legislation:
  - ✓ The Increasing Access to Mental Health in Schools Act (S. 1811), introduced by Sen. Tester (D–MT), which would expand mental health services in low-income schools by supporting partnerships between institutions of higher education and local education agencies to increase the number of school-based mental health professionals;
  - ✓ The Mental Health Services for Students Act (S. 1841), introduced by Sen. Tina Smith (D–MN), which would build partnerships between local educational agencies, tribal schools, and community-based organizations to provide school-based mental health care for students and provide resources for the entire school community on warning signs of mental health crises; and
  - ✓ A Senate counterpart to the Comprehensive Mental Health in Schools Pilot Program Act (H.R. 3549), which would create a new 4-year grant program to help schools that predominantly serve low-income students with building their capacity to address students' mental and behavioral well-being.
- *Address Inequities in Access to Mental and Behavioral Health Services.* The COVID–19 pandemic both highlighted and exacerbated longstanding disparities in access to mental health services, particularly amongst individuals from communities of color. Psychological science continues to inform innovative solutions to combat challenges related to health equity including, for example, guidance on facilitating transparent and thoughtful conversations between community leaders and individuals to enable informed decisions about vaccine behaviors. As a critical first step in remedying these disparities, AP A hopes this Committee will take up and pass H.R. 1475, the Pursuing Equity in Mental Health Act adopted by the House last month. Among other provisions, this bill would authorize funding to support health equity research, build

outreach programs to reduce the stigma of seeking mental health treatment, and develop a training program for providers.

APA stands ready to assist the Committee in finding impactful bipartisan solutions to expand the nation's mental and behavioral health system to serve all in need of these services. Please contact Andrew Strickland, J.D. at astrickland@apa.org if our association can serve as a resource.

References

Ahmad F.B., Rossen L.M., Sutton P. Provisional drug overdose death counts. Na- tional Center for Health Statistics. 2021. Accessed at *https://cdc.gov/nchs/ nvss/ vsrr/drug-overdose-data.htm.*

American Psychological Association (August 2020). Psychology's Understanding of the Challenges Related to the COVID–19 Global Pandemic in the United States. *https://www.apa.org/about/policy/covid-statement.pdf.*

American Psychological Association (2021). Stress in America Press Room. *https:// www.apa.org/news/press/releases/stress?tab=2.*

De Crescenzo et al., PLoS Medicine 2018; 15(12): e1002715.

Gallup (June 16, 2020). U.S. Parents Say COVID–19 Harming Child's Mental Health. *https://news.gallup.com/poll/312605/parents-say-covid-harming-child- mental-health.aspx.*

Gold, J.A., Rossen, L.M., Ahmad F.B., et al. Race, Ethnicity, and Age Trends in Persons Who Died From COVID–19—United States, May–August 2020. MMWR Morb

Mortal Wkly Rep 2020; 69:1517–1521. DOI: *https://www.ncbi.nlm.nih.gov/pmc/ articles/PMC7583501/.*

Nuamah, S., Good, R., Bierbaum, A., and Simon, E. (2020). School closures always hurt. They hurt even more now. Education Week. Retrieved from *https://www.edweek.org/ew/articles/2020/06/09/schoolclosures-always-hurt-they-hurt- even.html.*

U.S. Government Accountability Office, March 31, 2021. Behavioral Health: Patient Access, Provider Claims Payment, and the Effect of the COVID–19 Pandemic. *https://www.gao.gov/assets/gao-21-437r.pdf.*

Vogel, M.E., Kanzler, K.E., Aikens, J.E., and Goodie, J.L. (2017). Integration of behavioral health and primary care: Current knowledge and future directions. *Journal of Behavioral Medicine,* 40(1), 69–84.

Volkow, N. National Institute on Drug Abuse, 2021 "U.S. Overdose Deaths Involving Psychostimulants (Mostly Amphetamine), by Race" [Powerpoint presentation]. Accessed at *https://www.apa.org/members/content/ methamphetamine-addiction.*

Association for Behavioral Health and Wellness

1325 G Street, NW, Suite 500
Washington, DC 20005
https://abhw.org/
June 15, 2021

Dear Chairman Wyden and Ranking Member Crapo:

The Association for Behavioral Health and Wellness (ABHW) appreciates the opportunity to provide comments for the record on the hearing: ''Mental Health Care in America: Addressing Root Causes and Identifying Policy Solutions'' that took place Tuesday, June 15, 2021. We appreciate the Committee's leadership on and dedication to addressing behavioral health issues.

ABHW serves as the national voice for payers that manage behavioral health insurance benefits. ABHW member companies provide coverage to approximately 200 million people in both the public and private sectors to treat mental health (MH) and substance use disorders (SUDs), and other behaviors that impact health and wellness.

Overarchingly, our organization's goals aim to increase access, drive integration, support prevention, raise awareness, reduce stigma, and advance evidence-based treatment and quality outcomes. Furthermore, through our policy work, we strive to promote equal access to quality treatment and address the stark inequities created by systemic racism. We are deeply concerned about health disparities in this country in the areas of MH and SUD services and are committed to addressing systemic racism in the healthcare system. We applaud the Committee's commitment to health equity and look forward to working with you to improve behavioral health services in this country.

Behavioral health services have become increasingly important as a result of social isolation, job loss, illness and death, and domestic violence related to COVID–19 and we suspect the utilization of such services will continue long after the public health emergency (PHE) is lifted. Addressing the following issues can play a critical role in expanding access to MH and SUD services and provide long lasting improvements to our nation's behavioral health system.

- Expand the use of telehealth for MH and SUD services.
- Increase access to medication-assisted treatment (MAT).
- Support suicide prevention efforts and increase focus on crisis services.
- Eliminate the Institution for Mental Diseases (IMD) Medicaid exclusion.
- Develop a clear, universal compliance standard related to mental health and addiction parity.
- Ensure health coverage for individuals released from jails and prisons.
- Align 42 CFR Part 2 with the Health Insurance Portability and Accountability Act (HIPAA).

As you further examine behavioral health issues, we urge you to consider and include the following:

Expand the use of telehealth for MH and SUD services. We appreciate the current guidance and flexibilities in response to the PHE and request that the flexi bilities continue for at least one year after the PHE is lifted. These long overdue changes to telehealth policies have allowed payers and providers to ensure people can access necessary MH and SUD services in midst of physical distancing. ABHW members support extending flexibilities past the PHE and simultaneously collecting and analyzing data before making permanent changes. As the need for behavioral health services continues to grow, we urge Congress to support the following policy changes:

- *Eliminate the new in-person visit requirement for mental health services:* We applaud the recent changes made to remove geographic and originating site restrictions on originating sites for mental health services, allowing beneficiaries across the country to receive virtual care from a location of their choosing. However, these changes were accompanied by a new requirement, mandating that an individual must have an in-person visit no less than six months before he or she is eligible to receive mental health services via telehealth. Given that many individuals with mental health issues may not physically be able to leave the home, we urge you to support the Telemental Health Care Access Act, S. 2061/H.R. 4058, which removes the in-person requirement visit prior to receiving Medicare telehealth services for mental health.

- *Expand cross state licensure:* During the pandemic, all 50 states have used emergency authority to waive certain aspects of state licensure laws, thus providing widespread access to care. We encourage efforts for states to foster cross state licensure reciprocity to support increased access to services. We also propose convening a task force of federal and state leaders to examine this issue and outline recommendations on changes that would increase access to behavioral health services.
- *Examine audio-only telehealth services.* ABHW supports patient access to audio- only behavioral health services for the duration of the PHE. However, before audio-only services are made permanent, ABHW strongly suggests that the appropriate regulatory agencies conduct research as to whether or not behavioral health services provided via audio-only are an effective long-term strategy to provide quality, evidence-based, and clinically appropriate care. One way to do this would be to create an audio-only modifier so that it can be used in effectiveness research to differentiate between audio-visual and audio-only services.
  Currently, it is unclear whether audio-only is appropriate for all behavioral health treatments. Specifically, ABHW advocates for audio-only services to be evaluated in partial hospitalization programs, applied behavioral analyses, psych testing, and group therapy before they are reimbursed permanently. Ultimately, audio-only behavioral health treatments should have safeguards built around them and should not be a primary or default avenue for care. Post PHE, audio-only should only be used after it has proven to be effective and is deemed to be in the individual's best interest (for example, the patient has limited broadband access and difficulty accessing video technology).

Increase access to medication assisted treatment (MAT). Research has shown that MAT is the most effective intervention to treat opioid use disorders (OUDs) as it significantly reduces illicit opioid use compared to nondrug approaches and increased access to MAT can reduce overdose fatalities.[89] As such, ABHW supports the following policy changes to increase MAT access.

---

[89] Medication-Assisted Treatment Improves Outcomes for Patients with Opioid Use Disorder, Pew Fact Sheet, November 22, 2016.

- *Eliminate the X-waiver.* During the COVID–19 pandemic, overdoses and related deaths continue to rise, making access to MAT crucial. HHS recently published a Notice which allows providers to treat up to 30 patients using MAT without first obtaining the X-waiver. While this is a step in the right direction to treat OUDs, more must be done. As such, we ask that Congress pass the Mainstreaming Addiction Treatment (MAT) Act, S. 445/H.R. 1384. This bipartisan legislation would remove the federal rules established by the DATA 2000 Act that require health care practitioners to obtain a waiver (X-waiver) from the Drug Enforcement Administration (DEA) before prescribing buprenorphine to treat OUDs. The legislation would remove a major hurdle to prescribing MAT, impact existing nationwide shortage of treatment providers, and expand access to OUD treatment.
- *Eliminate the in-person evaluation requirement.* Given that not all individuals with SUDs are able to have an initial in-person visit with a provider due to behavioral health provider shortages or physical difficulty traveling, ABHW advocates for actions which would eliminate the in-person evaluation requirement before a provider can prescribe MAT via telehealth. The Ryan Haight Act, originally passed to combat the rise of rogue online pharmacies, requires an in-person evaluation before a provider can prescribe MAT via telehealth. This safeguard likely suppresses the use of MAT because under current law, the evaluation requirement cannot be fulfilled via a telehealth visit.[90] While the Ryan Haight Act allows for providers to use telemedicine when engaged in the ''practice of medicine,'' it is nearly impossible for providers to do so. The definition of ''practice of telemedicine'' includes seven categories in which a provider could meet the in-person requirement through a virtual care platform, including under a special registration granted by the DEA. However, the DEA never created that registration process. With the Special Registration for Telemedicine Act of 2018, which was part of the Substance Use-Disorder Prevention that Promotes Opioid Recovery and Treatment (SUPPORT) Act, the DEA had until October 24, 2019, to outline rules for providers with a special registration to prescribe

---

[90] Kayla R. Bryant, *Health Law Daily Wrap up, Strategic Perspectives: States Fail to Fully Use Telemedicine to Fight the Public Health Crisis,* Wolters Kluwer (September 28, 2018), p. 2.

controlled substances. That deadline passed without action, severely impeding those with OUDs from receiving the care they need.

As such, we recommend that Congress urge the DEA to move forward with promulgating the telemedicine special registration process rule, as mandated by federal law, to enable providers to prescribe MAT to patients with SUDs by employing telemedicine.

Support suicide prevention efforts and increase focus on crisis services. Last year Congress passed the National Suicide Hotline Designation Act of 2019, making the National Suicide Prevention Lifeline an easy to remember three-digit number, 9-8-8. The need for Americans to have readily available access to mental health crisis services through a ubiquitous number like 9-8-8 is more urgent than ever. We urge Congress to work with the Federal Communications Commission (FCC) to ensure the timely implementation of 9-8-8 by July 2022. Incidences of mental health crises and suicide attempts have been increasing annually, and are exacerbated by the COVID–19 pandemic.

In addition to swiftly creating the crisis line, it is equally important that the crisis line have adequate resources so that it can operate effectively and ensure that all Americans can access it. Since demand will undoubtedly increase for services of the crisis line, there will need to be significant investment after the initial implementation to expand capacity and provide services consistently for mental health crises. Therefore, we ask Congress to pass H.R. 2981, the Suicide Prevention Lifeline Improvement Act of 2021. This legislation would require increased coordination, data sharing, and provide more funding to support community-based crisis service delivery. ABHW supports an evidence-based continuum of crisis care for individuals experiencing a behavioral health crisis, and look forward to working with Congress to promote access to quality crisis services.

Eliminate the Institution for Mental Diseases (IMD) Medicaid exclusion. We urge Congress to remove policy barriers that limit beneficiary access to needed and appropriate MH and SUD care. This includes ending the IMD exclusion, which prohibits Medicaid reimbursement for adults under the age of 65 in residential behavioral health facilities with more than 16 beds. Although the IMD exclusion cannot be fully eliminated without Congressional action, the Administration could increase access and improve appropriate care through expanded use of waivers under section 1115, which would enable states to more broadly cover IMD services. Further, as we have witnessed, national hospital capacity has been pushed to its limits during the COVID–19 pandemic. Waiving the IMD exclusion to Medicaid funding for inpatient behavioral health treatment would free up beds in local hospitals, allowing them to better manage the surge capacity in both inpatient and emergency departments to care for COVID–19 patients. Additionally, new legislation was introduced this year by Representative Napolitano, the Increasing Behavioral Health Treatment Act, H.R. 2611. This legislation would remove the IMD exclusion for states that have submitted a plan to: increase access to outpatient and community-based behavioral health care; increase availability of crisis stabilization services; and improve data sharing and coordination between physical health, mental health and addiction treatment providers and first-responders. We urge Congress to pass this important legislation.

Develop a clear, universal compliance standard related to mental health and addiction parity. ABHW member companies continue to invest significant time and resources to understand and implement Mental Health Parity and Addiction Equity Act (MHPAEA). Our member companies have teams of dozens of people working diligently to implement and provide MH/SUD parity benefits to their consumers. We have also had numerous meetings with the regulators to help us better comprehend the regulatory guidance and to discuss how plans can operationalize the regulations.

While parity has progressed since its adoption in meaningful ways and access to MH and SUD treatment providers has greatly expanded, systemic issues continue to be a challenge due to other non-parity factors such as the looming shortage of physicians (both psychiatrists as well as other MH and SUD providers). Examples of key changes since the parity law and regulations were enacted include: the fact that routine MH outpatient treatment no longer habitually requires prior authorization or has explicit quantitative treatment limits; evidence-based levels of care for MH conditions are no longer subject to blanket exclusions (e.g., residential treatment for eating disorders); and transparency, documentation, attention to medical necessity criteria all have improved.

However, despite these gains and the parity language in the 21st Century Cures Act, aspects of the law and regulations remain overly complex and technical. As a result, compliance has become a moving target through a patchwork of conflicting and changing guidance. There is new parity language in Section 203 of the recently passed Consolidated Appropriations Act of 2021, and we hope that the regulations related to these parity provisions will provide the clarity payers need to appropriately implement MHPAEA. We strongly support the flexibility built into the law, yet there has been a proliferation of different compliance approaches, tools, and interpretations, which continues to lead to confusion in implementation, is costly for stakeholders, and ultimately hinders patient care. We believe this Administration can re-invigorate efforts to clarify and improve the application of the law for the benefit of all.

Strengthen and expand the behavioral health workforce. We appreciate your support to expand access to care, and address ongoing workforce shortages across the country in order to help ensure people who need MH and/or SUD treatment get the care they need. As one first step, we ask that the Administration and Congress work to increase funding to behavioral health providers so that we have an adequate workforce to meet the increasing need for MH and SUD services. We recommend expanding eligible Medicare providers to include marriage and family therapists (MFTs), mental health counselors (MHCs), and certified peer support specialists.

- *Medicare coverage of mental health counselors and marriage and family therapists.* Recognition of MHCs and MFTs as Medicare providers would increase the pool of eligible mental health professionals by over 200,000 licensed practitioners. Studies have shown that these providers have the highest success and lowest recidivism rates with their patients as well as being the most cost effective.[91] We encourage you to work with Congress to pass the Mental Health Access Improvement Act (S. 828, H.R. 432), which recognizes MHCs and MFTs as covered Medicare providers, helps address the critical gaps in care, and ensures access to needed services.
- *Medicare coverage of peer support services.* Certified peer support specialists can be vital in providing support to people living with mental health conditions and SUDs. These paraprofessionals are individuals with lived experience of recovery from a MH disorder or SUDs. This evidence-based practice helps individuals navigate the often-confusing health care system, get the most out of treatment, identify community resources, and develop resiliency. Due to the COVID–19 pandemic, engagement with treatment and care has been disrupted, but finding and utilizing support in a timely manner can help mitigate negative health outcomes of the disruption. Recently,

---

[91] D. Russell Crane and Scott H. Payne, ''Individual Versus Family Psychotherapy in Managed Care: Comparing the Costs of Treatment by the Mental Health Professions,'' Journal of Marital and Family Therapy 37, no. 3 (2011): 273-289.

the Promoting Effective and Empowering Recovery Services in Medicare (PEERS) Act of 2021, H.R. 2767/S. 2144, was introduced. This legislation is an important step in recognizing the unique role of peer support specialists in helping individuals better engage in services, man age physical and mental health conditions, build support systems, and, ultimately, live self-directed lives in their communities.

Ensure health coverage for individuals released from jails and prisons. ABHW strongly supports H.R. 955/S. 285, the Medicaid Reentry Act of 2021, to grant Medicaid eligibility to incarcerated individuals 30 days prior to their release to promote the health care needs of individuals transitioning back into communities. According to the Bureau of Justice Statistics, more than half of those in the criminal justice system suffer from a mental illness. Of those with serious mental illness, approximately 75 percent also have a co-occurring SUD. Allowing incarcerated individuals to receive services covered by Medicaid 30 days prior to their release from jail or prison will expand access to vital mental health and addiction services. Equipping individuals with timely access to addiction, mental health, and other health-related services before release, will facilitate the transition to community-based care upon release that is necessary to help break the cycle of recidivism. This is even more critical in the midst of the COVID–19 pandemic.

Issue regulation for 42 CFR Part 2. We look forward to the promulgation of the next 42 CFR Part 2 (Part 2) rule pursuant to the Coronavirus Aid, Relief, and Economic Security (CARES) Act of 2020. Part 2, which governs the confidentiality of SUD records, sets requirements limiting the use and disclosure of patients' SUD records from certain substance use programs, including the cumbersome requirement of a signed consent by the patient each time the SUD record is to be shared. The CARES Act brings Part 2 into significant alignment with the Health Insurance Portability and Accountability Act of 1996 (HIPAA). Changes in the CARES Act permit a patient to provide one written consent to disclose their Part 2 information for all future treatment, payment, and health care operations (TPO), unless the patient revokes consent. Additionally, under the CARES Act, breaches in a Part 2 program trigger patient notification, Part 2 programs are now subject to HIPAA civil and criminal penalties, and discrimination against Part 2 program patients is prohibited. This legislation culminates years of work from a broad range of organizations, and it represents a number of critical compromises.

Attached you will find recommendations from the Partnership to Amend 42 CFR Part 2 (Partnership), which we have previously shared with the U.S. Department of Health and Human Services (HHS), the Substance Abuse and Mental Health Services Administration (SAMHSA) as well as the Office for National Drug Control Policy (ONDCP). The Partnership, founded by ABHW, brings together a broad spectrum of the healthcare industry to advocate for aligning Part 2 with HIPAA. We urge HHS to ensure that the requirements for Part 2 stated in the CARES Act are reflected in the next Part 2 Rule.

Thank you for the opportunity to provide suggestions to address important behavioral health policies. If you have any questions or would like to discuss ABHW's policy priorities please contact Maeghan Gilmore, Director of Government Affairs, at gilmore@abhw.org or 202-503-6999.

Sincerely,
Pamela Greenberg,
MPP President and CEO

Center for Fiscal Equity

14448 Parkvale Road, Suite 6
Rockville, MD 20853 fiscalequitycenter@yahoo.com

Statement of Michael G. Bindner

Chairman Wyden and Ranking Member Crapo, thank you for the opportunity to submit these comments for the record.

It seems like we covered this ground last month in the subcommittee, but looking at the budget comments and appropriations history, I see that there is much to pull together. This is a very ambitious title. While I can trace my mental illness to an adrenal tumor and some have a genetic predisposition to disease, while others arrive at dysfunction through abuse, neglect or drug use, I suspect we won't cover everything in the 90 or so minutes that this hearing will last.

Mental health care and addiction services have actually stood up rather well during the pandemic. Zoom, and similar platforms, have stepped in nicely to continue face to face care where needed. Phone appointments and video calls have also worked in family practice settings where medication management is the only task.

Managing my prescriptions and assisting my housemate in managing his contacts with his are much easier than a trip to our respective mental health providers.

There is one area of major concern that must be addressed, although I am not sure how we can go about it. During this crisis, before there was vaccine hesitancy, there was Zoom hesitancy. Some of our older members simply could not figure out or declined to use video calls to attend meetings.

I experienced this reticence myself, not wanting to download software to my phone that was unknown to me. In the beginning, I was also too ill to do much more than eat, be tired from eating, rest and then go back to bed. It was only the usual miracles experienced by those who are spiritually awake that had me download the software and attend a midnight meeting.

My housemate is not technically savvy. Without my help, and the use of my Chromebook, he would still be visiting his psychiatrist in person, where he would be taken into a room for a teleconference with his doctor.

He is a victim of the digital divide. It inhibits him (as well as the lack of a computer of his own) to seek English as a Second Language courses, which are free at Montgomery College (our local community college). His disability, which is matched by his lack of education and equipment hamper both his treatment and his ability to improve his skills.

This is where improvement is necessary. As I have stated in previous comments for the record, paying a stipend to undertake both computer and basic literacy training is an essential incentive to seek it. Such stipends should not count against his disability payments. If they did, they would be a disincentive toward learning. It is a conservative meme that poverty leads to self-improvement. Research has shown that the opposite is the case. It certainly is for him.

And yes, better broadband in some areas of the country would be helpful, although this would not solve the problem of digital illiteracy, especially among vulnerable populations. Most people have access to the Internet through their cable companies, although those that do not should be given free access paid for by higher cable fees.

During the pandemic many mentally ill SSDI beneficiaries were not going out much and did not have many places to go. Libraries and movie theaters have been closed. Some were working in tense situations and need a vacation.

Those of us receiving SSDI benefits are spending more on food of late. Let me illustrate.

Even before the pandemic, my SSDI was inadequate for food, medicine, clothing and cable. If I owned a vehicle, there is no way I could maintain it or even buy gas. I have an above average benefit, high enough to be ineligible for SNAP or Medicaid. Many are not so lucky, even on a good day.

In the last few months, days have not been so good. Were it not for stimulus payments, I would be running out of food as I write this and would not have just bought new clothes, from socks and underwear to a jacket I can wear when the Committee finally asks me to testify in person. As it is, I will need to use the last $600 from my December payment (which should have come through Social Security) to attend my upcoming high school reunion. While I have wifi, I cannot afford cable and a car is still out of reach.

Let me underline a point. In most months, new underwear is not an option, I rely on free bus rides due to the pandemic and subsidies from Ride On and there is never enough money in that last week before the check comes. When it does arrive, the cupboard is bare.

Double underline: food prices are skyrocketing. Part of the problem may be too much money chasing too few goods, but retirees and the disabled find (our)selves between a rock and a hard place. We need a COLA and we need it now. Most of us cannot even afford cola. *Because this is a short term emergency due to the Pandemic, it should be funded out of the general fund until the normal process kicks in for next year.*

The important point is that, if wage growth is considered inflation, the retired and disabled can be given not only a Cost of Living Adjustment, but also have their income history rebased for inflation. Even with Chained CPI, such an increase will take the financial pressure off of many such households, including mine.

Home and Community-Based Health Care are addressed in the President's Budget. Home and community-based care should be funded by goods and services taxes as part of a newly created Medicare Part E. Senior Medicaid should be entirely federalized, with other clients insured through the President's proposal for a public option.

President Reagan's New Federalism proposal would have removed Medicaid from state budgets in exchange for ending or block granting other federal programs. This was a good idea then and a better idea now. Medicaid Part E should be created to both relieve states and the District of Columbia (or Washington, Douglass Commonwealth) from providing Medicaid for seniors and the Disabled and seeing to the enforcement of practice standards for nursing homes who receive these funds.

For workforce development and general recovery, Psychiatric Rehabilitation Programs, such as the Center for Behavioral Health in Rockville and Cornerstone Montgomery in Gaithersburg are essential. To make them more attractive, and to increase our ability to manage—especially in the period before disability programs kick in, participation should be paid at the minimum wage.

People will participate in this care more frequently if their opportunity costs are met. Those with less than a full education should receive it through public and private providers and also be paid to do so.

Health care currently provided through Medicaid should be dual eligible for everyone, regardless of income and before it kicks in entirely be a public option. Instead of using a larger system, clients should have the option of receiving coverage through the PRP provider's employee plan.

Low wages are endemic among the mentally ill. We need a raise, along with the rest of the working poor (and not so poor—who make more when the minimum goes up). The Minority proposed a $10 wage as a counter-offer to $15. A $12 wage for a 40 hour week puts us at parity to 1965, when the wage peaked and the war over wages started with the Kennedy-Johnson tax cuts. An $11 wage with a 32 hour week is also acceptable. With increased productivity, the work week should be shorter. The minimum wage should be indexed to inflation, including during any transitional period—which should have the goal of $18 per hour ($15 is a 20th Century goal).

Not raising minimum wages has been justified by the reactionary sector that claims that in the end, the market will sort everything out. The perception that doing the right thing makes a business non-competitive is the reason we enact minimum wage laws and should require mandatory leave. Because the labor product is almost always well above wages paid, few jobs are lost when this occurs. Higher wages simply reduce what is called the labor surplus, and not only by Marx. Any CFO who cannot calculate the current productive surplus will soon be seeking a job with adequate wages and sick leave.

The requirement that this be provided ends the calculation of whether doing so makes a firm non-competitive because all competitors must provide the same benefit. This applies to businesses of all sizes. If a firm is so precarious that it cannot survive this change, it is probably not viable without it.

Mentally ill people deserve to have families, just as others do. Increasing the child tax credit is as essential to us as to anyone. The child tax credit level passed in the American Recovery Act should be made permanent and doubled, with distribution through private sector payrolls, unemployment insurance benefits, emergency benefits for families and paid participation in educational programs.

There are two avenues to distribute money to families. The first is to add CTC benefits to unemployment, retirement, educational (TANF and college) and disability benefits. The CTC should be high enough to replace survivor's benefits for children.

The second is to distribute them with pay through employers. This can be done with long term tax reform, but in the interim can be accomplished by having employers start increasing wages immediately to distribute the credit to workers and their families, allowing them to subtract these payments from their quarterly corporate or income tax bills.

In recent decades, the problem of veteran disability determinations has remained troubling, with the Pandemic complicating processing. When a job gets too big to manage with staff, two options remain—contract out as much work as possible, including consolidating case files and making easy determinations—and sharing responsibility for processing with the Department of Defense. The handoff from DoD to DVA should be seamless.

The mental health and housing needs of veterans, both recent and lingering, is endemic. This is another area where coordination with DoD would prove helpful. This help must go beyond management and computer systems and include the human element of soldiers, veterans using services and those who need services can interact on a less formal, but not unprogrammed basis.

The DVA and DoD must both actively facilitate this and join state and local governments in reaching out to those who suffer, from active duty soldiers to veterans both receiving and in need of services. For those mentally ill or addicted veterans who do not trust the system, less restrictive systems should be developed—including providing camping supplies and a place to camp and a more permissive attitude to active drinking and drug use until help is sought. Such systems do not encourage use. No addict needs encouragement. They build the trust that makes recovery possible.

The largest provider of mental health services (including to veterans) is the correctional system. Job one is to shift from correctional modalities to new methods featuring mental health, education (including ESL programs) and addiction medicine. Warehousing young males of any race, but particularly African-Americans multiplies societal pathologies. While some forms of illness, such as sexual violence and physical violence or murder may require higher security, others can be treated as patients rather than criminals.

The Department of Justice can take the lead in both practice and in developing best practices for state correctional systems. Part of this would be specialized facilities based on the type of crime committed.

For example, sex offenders would be in facilities of their own. Those who remain dangerous post-sentence would still be detained until they are no longer dangerous. Such decisions must be based on science, not the desire for further punitive measures.

This change would migrate to local law enforcement, i.e., policing.

A pilot program could be developed to respond to certain incidents (especially those involving mental illness or alcohol) with immediate dispatch of emergency medical teams. This would require more ambulances, more mental health facilities and a pause in applying restraints until medical personnel arrive.

Funding more hospitals and ambulances would be part of this, possibly with some form of federal grant program. Private corrections facilities can also be transformed into contracted medical facilities with security contracting provided as a subcontract to mental health systems, both secular and religious. Catholic Health Association members come to mind. Both public and private educational systems would be an integral part of such facilities and be treated as an essential function, rather than the first item cut when states wish to minimize their spending by essentially torturing (and dehumanizing) inmates.

New standards of individual and societal protection must be developed. Improved standards of care and security will require much more funding than state and local governments are willing to commit to. This simply drives the problem to the correctional system, which is the largest provider of mental healthcare in this nation. The term for this practice is pennywise and pound-foolish.

It is too easy to get out of treatment and too hard to get it. Hospitalization for medication management is sometimes needed but rarely given. Often, people are released before a stable routine is established, including management of side effects. It is hard to create a good care plan in a five day hold. For both mental illness and alcoholism, it must be harder to simply sign out without a real prospect for long-term recovery. Again, the term is penny wise and pound foolish.

A final reform, which will save money and resources, is to create a plea in criminal cases of guilty by reason of insanity. Those who enter this plea would be confined in the facilities detailed above for at least the minimum sentence for their offences, with no release after that if the subject remains a danger to society.

If relapse occurs or treatment protocols are evaded after release, rehospitalization must be automatic and last until a treatment program is more deeply ingrained. There should, of course, be protections on both sides in the decision to release subjects—both for the protection of the rights of subjects who made be held for punitive, rather than hygienic reasons and, as importantly, the interests of the victims of crime, including but not limited to the possibility of physical danger. Sometimes, exile should be a part of release.

Thank you for the opportunity to address the committee. We are, of course, available for direct testimony or to answer questions by members and staff.

Eating Disorders Coalition for Research, Policy, and Action

PO Box 96503–98807
Washington, DC 20090

Statement of Allison Ivie, MPP, MA, Government Relations Representative

Chairman Wyden, Ranking Member Crapo, and members of the U.S. Senate Committee on Finance, thank you for holding this important hearing entitled, ''Mental Health Care in America: Addressing Root Causes and Identifying Policy Solutions'' to ensure the nation has the services and supports in place to care for individuals across the nation with mental illness and addiction, including those with eating disorders.

The Eating Disorders Coalition for Research, Policy, and Action (EDC) is a nonprofit organization comprised of patient and caregiver advocates, treatment providers, advocacy organizations, and academics, aimed to advance the recognition of eating disorders as a public health priority throughout the U.S. By promoting federal support for improved access to care, the EDC seeks to increase the resources available for education, prevention, and improved training, as well as for scientific research on the etiology, prevention, and treatment of eating disorders.

As the number of new COVID–19 cases continues to decline, eating disorders diagnoses continue to climb. Research indicates a 30 percent increase in eating disorder diagnoses since March 2020 compared with data in previous years.[92] *EDC members, the National Eating Disorders Association has seen a 53 percent increase in their call volume to their helpline since March 2020 and the Alliance for Eating Disorders Awareness has already served 7,000 individuals representing all 50 states and 32 countries and provided approximately 50,000 referrals for treatment since January 2021.* This is just a sampling of the magnitude of services our coalition members are doing to support individuals and families in need. Despite this incredible work, we know there is still work to be done to improve the care for individuals with eating disorders.

Eating disorders are serious mental illnesses that affect 28.8 million Americans over the course of their lifetime.[93] They have the second highest mortality rate of any psychiatric illness, with one death occurring every 52 minutes as a direct result of an eating disorder.[94] *Without access to comprehensive treatment, eating disorders create great economic distress, costing the U.S. economy $64.7 billion annually with the federal government shouldering $17.7 billion of that cost.*[95] Ensuring comprehensive coverage for eating disorders treatment has the potential to mitigate disease progression or relapse into higher levels of treatment. *Without access and/or coverage to treatment, higher levels of eating disorders treatment cost the U.S. $29.3 million in emergency room visits* and $209.7 million in inpatient hospitalizations annually.[96]

Eating disorder prevalence rates among the senior and disabled populations are similar to the general population at approximately 3 percent to 6 percent.[97,98] However, older Americans with eating disorders are

---

[92] Tanner, Lindsay. (May 23, 2021). Pandemic has fueled eating disorders surge in teens, adults. Associated Press. Retrieved from: *https://apnews.com/article/coronavirus-pandemic-virus-lifestyle-eating-disorders-health-27c9d5680980b1452f7e512db4d9f825.*

[93] eloitte Access Economics. The Social and Economic Cost of Eating Disorders in the United States of America: A Report for the Strategic Training Initiative for the Prevention of Eating Disorders and the Academy for Eating Disorders. June 2020. Available at: *https://www.hsph.harvard.edu/striped/report-economic-costs-of-eating-disorders/.*

[94] *Ibid.*

[95] *Ibid.*

[96] *Ibid.*

[97] Peat, Christine; Peyerl, Naomi; and Muehlenkamp, Jennifer. (2010). Body Image and Eating Disorders in Older Adults: A Review. *The Journal of General Psychology*, 135:4, 343–358.

[98] Mangweth-Matzek B, Hoek HW. Epidemiology and treatment of eating disorders in men and women of middle and older age. Curr Opin Psychiatry. 2017;30(6):446–451. doi: 10.1097/YCO.0000000000000356.

particularly serious as chronic disorders or diseases may already compromise their health.[99] Inadequate nutrition as a result of their eating disorder can result in memory deficits; cognitive decline; decubitus ulcers; impaired healing of sores, wounds, or infections; and dizziness, disorientation, and falls, which can initiate a cascade of patho-physiological events leading to a 30 percent to 40 percent mortality rate.[100] *Tragically, 78 percent of deaths from anorexia nervosa occur in the elderly.*[101]

Prevention and early intervention are the best tools to prevent disease progression for those with mental illness or substance use disorders. Given the complexity of eating disorders, a multidisciplinary treatment team that includes a medical provider, psychiatrist, psychologist, and registered dietitian is considered to be the four key provider components for comprehensive eating disorders treatment. The exponential rise in eating disorders as a consequence of the pandemic further underscores the importance of early intervention.

Unfortunately, Medicare does not provide outpatient coverage for medical nutrition therapy (MNT) for individuals with eating disorders. This coverage only applies to beneficiaries that are diagnosed with diabetes or end stage renal disease. This lack of coverage leaves individuals susceptible to disease progression and in need of a higher, costlier level of treatment. According to the American Dietetic Association, nutritional therapy conducted by a registered professional is an ''essential component'' for the treatment of patients with anorexia nervosa, bulimia nervosa, and other eating disorders.[102] Research shows mental health interventions for eating disorders may not be successful if the underlying nutritional issues haven't been addressed first, since nutritional deficiency causes cognitive issues (e.g., depression) that can impede recovery.[103] Nutrition counseling guides patients in identifying problematic behaviors and setting realistic and achievable nutrition related goals to support clients in making behavior changes. Nutrition education includes conversations about discrepancies between knowledge,

---

[99] Peat, Christine; Peyerl, Naomi; and Muehlenkamp, Jennifer. (2010). Body Image and Eating Disorders in Older Adults: A Review. *The Journal of General Psychology,* 135:4, 343–358.

[100] Dudrick, Stanley. (2013). Older Clients and Eating Disorders. *Today's Dietitian,* 15:11, 44.

[101] Dudrick, S. (2014). Older clients and eating disorders. *Today's Dietitian,* 15(11), 44.

[102] Ozier, AD; and Henry, BW. ''Position of the American Dietetic Association: Nutrition intervention in the treatment of eating disorders.'' *NCBI/NLM/NIH. https://www.ncbi.nlm.nih.gov/ pubmed/21802573.*

[103] Rosen, David. (2010). Clinical Report—Identification and Management of Eating Disorders in Children and Adolescents. American Academy of Pediatrics, 126:6.

beliefs and behaviors, ultimately empowering the patient to normalize eating and make healthier decisions.[104]

Fortunately, Congress has legislation to address this gap in coverage with a bipartisan bill entitled, the Nutrition Counseling Aiding Recovery for Eating Disorders Act or the *Nutrition CARE Act (H.R. 1551/S. 584)* led by Senators Maggie Hassan (D–NH) and Lisa Murkowski (R–AK) and Representatives Judy Chu (D–CA– 27), Jackie Walorski (R–IN–02) and Lisa Blunt Rochester (D–DE–AL). *The legislation would provide Medicare Part B coverage for medical nutrition therapy for beneficiaries diagnosed with an eating disorder at the same coverage levels beneficiaries with diabetes and end stage renal disease receive.*

This legislation is a small, critical step in ensuring the federal government is meeting the mental health needs of Americans across the lifespan. We urge the U.S. Senate Committee on Finance, Health Subcommittee to move this bill forward for consideration to the full committee as we work together to support the 2 to 2.5 million Medicare beneficiaries with eating disorders that could benefit from the Nutrition CARE Act.

Thank you for your consideration.

Sincerely,

Eating Disorders Coalition for Research, Policy, and Action Members in Formation:

Academy for Eating Disorders	Reston, VA
Academy of Nutrition and Dietetics	Chicago, IL
Alliance for Eating Disorders Awareness	West Palm Beach, FL
Alsana: Eating Disorders Treatment and Recovery Centers	Ballwin, MO
Bannister Consultancy	Durham, NC
BE REAL USA	Chicago, IL
Cambridge Eating Disorder Center	Cambridge, MA
Center for Change	Orem, UT
Center for Discovery	Los Alamitos, CA
Eating Disorder Coalition of Iowa	Clive, IA

[104] Ruiz-Prieto, Inmaculada; Bolanos-Rios, Patricia; and Jauregui-Lobera, Ignacio. (2013). Diet Choice in weight-restored patients with eating disorders; progressive autonomy by nutritional education. *Nurtricion Hospitlaria,* 28:5, 1725–1731.

Eating Disorder Hope	Redmond, OR
Eating Recovery Center	Denver, CO
Farrington Specialty Centers	Fort Wayne, IN
Gail R. Schoenbach FREED Foundation	Warren, NJ
International Association of Eating Disorders Professionals	Pekin, IL
International Federation of Eating Disorders Dietitians	Dallas, TX
Laureate Eating Disorders Program	Tulsa, OK
Monte Nido and Affiliates	Miami, FL
Montecatini	Carlsbad, CA
Moonshadow's Spirit	Webster, NY
Multi-Service Eating Disorders Association	Newton, MA
National Eating Disorders Association	New York, NY
Park Nicollet Melrose Center	St. Louis Park, MN
Project HEAL	Brooklyn, NY
REDC Consortium	St. Paul, MN
Rogers Behavioral Health	Oconomowoc, WI
Rosewood Centers for Eating Disorders	Wickenburg, AZ
Stay Strong Virginia	Chesterfield, VA
Strategic Training Initiative for the Prevention of Eating Disorders	Boston, MA
SunCloud Health	Northbrook, IL
The Donahue Foundation	Richmond, VA
The Emily Program	St. Paul, MN
The National Association of Anorexia Nervosa and Associated Eating Disorders	Chicago, IL
The Renfrew Center	Pittsburgh, PA
Veritas Collaborative	Durham, NC
Walden Behavioral Care	Waltham, MA
WithAll	St. Louis Park, MN
Wrobel and Smith, PLLP	St. Paul, MN

Healthcare Leadership Council

750 9th St., NW, Suite #500
Washington, DC 20510

June 21, 2021

The Honorable Ron Wyden
Chair
U.S. Senate
Committee on Finance
Washington, DC 20510

The Honorable Mike Crapo
Ranking Member
U.S. Senate
Committee on Finance
Washington, DC 20510

Dear Chair Wyden and Ranking Member Crapo:

On behalf of the Healthcare Leadership Council (HLC), we thank you for holding a hearing on, ''Mental Health Care in America: Addressing Root Causes and Identifying Policy Solutions.''

HLC is a coalition of chief executives from all disciplines within American healthcare. It is the exclusive forum for the nation's healthcare leaders to jointly develop policies, plans, and programs to achieve their vision of a 21st century healthcare system that makes affordable high-quality care accessible to all Americans. Members of HLC—hospitals, academic health centers, health plans, pharmaceutical companies, medical device manufacturers, laboratories, biotech firms, health product distributors, post-acute care providers, home care providers, and information technology companies—advocate for measures to increase the quality and efficiency of healthcare through a patient-centered approach.

The COVID–19 health pandemic has created significant barriers to accessing mental health services. A January study found that over 40% of adults have reported struggling with anxiety or depression since the beginning of the pandemic.[105] The impact of COVID on mental health is expected to continue to be a challenge in the coming years. We applaud Congress for providing over $4 billion in the Consolidated Appropriations Act and $3.8 billion in the American Rescue Plan Act for mental health services. These investments will provide much-needed assistance to struggling communities.

We encourage the Committee to examine ways to improve access to mental health services, particularly via telehealth options. A recent survey found that approximately 50% of patients using telehealth services were

[105] Nirmita Panchal et al., The Implications of COVID–19 for Mental Health and Substance Abuse, Kaiser Family Foundation (February 10, 2021), *https://www.kff.org/coronavirus-covid-19/issue-brief/the-implications-of-covid-19-for-mental-health-and-substance-use/.*

seeking behavioral health treatment.[106] Providing mental health treatment via telehealth provides a unique opportunity to reach underserved patients. Estimates have found that up to 60% of patients do not arrive for their behavioral health appointments.[107] By using telehealth solutions to deliver such care, providers have been able to deliver much needed assistance to patients in their homes. Patient satisfaction in receiving behavioral health treatment via telehealth[108] has shown that providers can innovate in care delivery without sacrificing quality.

The COVID–19 health pandemic has also exacerbated the substance use disorder (SUD) crisis in the United States. From May 2019–June 2020, the number of deaths related to drug overdoses rose 20% and a record number of Americans died from overdoses.[109] Preliminary data expects 2020 to be the worst year on record for drug overdoses.[110] In order to respond to this crisis, Congress and federal agencies took swift action to ensure patients struggling with SUDs received proper care. We applaud the Drug Enforcement Agency's (DEA) decision to temporarily waive in-person requirements to prescribe controlled substances. This has allowed patients to continue to receive important medications, particularly buprenorphine. HLC also thanks the Centers for Medicare and Medicaid Services (CMS) for finalizing regulations mandated under the SUPPORT Act that require providers to use electronic prescribing for controlled substances (EPCS). Requiring EPCS puts a more advanced monitoring system in place to ensure that controlled substances are only prescribed when necessary and allows for relevant authorities to monitor potential trends. We encourage Congress to work with federal agencies to further implement flexibilities that would allow patients to receive

---

[106] Shira Fischer et al., The Transition to Telehealth During the First Months of the COVID–19 Pandemic, RAND Corporation (January 8, 2021), *https://link.springer.com/content/pdf/10.1007/s11606-020-06358-0.pdf.*

[107] Eric Berger, No-Cancel Culture: How Telehealth Is Making It Easier to Keep that Therapy Session, *Kaiser Health News* (May 24, 2021), *https://khn.org/news/article/no-cancel-culture- how-telehealth-is-making-it-easier-to-keep-that-therapy-session/.*

[108] Joe Gramigna, Patient satisfaction high for psychiatric telehealth platforms in partial hospital program, Healio (March 25, 2021), *https://www.healio.com/news/psychiatry/ 20210325/patient-satisfaction-high-for-psychiatric-telehealth-platforms-in-partial-hospital-program.*

[109] Usha Lee McFarling, As the pandemic ushered in isolation and financial hardships, overdose deaths reached new heights, STAT News (February 16, 2021), *https://www.statnews.com/2021/02/16/as-pandemic-ushered-in-isolation-financial-hardship-overdose-deaths-reached-new-heights/.*

[110] Chris Sweeney, A crisis on top of a crisis: COVID–19 and the opioid epidemic, Harvard T.H. Chan School of Public Health (February 16, 2021), *https://www.hsph.harvard.edu/news/features/a-crisis-on-top-of-a-crisis-covid-19-and-the-opioid-epidemic/.*

medications through the duration of the public health emergency (PHE) while maintaining robust safety and monitoring programs.

HLC appreciates your work on improving mental health outcomes for patients and looks forward to working with you on future solutions. Please feel free to contact Tina Grande at 202–449–3433 or tgrande@hlc.org with any questions.

Sincerely,
Mary R. Grealy President

HR Policy Association, American Health Policy Institute, and National Alliance of Healthcare Purchaser Coalitions

June 15, 2021

The HR Policy Association, the American Health Policy Institute, and the National Alliance of Healthcare Purchaser Coalitions appreciate the Committee holding this important hearing on behavioral and mental health care issues.

The HR Policy Association is the leading organization representing chief human resource officers of over 390 of the largest employers in the United States. Collectively, their companies provide health care coverage to over 20 million employees and dependents in the United States. The American Health Policy Institute, a part of HR Policy Association, examines the challenges employers face in providing health care to their employees and recommends policy solutions to promote affordable, high-quality, employer-based health care. The Institute serves to provide thought leadership grounded in the practical experience of America's largest employers.

The National Alliance of Healthcare Purchaser Coalitions (National Alliance) is the only nonprofit, purchaser-led organization with a national and regional structure dedicated to driving health and health care value across the country. Its members represent private and public sector, nonprofit, and Taft-Hartley organizations, and more than 45 million Americans, spending $300 billion annually on healthcare.

The National Alliance, HR Policy Association and the American Health Policy Institute are also part of The Path Forward initiative to execute a disciplined, private sector approach to systematically and measurably improve five established best practices of mental health and substance use care. Below are our policy recommendations to improve access to behavioral and mental health care services.

Sincerely,

D. Mark Wilson
President and CEO,
American Health
Policy Institute
Vice President, Health
and Employment Policy
HR Policy Association
1001 19th St. North, Suite 1002
Arlington, VA 22209

Michael Thompson
President and CEO
National Alliance of Healthcare
Purchaser Coalitions
1015 18th Street, NW, Suite 705
Washington, DC 20036

Collaborative Care Model (CoCM)

While employer health plans and Medicare reimburse providers in collaborative care practices, behavioral health is not broadly integrated with primary care. Because behavioral health conditions often initially present themselves in primary care settings, this lack of integration leaves patients with undiagnosed or poorly managed behavioral health conditions. Increasing the number of collaborative care practices would improve access to behavioral health services, increase the effectiveness of treatment, and reduce disparities in identification of behavioral health issues. Over 70 randomized controlled trials have demonstrated collaborative care models are more effective and cost efficient than usual care.[111]

Policy Recommendations

Allocate funds to support a change effort to provide technical assistance, training and startup funds to allow for large scale adoption for collaborative care across the country. Collaborative care can be delivered virtually or by in

[111] https://www.chcs.org/media/HH_IRC_Collaborative_Care_Model__052113_2.pdf.

person care managers meaning this model can deliver to large medical groups or small and rural primary care practices.

1) CMS should establish a national Technical Assistance (TA) center and regional extension centers to assist primary care practices in implementing the CoCM.
2) Incentivize behavioral health care providers to adopt electronic health record technology that is interoperable with general health care providers into their practices.
3) Expand research on promising integrated care models.

TeleBehavioral Healthcare (TBH)

Background—During the COVID–19 pandemic, Medicare rules related to TBH have been liberalized resulting in an exponential growth in the use of TBH, including enabling cross-state care which has been critical to underserved areas and rural communities. However, the requirements for employer health plans around how TBH is provided and reimbursed remain far too restrictive and result in access and quality disparities. TBH has the potential to overcome patient stigma and improve access and efficiency of care for BH services. We know that since the COVID–19 public health emergency, there has been a significant increase in patients keeping their appointments. In general, when patients keep their first appointment, they are more likely to keep subsequent appointments; and when patients are satisfied with treatment, they are more likely to continue with their course of therapy. Research also suggests that TBH results in better medication compliance, fewer visits to the emergency department, fewer patient admissions to inpatient units, and fewer subsequent readmissions. However, many older adults and people with disabilities, lack access to video-enabled devices or struggle to use the more complex video-enabled devices even if they have them. Likewise, many in racial/ethnic and low-income communities lack access to broadband or video-enabled devices, which only expands the health inequities in the U.S.

Policy Recommendations

1) Eliminate cross-state border restrictions on TBH on a permanent basis for Medicare, employer and commercial plans. Licensing

requirements should be based on the location of the provider not the patient.

2) Enable patient access to TBH without having the first provider appointment be in person.
3) Make permanent the allowance of first-dollar coverage of telehealth in high deductible health plans. Specifically, Congress should pass the Telehealth Expansion Act of 2021 (S. 1704).
4) Allow employers to offer standalone ''excepted benefit'' telehealth benefits.
5) Adopt technology-neutral requirements, permitting use of different types of technology platforms for telehealth services.
6) Establish a uniform set of rules for multi-state telehealth benefit plans to eliminate state restrictions that block patients from telehealth benefits.

The HR Policy Association, the American Health Policy Institute, and the National Alliance welcome any opportunity to provide input and speak in further detail about improving access to behavioral and mental health care services. We look forward to working with you on this important topic.

The Partnership to Amend 42 CFR Part 2

April 13, 2021 Robinsue Frohboese
Acting Director and Principal Deputy Office for Civil Rights
U.S. Department of Health and Human Services
200 Independence Avenue, SW
Room 509F, HHH Building Washington, DC 20201

Dr. Neeraj Gandotra Chief Medical Officer
Substance Abuse and Mental Health Services Administration
5600 Fishers Lane
Rockville, MD 20852
Re: 42 CFR Part 2—Recommendations for Next Rule

Dear Ms. Frohboese and Dr. Gandotra,

The Partnership to Amend 42 CFR Part 2 (Partnership), writes to provide recommendations for the U.S. Department of Health and Human Services'

(HHS) Office for Civil Rights (OCR) and the Substance Abuse and Mental Health Services Administration (SAMHSA) to consider when drafting the new rule for the 42 CFR Part 2 (Part 2) provisions in the Coronavirus Aid, Relief, and Economic Security Act (CARES Act). We have appreciated working with HHS and SAMHSA on Part 2 in the past and welcome the opportunity to partner with both SAMHSA and OCR on this important issue moving forward.

The Partnership is a coalition of nearly 50 organizations committed to aligning Part 2 with the disclosure requirements of the Health Insurance Portability and Accountability Act (HIPAA) for the purposes of treatment, payment, and health care operations (TPO).

This is a time of unprecedented urgency. First, the Centers for Disease Control and Prevention's preliminary estimate is that more than 81,000 Americans died of drug overdose in 2020. Second, federal health officials believe the drug crisis is only being amplified by months of social isolation, high unemployment, and diversion of public health resources, all a result of the COVID–19 pandemic.[112] Given this alarming correlation, an important part of responding to the COVID–19 pandemic will be to simplify coordination of care for substance use disorders (SUDs), which ultimately will prevent gaps and expand access to care. Furthermore, we anticipate SUDs may continue to rise even after the COVID–19 pandemic is over, reflecting the extreme toll it has taken on Americans. As such, we believe quickly issuing the proposed rule-making, as required by section 3221 of the CARES Act, will both help curb the SUD epidemic and also strongly supports the incoming Biden-Harris Administration's Build Back Better strategy.

Previous requirements in the Part 2 regulation led to segmented data, interrupted flow of that data, and ultimately hindered informed diagnosis, treatment, and implementation of an individual's care plan and access to care. The CARES Act takes great strides to remedy these issues by promoting partial alignment between Part 2 and HIPAA, though the two privacy frameworks remain distinct, particularly for consent purposes. Nevertheless, the law clearly strives to bring Part 2 in line with HIPAA, a fact being embraced by industry thought leaders. For example, the Medicaid and CHIP Payment and Access Commission (MACPAC) noted during its December

[112] Dan Goldberg and Brianna Ehley, Biden's other health crisis: A resurgent drug epidemic, Politico, November 28, 2020.

2020 meeting that the CARES Act ''[p]ermanently aligns 42 CFR Part 2 and HIPAA.''[113]

Additionally, and most importantly, the Partnership staunchly supports patient privacy. We are acutely aware that even if the sharing of information is made easier, it has limited utility without continued strong protections for patient privacy. Without trust, patients may not seek the care they need to treat SUDs. We are also aware that individuals may be concerned that SUD records will be used against them by law enforcement.

These are significant concerns. However, the CARES Act protects patient rights in two important ways. First, it allows an individual to revoke his or her consent to sharing SUDs records, giving patients control over their information.[114] Second, SUD records are expressly prohibited by law from being used in civil, criminal, administrative, or legislative proceedings against a patient by any government authority (unless authorized by court order or patient consent). Furthermore, SUD records specifically cannot: (a) be entered into evidence in criminal prosecutions or civil actions; (b) form part of the record for a decision or otherwise be taken into account in government agency proceedings; (c) be used by a governmental agency for law enforcement purposes or investigations; or (d) be used in a warrant application.[115]4 As such, we believe the changes made to Part 2 by the CARES Act will allow for smoother care coordination while simultaneously strengthening patient privacy.

As you begin drafting the next Part 2 rule, we submit the following for your consideration:

Original Consent Process. While the Confidentiality of Substance Use Disorder Patient Records Final Rule (final rule) issued in July 2020 takes an important step forward to address the issue of patient consent, we believe more needs to be done in this regard. The final rule allows an entity, instead of an individual, to be specified as the recipient of Part 2 records, which broadens the scope of the consent and incrementally relieves the burden on patients and providers. However, this is not enough because a new patient consent is needed each time there is a new entity where the Part 2 record needs to be

---

113 Aaron Pervin and Erin McMullen, Promoting Behavioral and Physical Clinical Integration Through EHRs, 2020. https://www.macpac.gov/wp-content/uploads/2020/12/Integrating-Clinical-Care-through-Greater-Use-of-Electronic-Health-Records-by-Behavioral-Health-Providers.pdf, last visited April 1, 2020.

114 Coronavirus Aid, Relief, and Economic Security Act (CARES Act), Pub. L. No. 116–136, section 3221(b)(1)(C).

115 Id. at section 3221(e).

disclosed. Fortunately, the CARES Act further simplifies the process by requiring only one consent, after which the Part 2 record can be used or disclosed by a covered entity or business associate for the purposes of TPO in accordance with the HIPAA regulations.

Additionally, please note that although the initial consent requirement was amended under section 3221 of the CARES Act to allow a general designation (instead of a specific practice), there still remains a roadblock in practice: the list of disclosures requirement in Part 2. Specifically, section 2.31 of Part 2 mandates that ''upon request, patients who have consented to disclose their patient identifying information using a general designation must be provided a list of entities to which their information has been disclosed pursuant to the general designation'' [emphasis added]. Due to the list of disclosures requirement, practitioners are often uncomfortable attempting to use the general designation in the consent.

Recommendation: Ensure that the consent requirements in the next rule are simple and straightforward so additional administrative processes are not imposed on patients, providers, or payers (including health plans and their subcontractors). The consent process should be easily folded into existing HIPAA compliance processes, preferably with the patient's acknowledgement of HIPAA practices and the patient's Part 2 consent incorporated into the same document at intake where feasible. Furthermore, include language to address the conflict with Part 2's list of disclosures requirement.

Transmission and Retransmission of Data. The CARES Act plainly states that once written consent is obtained, a Part 2 record may be transmitted and retransmitted for TPO in accordance with HIPAA regulations. No further consent should be required for TPO unless the patient revokes consent.

Recommendation: Include specific language directing covered entities and business associates to disclose and redisclose data in accordance with HIPAA regulations.

The final rule also requires physically separating records with Part 2 data. However, such physical separation is difficult once the data is transmitted, as very few integrated systems or Health Information Exchanges (HIEs) can manage the consent process for a completely separate database for Part 2 records. The separation of data not only creates an administrative burden, but also makes the data difficult to obtain by subsequent treating providers, ultimately hindering patient care. For example, we have heard anecdotes of physicians physically carrying two separate laptops for the purposes of compliance with the data segregation requirements.

Recommendation: Specify that once Part 2 data is transmitted or retransmitted with patient consent, there is no requirement to segregate a patient's Part 2 data from the rest of a HIPAA database, with the regulatory requirement for data segmentation terminating upon transmission or retransmission.

Revocation of Consent Provisions. The patient's ability to revoke consent is an important privacy protection supported by the Partnership. However, serious administrative issues arise when there is an expectation that a revocation be retroactively effective. Specifically, practices are now required, under the Promoting Interoperability program, to incorporate information from outside sources for medications, allergies, and other problems. If revocation is mandated to be retroactive, there is technically no way to go back and isolate this data from a patient's overall clinical record.

Furthermore, it is critical that the responsibility for managing the revocation remain with a designated entity. We believe that the management of the consent revocation should be the responsibility of the Part 2 treatment entity that contributed that data and that program would be responsible for seeing that the Part 2 data is not being transmitted either to another covered entity or business associate.

Recommendation: Specifically, state that the revocation of consent for Part 2 data transmission is effective only from the point of revocation going forward and that responsibility for the revocation should be limited to those who are so notified by the patient and their respective actions.

Scope of Part 2 Consent Process. SAMHSA's current guidance seems to indicate that a Part 2 consent should not impede the transmission of behavioral health data that does not originate with a Part 2 program. However, this is very different in practice as there is much confusion on how to handle behavioral health data. Providers hesitate to share behavioral health data because they are concerned that they may be violating Part 2 requirements related to consent.

Recommendation: OCR and SAMHSA should explore, in partnership with stakeholders, how to exclude behavioral health data from the Part 2 data and incorporate the findings into the rule and any subsequent frequently asked questions or guidance. Similarly, OCR and SAMHSA should explore, in conjunction with the States and stakeholders, policy mechanisms for promoting the use of behavioral health data for care coordination purposes when state privacy laws may impose restrictions beyond both Part 2 and HIPAA.

Research. The final rule permits disclosures for the purposes of research under Part 2 by a HIPAA covered entity or business associate to non-HIPAA covered individuals and organizations. However, the CARES Act does not specifically address disclosures for the purpose of research.

Recommendation: Include a provision in the next rule, consistent with the last rule, to ensure that disclosures for the purposes of research from a HIPAA covered entity to a non-HIPAA covered entity are permissible.

Patient Rights. The final rule does not address patient rights. However, in Section 422(j) of the CARES Act, it is stated that nothing in that section can be construed to limit patient rights related to privacy protections for protected health information as defined under Section 164.522 of the HIPAA Privacy Rule.

Recommendation: Include specific language to ensure that patient privacy rights are protected in accordance with the CARES Act and HIPAA.

Claims Data Access. Currently, HHS provides patients' claims data through various initiatives, including to organizations participating in alternative payment models. Accountable care organizations, for example, are provided claims data at least monthly, and sometimes weekly. But these data lack SUD-related information because of limits of Part 2.

Recommendation: We urge HHS to start providing SUD-related claims data to providers practicing in alternative payment models to help support their work in population health management.

Thank you for your time and consideration on this crucial issue. Please feel free to contact Deepti Loharikar, Director of Regulatory Affairs, Association for Behavioral Health and Wellness, at loharikar@abhw.org or (202) 505–1834 with any questions.

Sincerely,
Maeghan Gilmore, MPH
Chairperson, Partnership to Amend 42 CFR Part 2

Members of the Partnership

Academy of Managed Care Pharmacy • Alliance of Community Health Plans • American Association on Health and Disability • American Health Information Management Association • American Hospital Association • American Psychiatric Association • American Society of Addiction Medicine

American Society of Anesthesiologists • America's Essential Hospitals • America's Health Insurance Plans • AMGA • Association for Ambulatory

Behavioral Healthcare • Association for Behavioral Health and Wellness • Association for Community Affiliated Plans • Association of Clinicians for the Underserved • Blue Cross Blue Shield Association • The Catholic Health Association of the United States • Centerstone • College of Healthcare Information Management Executives • Confidentiality Coalition

Employee Assistance Professionals Association • Global Alliance for Behavioral Health and Social Justice • Hazelden Betty Ford Foundation • Healthcare Leadership Council • InfoMC • The Joint Commission • The Kennedy Forum • Medicaid Health Plans of America • Mental Health America • National Alliance on Mental Illness • National Association for Behavioral Healthcare • National Association for Rural Mental Health • National Association of ACOs • National Association of Addiction Treatment Providers • National Association of Counties • National Association of County Behavioral Health and Development Disability Directors • National Association of State Mental Health Program Directors • National Rural Health Association • Netsmart • OCHIN • Opioid Safety Alliance • Otsuka America Pharmaceutical, Inc. • Primary Care Collaborative • Pharmaceutical Care Management Association • Premier Healthcare Alliance • Population Health Alliance • Smiths Medical • Strategic Health Information Exchange Collaborative

Office of the United States Surgeon General

The Honorable Ron Wyden Chairman
U.S. Senate Committee on Finance Washington, DC 20510
The Honorable Mike Crapo Ranking Member
U.S. Senate Committee on Finance Washington, DC 20510

Dear Chairman Wyden and Ranking Member Crapo,

Thank you for your leadership and dedication to this critical issue. As you mention in your letter, the COVID–19 pandemic has not simply created a new mental health crisis, but rather exacerbated a longstanding crisis that continues to affect people across this country. I was deeply concerned about the mental health of our country before the pandemic, and my concerns have grown over the past year.

Before COVID–19, mental health conditions were widespread in the United States, and there was significant unmet need for mental health diagnosis and treatment among young people and adults. Drivers of this crisis before the pandemic included stigma, shortages in the mental health workforce, health disparities, limited investments in prevention, and treatment services that were too limited and insufficiently integrated with primary care. And the cost of this crisis is accumulated in both human suffering and financial losses, as people with mental illness incur higher health care spending for non-mental health associated conditions and billions of dollars in lost earnings per year.

The pandemic has added urgency to these challenges. Millions of people have experienced the trauma of family, friends, and neighbors dying or being hospitalized with COVID–19. Working people have lost jobs or had their hours cut. Parents, disproportionately mothers, have endured significant stress in caring for their children and adapting to virtual schooling. An estimated 40,000 children in America lost a parent to COVID–19, and millions of children have been isolated from their friends and supportive school environments. Patients dealing with anxiety, depression, addiction, and other illnesses have had their access to treatment disrupted. And health care workers have gone through unimaginable pain watching, in some cases, dozens of their patients die of this terrible disease. The statistics on substance misuse, which so often occurs alongside mental illness, are also heartbreaking:

More than 87,000 of our neighbors, friends, and family members died of a drug overdose over the past year—the highest number of yearly drug overdose deaths in recent memory.

Mental health has been an important issue for the Office of the Surgeon General dating back to 1999, when my predecessor, Dr. David Satcher, released the landmark Surgeon General's Report on Mental Health. As a nation, we've come a long way since then in raising awareness about mental health, helping reduce stigma and shame, and expanding access to mental health treatment.

But the pandemic has reminded us just how much more remains to be done.

We must expand access to mental health services, by supporting mental health telehealth programs, training more mental health professionals, enforcing the 2008 Mental Health Parity and Addiction Equity Act, and integrating mental health services with primary care. We must do more to protect our children, who at times struggle for years with undiagnosed mental illness, by increasing access to mental health diagnostic and treatment services and by investing in evidence-based social emotional learning programs. We must extend further help to those at risk for suicide, including transitioning to full national availability of 988 as the new national suicide prevention and mental health crisis number. And we must target our efforts to communities that have struggled with high rates of depression, anxiety, and suicide—including health care workers whose alarmingly high rate of mental illness and burnout poses a threat to our ability to provide care to people throughout our nation. In all this work, we must prioritize equity, as we know that rural communities and communities of color face higher rates of mental health stigma and less access to treatment.

Perhaps most challenging of all, we must change the way we think about mental health. For too long, mental illness was a source of shame, and that shame prevented people from seeking help and compounded their suffering. Through our words, our actions, and our example, we can help people recognize that you are not broken or deficient if you are struggling with your mental health. Each of us can play a role in providing support to those who are suffering and in affirming their humanity. When we treat mental health with the same importance and urgency as physical health, when we apply ourselves as much to prevention programs as treatment efforts, when we set bold goals and hold ourselves to account, then we will see the change our nation needs.

We have many reasons to be hopeful. We have evidence-based programs, such as the Certified Community Behavioral Health Clinics, that are well-positioned to provide critical behavioral health services and expand access to care across the nation. We have school-based programs which have demonstrated their ability to reduce rates of mental illness and substance use disorders in a cost-effective manner. And we have millions of people across America whose lives have been touched by mental illness and who now want to be part of the solution. We can use this opportunity during the COVID–19 pandemic, when more people are talking about mental health and increased funding is being directed to address mental health issues, to act and take bold steps to improve the mental health of our country.

Responding to the mental health needs across America should be a central focus both during and after this pandemic, and I appreciate the attention you and others in Congress have brought to this issue. I know the road ahead is steep. We have much work to do. And we are still making our way through a difficult pandemic. But the progress we have made gives me faith in what is yet to come.

As the Committee moves forward under your leadership, HHS is committed to working with the Senate Finance Committee—and all of

Congress—to address America's mental health crisis. Thank you for the opportunity to weigh in on such an important issue. I look forward to learning from you and partnering with you in the months ahead to tackle the nation's mental health crisis.

Sincerely,

Vivek Murthy, M.D., M.B.A.
U.S. Surgeon General
Vice Admiral, U.S. Public Health Service

Chapter 2

Mental Health Parity and Coverage in Private Health Insurance: Federal Requirements*

Vanessa C. Forsberg

Summary

Given that most people in the United States have private health insurance, and given the prevalence of mental health and substance use disorders (MH/SUDs) in the United States, there is considerable congressional interest in understanding private coverage of MH/SUD benefits, including diagnostic and treatment services.

This report explains federal requirements related to coverage of MH/SUD benefits, as well as federal mental health parity requirements. It discusses the applicability of these requirements to different types of group and nongroup private health insurance plans.

Benefit coverage requirements generally address whether a plan must cover certain health care services or items. The two federal requirements most relevant to private health insurance coverage of MH/SUD benefits are as follows:

- Certain plans must offer a core package of 10 categories of *essential health benefits* (EHB), one of which is "mental health and substance use disorder services, including behavioral health treatment." States, rather than the federal government, generally specify the benefit coverage requirements within the EHB categories.

---

* This is an edited, reformatted and augmented version of Congressional Research Service Publication No. R47402, dated February 1, 2023.

In: Healing Minds
Editor: Wilburn M. Conner
ISBN: 979-8-89530-893-6

- Most plans must cover specified preventive services and items without cost sharing. These include various MH/SUD screenings as recommended for particular populations, such as men and/or women of certain ages, pregnant and postpartum persons, adolescents, and children.

There is no federal requirement that all private health insurance plans cover a set of specific MH/SUD benefits—or medical/surgical (M/S) benefits—beyond what is described in this report.

Mental health parity requirements do not mandate that plans cover MH/SUD benefits. However, when an applicable plan (i.e., a plan otherwise subject to parity law) *does* cover both MH/SUD benefits and M/S benefits, parity law generally prohibits the imposition of more restrictive limitations on MH/SUD benefits than on M/S benefits. Statutory and regulatory parity requirements focus primarily on whether and how plans may impose the following types of coverage limits on their MH/SUD benefits, within six classifications of benefits.

- Aggregate Lifetime Limits and Annual Limits: Dollar limits on plans' coverage of benefits
- Financial Requirements: Consumer cost-sharing requirements for covered benefits (e.g., co-payments)
- Quantitative Treatment Limitations (QTLs): Numeric benefit coverage limits (e.g., number of days or visits covered)
- Nonquantitative Treatment Limitations (NQTLs): Non-numeric benefit coverage limits (e.g., utilization review requirements)

The six classifications of benefits are (1) in-network inpatient, (2) out-of-network inpatient, (3) in-network outpatient, (4) out-of-network outpatient, (5) emergency care, and (6) pharmacy. In short, parity statute and regulations prohibit plans from imposing more restrictive limits on MH/SUD benefits than on M/S benefits, in terms of each type of coverage limit listed above, within each of these benefit classes. Parity law also includes information disclosure and documentation requirements on plans, and oversight and reporting requirements on federal agencies.

A brief legislative history explains changes regarding the above requirements that were made by the Paul Wellstone and Pete Domenici Mental Health Parity and Addiction Equity Act of 2008 (MHPAEA), the Patient Protection and Affordable Care Act (ACA, as amended) in 2010, and other relevant laws including the Consolidated Appropriations Act, 2023 (CAA 2023), enacted in December 2022. Additional legislative history information is in a summary table in the appendix of this report (Table A-1).

Introduction

Mental health conditions and substance use disorders are common in the United States. According to estimates from the Substance Abuse and Mental Health Services Administration (SAMHSA) derived from the 2021 National Survey on Drug Use and Health, 82.5 million adults in the United States reported having had either a mental health condition or a substance use disorder in 2021.

Participation in treatment for these conditions is also common. In 2021, 46.5 million adults reported that they had received mental health treatment and 4 million adults reported that they had received substance use treatment in the past year.[1]

Given that most people in the United States have private health insurance,[2] there is considerable congressional interest in understanding private coverage of mental health and substance use disorder (MH/SUD) benefits, including diagnostic and treatment services. This report explains federal requirements related to coverage of MH/SUD benefits, as well as federal mental health parity requirements, with respect to private health insurance.[3]

- *Benefit coverage requirements* generally address whether a plan must cover certain health care services or items. The two federal provisions most relevant to private health insurance coverage of MH/SUD benefits are the requirements that (1) certain plans cover a set of essential health benefits (EHB) and (2) most plans cover certain preventive services without cost sharing. For example, per EHB requirements, plans must offer a core package of 10 categories of

---

[1] Estimates in this paragraph are from pp. 41, 58, and 51, respectively, of Substance Abuse and Mental Health Services Administration (SAMHSA), *Key Substance Use and Mental Health Indicators in the United States: Results from the 2021 National Survey on Drug Use and Health*, January 2023, at https://www.samhsa.gov/data/report/2021-nsduh- annual-national-report. See the SAMHSA report for additional details, other estimates, and data sources and methodology. These data are not specific to individuals with private health insurance.

[2] See CRS In Focus IF10830, *U.S. Health Care Coverage and Spending*, for overviews of different sources of health coverage in the United States, including private health insurance, Medicare, and Medicaid.

[3] Mental health and substance use are often collectively referenced as *behavioral health*, but this report generally does not use this term, given specific references in relevant private health insurance requirements to mental health and/or substance use conditions and/or benefits.

health benefits, one of which is "mental health and substance use disorder services, including behavioral health treatment."[4]

- *Mental health parity requirements* do not mandate that plans cover MH/SUD benefits. However, when an applicable plan (i.e., a plan otherwise subject to parity law) *does* cover MH/SUD benefits and medical/surgical (M/S) benefits, parity law generally prohibits the imposition of more restrictive limitations on MH/SUD benefits than on M/S benefits.

This report explains these MH/SUD benefit coverage and parity requirements, as well as the types of private health insurance plans subject to such requirements. It includes a brief review of relevant legislative history—including changes enacted in December 2022—and a discussion and examples of required federal agency activities (e.g., oversight and reporting).

The report's focus is federal private health insurance requirements; it does not compare state requirements or actual plan variations in coverage. This report also does not address mental health benefits in public programs such as Medicare and Medicaid.

Legislative History

EHB and preventive services coverage requirements were enacted in 2010 via the Patient Protection and Affordable Care Act (ACA, as amended).[5]

The first federal mental health parity law, the Mental Health Parity Act of 1996 (MHPA), applied limited parity requirements to certain group health plans.[6] The Paul Wellstone and Pete Domenici Mental Health Parity and Addiction Equity Act of 2008 (MHPAEA) expanded on MHPA's private health insurance parity requirements. Five laws have since amended MHPAEA and federal parity law with regard to private health insurance: the ACA in 2010; the Helping Families in Mental Health Crisis Reform Act of 2016 (Division B of the 21st Century Cures Act of 2016, or the Cures Act); the SUPPORT for Patients and Communities Act (SUPPORT Act), enacted in 2018; the Consolidated Appropriations Act, 2021 (CAA 2021), enacted in

---

[4] 42 U.S.C. §18022(b)(1)(E).

[5] See *Table A-1* for full citations of and relevant details regarding all legislation in this section.

[6] See "Plans Subject to Coverage and Parity Requirements" for more information about plan types and applicability of parity law.

2020; and the Consolidated Appropriations Act, 2023 (CAA 2023), enacted in 2022.

Over time, the legislative changes have increased the scope of parity law to include substance use disorder benefits in addition to mental health benefits; expanded the required areas of parity and addressed classification of benefits; expanded federal parity law's applicability to most types of private health insurance plans; and specified that if an applicable plan covers eating disorder treatment, such coverage is subject to parity requirements. In addition, multiple changes have aimed to improve plans' understanding of and compliance with parity requirements and increase federal enforcement of and reporting on parity requirements. Although MHPAEA has been amended multiple times, the body of federal parity law is still commonly called MHPAEA.[7]

In general, the Departments of Health and Human Services (HHS), Labor, and the Treasury (in this report, the Tri-Agencies) coordinate enforcement with respect to federal private health insurance requirements.

Benefit Coverage Requirements

MH/SUD benefits may include services, such as office visits or hospital stays, or items, such as prescription medications. MH/SUD benefits may be furnished by a range of providers (e.g., psychiatrists, psychologists, psychiatric nurses, licensed professional counselors) and via various settings and modalities (e.g., inpatient, outpatient, telehealth).

The two federal provisions most relevant to private health insurance coverage of MH/SUD benefits are the requirements that (1) certain plans cover a set of EHB and (2) most plans cover certain preventive services without cost sharing.[8] These requirements are explained below (see *"Plans Subject to*

---

[7] Most of the private health insurance parity requirements from the above laws are codified as similar provisions in three separate federal statutes the Public Health Service Act (PHSA) Section 2726, at 42 U.S.C. §300gg-26; the Employee Retirement Income Security Act (ERISA) Section 712, at 29 U.S.C. §1185a; and the Internal Revenue Code (IRC) Section 9812, at 26 U.S.C. §9812. This report generally uses the PHSA citations.

[8] Other types of federal requirements—those not specific to mental health and substance use disorder (MH/SUD) benefit coverage or parity—also may be relevant. See, for example, "Requirements Related to Health Care Providers" in CRS Report R45146, *Federal Requirements on Private Health Insurance Plans*, and network adequacy requirements in the "Qualified Health Plans" section of CRS Report R44065, *Overview of Health Insurance Exchanges*.

Coverage and Parity Requirements" regarding the requirements' applicability to different types of private plans).

There is no federal requirement that all private health insurance plans cover a set of specific MH/SUD benefits (or M/S benefits), beyond what is described below.

Coverage of the Essential Health Benefits

Certain plans must cover a core package of 10 categories of health care benefits, known as the essential health benefits.[9] One category of EHB is "mental health and substance use disorder services, including behavioral health treatment."[10] Other EHB categories also may include benefits relevant to MH/SUD.[11] For example, current EHB prescription drug coverage regulations effectively require applicable plans (those subject to EHB requirements) to cover at least one form of naloxone, a drug that can treat opioid overdoses.[12]

States, rather than the federal government, generally specify the benefit coverage requirements within the EHB categories. Current regulation allows each state to select an EHB benchmark plan, within certain parameters. The benchmark plan serves as a reference for applicable plans in that state, which must provide EHB coverage that is "substantially equal" to such coverage in the benchmark plan, as specified in regulations.[13] Because states select their own EHB benchmark plans, EHB coverage may vary considerably from state to state.[14]

---

[9] 42 U.S.C. §300gg-6; 42 U.S.C. §18022; 45 C.F.R. §156.115.

[10] 42 U.S.C. §18022(b)(1)(E).

[11] The 10 essential health benefit (EHB) categories are (1) ambulatory patient services; (2) emergency services; (3) hospitalization; (4) maternity and newborn care; (5) mental health and substance use disorder services, including behavioral health treatment; (6) prescription drugs; (7) rehabilitative and habilitative services and devices; (8) laboratory services; (9) preventive and wellness services and chronic disease management; and (10) pediatric services, including oral and vision care.

[12] Department of Health and Human Services (HHS), "Patient Protection and Affordable Care Act; HHS Notice of Benefit and Payment Parameters for 2019," 83 *Federal Register* 16930, April 17, 2018. See footnote 64, referencing 45 C.F.R. §156.122(a)(1) and other sections of regulation.

[13] 45 C.F.R. §156.115(a)(1).

[14] For more information on the process for defining the EHB, and for links to state benchmark plans, see Centers for Medicare & Medicaid Services (CMS), Center for Consumer Information and Insurance Oversight (CCIIO), "Information on Essential Health Benefits (EHB) Benchmark Plans," at https://www.cms.gov/ cciio/resources/data- resources/ehb.

Federal law permits consumer cost sharing (e.g., deductibles, coinsurance, and co-payments, up to an annual out-of-pocket limit) for most categories of EHB. Coverage and cost sharing for EHB furnished by out-of-network providers may vary, subject to applicable federal and state requirements.[15] Certain federal limits on cost sharing, such as a prohibition on lifetime and annual coverage limits, apply to the EHB.[16]

Coverage of Certain Preventive Services Without Cost Sharing

There is also a federal requirement that most plans cover specified preventive services and items without cost sharing.[17] These services and items include, at a minimum, four categories of preventive benefits recommended by specified entities, such as the United States Preventive Services Task Force (USPSTF). The recommendations include various MH/SUD screenings for specified populations, such as men and/or women of certain ages, pregnant and postpartum persons, adolescents, and children.[18]

The recommended benefits are meant to be preventive in nature—that is, provided to specified populations without regard to the presence of a diagnosis or particular symptoms. Preventive benefits include, for example, depression screenings for the general adult population as recommended by the USPSTF.

---

[15] In general, beginning with each plan year, an enrollee pays 100% of costs for covered health care benefits until the costs meet a certain threshold amount called a deductible. Exceptions apply. After that, the enrollee pays coinsurance (a percentage amount) or co-payments (a flat amount) for covered benefits, and the plan pays the rest. If an enrollee's spending meets an annual out-of-pocket limit, the plan generally will pay 100% of covered costs for the remainder of the plan year. See CRS Report RL32237, *Health Insurance: A Primer* for further explanations of cost sharing, including when benefits are furnished by out-of-network providers.

[16] Plans are prohibited from setting lifetime or annual dollar limits on their coverage of the EHB, generally whether provided in network or out of network. This prohibition applies to individual and fully insured small-group plans, which are subject to EHB requirements. It also applies to large-group and self-insured plans; because these plans are not required to cover EHB, regulations address how the plans may define their benefits for purposes of this requirement. See CRS Report R45146, *Federal Requirements on Private Health Insurance Plans*, for additional information on this and other federal requirements relevant to consumer cost sharing.

[17] 42 U.S.C. §300gg-13; 45 C.F.R. §147.130.

[18] For the preventive benefits that must be covered (1) for all adults, (2) additionally for women, and (3) for children and adolescents, from across the four categories of recommendations, see HealthCare.gov, "Preventive Health Services," at https://www.healthcare.gov/preventive-care-benefits/. For more information on the coverage requirement and recommendation categories, see CRS Report R45146, *Federal Requirements on Private Health Insurance Plans*.

If an individual has symptoms and needs a certain screening (e.g., a depression screening) for purposes of diagnosis, that screening may not necessarily be covered without cost sharing per this federal requirement. The same is true if a screening identifies a condition that needs further treatment. However, the plan may cover diagnostic screenings and treatments (with or without cost sharing), including due to other applicable federal requirements (e.g., EHB) or state requirements.

Mental Health Parity Requirements

Federal parity law does not require private health insurance plans to cover MH/SUD benefits, when such coverage is not otherwise required by federal or state law. However, when an applicable plan covers both MH/SUD benefits and M/S benefits,[19] federal parity law generally prohibits the imposition of more restrictive limits on MH/SUD benefits than on M/S benefits, as specified below and summarized in *Table 1.* Parity law also includes information disclosure and other requirements discussed later in this section.

Although this body of law is commonly referred to as mental health parity, and although initial parity law did apply only to mental health benefits, current parity law applies to both mental health and substance use disorder benefits (to the extent they are covered).

Parity Law Definitions of MH/SUD Benefits

The question of whether a covered benefit is considered an MH/SUD benefit can have implications for the applicability of parity requirements. Within mental health parity statute, the definition of mental health benefits is "benefits with respect to services for mental health conditions, as defined under the terms of the plan and in accordance with applicable Federal and State law" (emphasis added).[20] Similarly, the definition of substance use disorder benefits references benefits with respect to services for substance use disorders. The terms mental health conditions and substance use disorders are not further defined in mental health parity statutory language.

---

[19] Regarding applicable plans, see "Plans Subject to Coverage and Parity Requirements."

[20] See 42 U.S.C. §300gg-26(e) for these definitions of mental health benefits and substance use disorder benefits.

In parity regulations, the definitions of mental health benefits and substance use disorder benefits include additional clarifications. For example, the regulatory definition of mental health benefits states that "any condition defined by the plan or coverage as being or as not being a mental health condition must be defined to be consistent with generally recognized independent standards of current medical practice (for example, the most current version of the Diagnostic and Statistical Manual of Mental Disorders (DSM), the most current version of the ICD, or State guidelines)."[21]

In general, parity law does not further specify that any particular type of benefits be considered MH/SUD benefits. However, a provision of the Cures Act specified that parity requirements

apply to eating disorder benefits, if these benefits are covered.[22] (See also the discussion below of "Coverage of MH/SUD Benefits in the Six Classifications.")

Parity Requirements Related to Coverage Limits and Benefit Classifications

Parity Requirements and Parity Tests

Statutory and regulatory parity requirements focus primarily on whether and how plans may impose certain types of coverage limits on their MH/SUD benefits, within six classifications of benefits. Parity law provides different tests to determine compliance with the various requirements.

Parity requirements apply to the following types of coverage limits:[23]

- Aggregate Lifetime Limits and Annual Limits: Dollar limits on plans' coverage of benefits
- Financial Requirements: Consumer cost-sharing requirements for covered benefits (e.g., co-payments)

---

[21] 45 C.F.R. §146.136(a). The ICD is the Internal Classification of Diseases. Also see the Department of Labor (DOL), HHS, and Department of the Treasury, "Self-Compliance Tool for the Mental Health Parity and Addiction Equity Act (MHPAEA)," updated October 2020, at https://www.dol.gov/sites/dolgov/files/EBSA/laws-and-regulations/laws/ mental-health-parity/self-compliance-tool.pdf (hereinafter referred to as Tri-Agency Self-Compliance Tool 2020).

[22] 42 U.S.C. §300gg-26, Statutory Note, "Clarification of Existing Parity Rules."

[23] 42 U.S.C. §300gg-26(a)(1, 2, 3) and 45 C.F.R. §146.136(a-c).

Table 1. Parity requirements related to coverage limits (Private Health Insurance)

Coverage Limits Subject to Parity Law[a]	Definition of Coverage Limit in Parity Law	Test for Determining Parity Compliance
Aggregate Lifetime Limits	Dollar limitations on the "total amount" the plan will pay for specified benefits for a "coverage unit" (e.g., an enrollee or family).	If a plan *does not* include aggregate lifetime or annual limits on *substantially all* medical/ surgical (M/S) benefits, it may not impose *any* such limits on mental health/substance use disorder (MH/SUD) benefits.[b]
Annual Limits	Dollar limitations on the total amount the plan will pay for specified benefits "in a 12- month period" for a coverage unit.	
Financial Requirements	Cost-sharing requirements for coverage units such as co-payments and coinsurance, and "cumulative financial requirements" such as deductibles and out-of-pocket maximums.	A plan may not impose a financial requirement or QTL on MH/SUD benefits that is "more restrictive than the *predominant* financial requirement or treatment limitation of that type applied to *substantially all* [M/S] benefits" in the same classification.[c]
Quantitative Treatment Limitations (QTLs)	Numeric benefit coverage restrictions or plan attributes, such as limits on the number of days or visits covered.	
Nonquantitative Treatment Limitations (NQTLs)	Non-numeric benefit coverage restrictions or plan attributes. Examples of NQTLs include "medical management standards (e.g., limits based on medical necessity or if a treatment is experimental)"; drug formularies; step therapy requirements; and "standards for provider admission to participate in a network, including reimbursement rates."	A plan may not impose an NQTL on MH/SUD benefits unless "any processes, strategies, evidentiary standards, or other factors" used in applying the NQTL to MH/SUD benefits are *"comparable to, and are applied no more stringently than,"* the processes, etc., used in applying the limitation with respect to M/S benefits in the same classification.[d]

Source: CRS analysis of statutory and regulatory provisions at 42 U.S.C. §300gg-26 and 45 C.F.R. §146.136. Quoted language in the table is from these provisions. For example, see the definitions of aggregate lifetime limits and annual limits at 42 U.S.C. §300gg-26(e), and see examples of NQTLs at 45 C.F.R. §146.136(c)(4).

Notes: Certain emphases added (e.g., predominant and substantially all).

[a] As specified, these coverage limits for MH/SUD benefits must be no more restrictive than such coverage limits for M/S benefits, within each of six benefit classifications in which MH/SUD benefits are covered: (1) in-network inpatient, (2) out-of-network inpatient, (3) in-network outpatient, (4) out-of-network outpatient, (5) emergency care, and (6) pharmacy.

[b] Statutory and regulatory parity language also provide for situations in which a plan does include an aggregate lifetime or annual limit on substantially all M/S benefits or on different categories of benefits. However, given other federal provisions that prohibit most plans from imposing lifetime or annual limits on coverage (as specified by such provisions), parity regulations and guidance acknowledge that such situations are rare. See 45 C.F.R. §146.136(b) and Tri-Agency Self-Compliance Tool 2020, Section C.

[c] Regulations apply numerical standards to the terms predominant and substantially all, and establish a two-step mathematical test by which applicable plans can determine allowable restrictions on

MH/SUD benefits in each classification. To explain the two-step test via an example, an applicable plan may impose a deductible on its in-network inpatient MH/SUD benefits only if it also imposes a deductible on at least two-thirds (i.e., substantially all) of its in-network inpatient M/S benefits. If that is the case, the deductible for such MH/SUD benefits may not be higher than the deductible applied to more than half (i.e., the predominant) of the in- network inpatient M/S benefits. For further details, see 45 C.F.R. §146.136(c)(3)(i)(A), 45 C.F.R §146.136(c)(3)(i)(B)(1), and the Tri-Agency Self-Compliance Tool 2020, Sections D and E.

[d] For example, what are the standards by which a plan applied a medical necessity determination to MH/SUD benefits in a class, as compared with M/S benefits in that class? Or, what are the factors a plan used to set its provider reimbursement rates and otherwise establish its provider network for MH/SUD providers as compared with M/S providers? MH/SUD provider reimbursement rates need not be the same as M/S provider reimbursement rates, nor does parity law require any particular MH/SUD reimbursement rates, but parity guidance provides various "warning signs" to plans about provider reimbursement rates and related topics (see Tri-Agency Self-Compliance Tool 2020 Appendix II). For more information about NQTL parity requirements, see 45 C.F.R. §146.136(c)(4) and the Tri-Agency Self-Compliance Tool 2020, Section F.

- Quantitative Treatment Limitations (QTLs): Numeric benefit coverage limits (e.g., number of days or visits covered)
- Nonquantitative Treatment Limitations (NQTLs): Non-numeric benefit coverage limits (e.g., utilization review requirements)

The above are all types of coverage limits that a plan may impose on any benefit it covers (not just MH/SUD), subject to federal and state law. For example, a plan may specify that inpatient hospital stays for certain conditions are covered only when the plan has provided preauthorization to the enrollee or provider; this example would be a type of NQTL.

Parity requirements related to these coverage limits apply in each of six classifications of benefits that parity regulations have established: (1) in-network inpatient, (2) out-of-network inpatient, (3) in-network outpatient, (4) out-of-network outpatient, (5) emergency care, and (6) prescription drugs.[24]

In short, parity statute and regulations prohibit plans from imposing more restrictive limits on MH/SUD benefits than on M/S benefits, in terms of each type of coverage limit listed above, within each of these benefit classes. For example, a plan must ensure its NQTL requirements are no more restrictive for MH/SUD benefits than for M/S benefits for in-network inpatient services and, separately, for emergency care.[25]

---

[24] 45 C.F.R. §146.136(c)(2)(ii). Also see 42 U.S.C. §300gg-26(a)(4) regarding coverage of benefits furnished by out- of-network providers.

[25] See Tri-Agency Self-Compliance Tool 2020, Section B regarding the benefit classifications, including determining which class a benefit (such as certain "intermediate" services) belongs in and allowable subclassifications (e.g., outpatient office visits versus all other outpatient services).

The tests for determining parity compliance are specified in statute and regulation. For example, there is one test for quantitative parity requirements (including financial requirements and QTLs), a different test for NQTL parity requirements, and another test for aggregate lifetime and annual limits. Table 1 summarizes all of the parity requirements and their parity tests.

Coverage of MH/SUD Benefits in the Six Classifications

Besides their relevance to the specified coverage limits, the six classifications of benefits also are related to a coverage requirement for plans that are subject to parity law. Although parity law does not include a benefit coverage mandate in general, it does provide that if an applicable plan covers MH/SUD benefits in *any* of the six classifications, the plan must cover MH/SUD benefits in *all* of the classes in which it also covers M/S benefits.[26]

This does not necessarily require plans to cover particular MH/SUD benefits within a class, but it means a plan cannot exclude coverage of a whole class of MH/SUD benefits if the plan covers M/S benefits in that class. For example, if a plan provides any coverage of out-of-network outpatient M/S services, it also must cover some out-of-network outpatient MH/SUD services. By contrast, if a plan does *not* cover any M/S benefits in a class (which may be the case for inpatient or outpatient out-of-network benefits), the plan does not have to cover any MH/SUD benefits in that class.[27]

Parity Requirements Related to Disclosure and Documentation

Information Disclosure to Enrollees and Others

Applicable plans are required to disclose certain information related to medical necessity determinations and/or denials of payment, with respect to MH/SUD benefits, upon request by specified parties. Per parity statutory and regulatory provisions,[28]

---

[26] 45 C.F.R. §146.136(c)(2)(ii)(A). Also see 42 U.S.C. §300gg-26(a)(5), specific to coverage of MH/SUD benefits provided out-of-network, if medical/surgical benefits are covered out-of-network.

[27] See the Tri-Agency Self-Compliance Tool 2020, Section B, for further discussion and examples of this requirement, including as related to coverage of medication-assisted treatment for opioid use disorder.

[28] See 42 U.S.C. §300gg-26(a)(4) for requirements listed in both bullets, including quoted language. Also see 45 C.F.R.§146.136(d). As discussed in such parity regulations and in the Tri-Agency Self-Compliance Tool 2020, Section G, there are also relevant federal

- "*The criteria for medical necessity determinations*" made with respect to MH/SUD benefits must be disclosed to "any current or potential participant, beneficiary, or contracting provider upon request."
- "The reason for any denial ... of reimbursement or payment for services" with respect to MH/SUD benefits, including applicable medical necessity criteria as applied to that enrollee, must be disclosed to any participant or beneficiary who receives such a denial.

NQTL Comparative Analyses

As discussed above, applicable plans are prohibited from imposing more restrictive NQTLs (and other specified types of limits) on MH/SUD benefits than on M/S benefits.

Per the CAA 2021, plans also are required to "perform and document comparative analyses of the design and application of NQTLs" and to make such analyses available to the Tri-agency Secretaries or applicable state authorities, upon request (see "Federal Oversight of Parity Requirements" section below).[29] These analyses must include statutorily specified information, such as a description of all MH/SUD and M/S benefits to which each NQTL applies in each benefit classification, and demonstrations of compliance with NQTL parity standards.

Parity Requirements Related to Oversight and Reporting

Parity law includes oversight and reporting requirements for federal agencies. There are also newly authorized grants to states for parity enforcement.

Federal Oversight of Parity Requirements[30]

The Tri-Agency Secretaries must annually request and review at least 20 of the NQTL analyses described above from plans that "involve potential [parity]

---

requirements not specific to parity (e.g., 29 U.S.C. §1133 and 29 C.F.R. §2560.503-1, regarding claims procedures).

[29] 42 U.S.C. §300gg-26(a)(8)(A).

[30] For additional information about federal enforcement of private health insurance requirements in general, see CRS Report R46637, *Federal Private Health Insurance Market Reforms: Legal Framework and Enforcement*.

violations" or complaints of noncompliance, or in "any other instances in which the Secretary determines appropriate."[31]

Required follow-up actions are specified if more information is needed or parity violations are found.

In addition, per the Cures Act, if the Tri-Agency Secretaries determine a plan has violated parity requirements five times, the Secretaries must audit plan documents in the following plan year.[32]

Required Federal Reports, Rulemaking, Guidance, and Other Activities

The Tri-Agencies are required to submit annual and biannual reports to Congress on issues related to parity compliance, including the NQTL analyses discussed above.[33] Parity law also includes requirements for agency guidance (including a "compliance program guidance document" and "additional guidance" as specified), and other activities (e.g., a public meeting of stakeholders "to produce an action plan for improved federal and state coordination" related to enforcement of MHPAEA and state parity laws).[34] MHPAEA required Tri-Agency rulemaking on parity requirements.[35] Examples of reports, guidance, and other deliverables created to fulfill these requirements include the following:[36]

- A January 2022 Tri-Agency report to Congress meets several agency reporting requirements for the year, including the Departments' first required review of plans' NQTL comparative analyses and discussions of other compliance issues.[37]

---

[31] 42 U.S.C. §300gg-26(a)(8)(B).

[32] 42 U.S.C. §300gg-26, Statutory Note, "Improving Compliance."

[33] As required biannually (beginning in 2012) by MHPAEA: 29 U.S.C. §1185a(f). As required annually (beginning December 2021) by the CAA 2021: 42 U.S.C. §300gg-26(a)(8)(B)(iv). The Cures Act, as amended by the SUPPORT Act, also required annual reporting for five years on federal investigations into parity compliance. See Table A-1.

[34] See 42 U.S.C. §300gg-26(a)(6) regarding the "compliance program guidance document"; 42 U.S.C. §300gg-26(a)(7) regarding "additional guidance"; and Cures Act, Division B, Title XIII, §13002 regarding the action plan.

[35] MHPAEA, Division C, Title V, Subtitle B, §512(d).

[36] See additional resources, including prior-year reports to Congress, at DOL and HHS parity webpages: https://www.dol.gov/agencies/ebsa/laws-and-regulations/laws/mental-health-and-substance-use-disorder-parity; and https://www.cms.gov/CCIIO/Programs-and-Initiatives/Other-Insurance-Protections/mhpaea_factsheet.

[37] DOL, HHS, and the Treasury, Realizing Parity, Reducing Stigma, and Raising Awareness: Increasing Access to Mental Health and Substance Use Disorder Coverage, 2022 MHPAEA Report to Congress, January 2022, at https://www.dol.gov/sites/dolgov/files/EBSA/laws-and-regulations/laws/mental-health-parity/report-to-congress-2022-realizing-parity-reducing-stigma-and-raising-awareness.pdf.

- A Self-Compliance Tool (i.e., the compliance program guidance document), last updated in October 2020, is meant to help applicable plans, state regulators, and other stakeholders understand and comply with parity requirements.[38]
- Several Tri-Agency FAQs, issued between June 2017 and September 2019, are examples of the required additional guidance.[39] They addressed information disclosure requirements, NQTL parity requirements, and required agency activities (e.g., the stakeholder meeting and action plan).
- A November 2013 final rule implemented MHPAEA and ACA parity requirements.[40]

In addition, certain parity provisions have required Government Accountability Office (GAO) reports to Congress. GAO has published multiple reports on mental health parity and mental health access in private health insurance, for example in 2011,[41] 2019,[42] 2021,[43] and 2022.[44]

Grants to States for Parity Enforcement

The CAA 2023 established new HHS grants for states "to enforce and ensure compliance with" mental health parity requirements.[45] The act authorized to

---

[38] Tri-Agency Compliance Tool 2020, as cited at footnote 21.

[39] Tri-Agency FAQs 38, 39, and related documents (June 2017-September 2019), at CMS, CCIIO, "Fact Sheets and Frequently Asked Questions (FAQs)," at https://www.cms.gov/cciio/resources/fact-sheets-and- faqs#Mental_Health_Parity. Also see Tri-Agency FAQ 45 (April 2021) on the NQTL comparative analyses.

[40] Treasury, Internal Revenue Service; DOL, Employee Benefits Security Administration; and HHS, CMS, "Final Rules Under the Paul Wellstone and Pete Domenici Mental Health Parity and Addiction Equity Act of 2008; Technical Amendment to External Review for Multi-State Plan Program," 78 *Federal Register* 68239, November 13, 2013.

[41] Government Accountability Office (GAO), Mental Health and Substance Use: Employers' Insurance Coverage Maintained or Enhanced Since Parity Act, But Effect of Coverage on Enrollees Varied, GAO-12-63, November 30, 2011, at https://www.gao.gov/products/gao-12-63.

[42] GAO, Mental Health and Substance Use: State and Federal Oversight of Compliance with Parity Requirements Varies, GAO-20-150, December 13, 2019, at https://www.gao.gov/products/gao-20-150.

[43] GAO, Behavioral Health: Patient Access, Provider Claims Payment, and the Effects of the COVID-19 Pandemic, GAO-21-437R, March 31, 2021, at https://www.gao.gov/products/gao-21-437r.

[44] GAO, Mental Health Care: Access Challenges for Covered Consumers and Relevant Federal Efforts, GAO-22-104597, March 30, 2022, at https://www.gao.gov/products/gao-22-104597.

[45] 42 U.S.C. §300gg-94(c)(3).

be appropriated $10 million for each of the first five fiscal years beginning after the date of enactment, to remain available until expended, for purposes of awarding these grants. To be eligible for the grants, states must agree to request and review (an unspecified number of) the NQTL comparative analyses required of plans, as described above. The HHS Secretary is otherwise required to specify the timing, manner, and information requirements for state applications for the grants.

Plans Subject to Coverage and Parity Requirements

Broadly, private health insurance includes *group plans* of several types and *nongroup plans*. Federal private health insurance requirements may apply to some or all such plans.[46]

Group plans largely refer to health benefits provided to employees (and their dependents) by employers that sponsor such benefits. Employers and other group health plan sponsors may purchase coverage from a state-licensed insurer and offer it to their group (i.e., they may *fully insure*). Sponsors may instead finance coverage themselves (i.e., they may *self-insure*). Fully insured plans may be purchased in the large- or small-group markets. For purposes of private health insurance regulation, a *small group* is typically defined as a group of up to 50 individuals (e.g., employees) and a *large group* is typically defined as one with 51 or more individuals.

Consumers purchase *nongroup plans* directly from an insurer. In general, nongroup plans are fully insured. The nongroup market (also called the *individual market*) and the small-group market include plans sold on and off the health insurance exchanges—the individual exchanges and Small Business Health Options Program exchanges, respectively.[47]

Federal private health insurance requirements generally apply to some or all of the following types of plans: (1) fully insured group plans offered by large employers (i.e., large-group plans), (2) fully insured group plans offered

---

[46] For simplicity, this report refers to requirements on private health insurance *plans*, but such requirements are generally on the health insurance *issuers* that sell plans or the sponsors (such as employers) that offer plans.

[47] The exchanges are government-administered marketplaces in which consumers and small businesses can purchase private health insurance offered by participating insurers. Plans sold in the individual and Small Business Health Options Program exchanges must meet the requirements applicable to the nongroup and small-group markets, respectively. Additional requirements apply only to exchange plans. For more information, see CRS Report R44065, *Overview of Health Insurance Exchanges*.

by small employers (i.e., small-group plans), (3) self-insured group plans, and (4) nongroup plans. Federal requirements on self-insured group plans generally do not depend on group size; however, due to certain details regarding parity requirements, this report specifies the following variations: (3a) self-insured group plans offered by large employers and (3b) self-insured group plans offered by small employers.

Table 2 summarizes the applicability of EHB, preventive services, and mental health parity requirements to such plans. Additional discussion of parity applicability follows the table.

Table 2. Applicability of mental health parity and selected benefit coverage requirements to specified types of private health insurance plans

Type of Plan	Essential Health Benefits (EHB)	Preventive Services Without Cost Sharing	Mental Health Parity[a]
Fully Insured Group Plan (Large Employer)	NA	√	√ [b]
Fully Insured Group Plan (Small Employer)c	√	√	√ [d]
Self-Insured Group Plan (Large Employer)	NA	√	√ [b]
Self-Insured Group Plan (Small Employer)	NA	√	NA
Nongroup Plan[c]	√	√	√

Sources: CRS analysis of statutory and regulatory provisions. EHB: 42 U.S.C. §300gg-6; 42 U.S.C. §18022; 45 C.F.R. §156.115. Preventive Services: 42 U.S.C. §300gg-13; 45 C.F.R. §147.130. Parity: 42 U.S.C. §300gg-26, 45 C.F.R. §146.136.

Notes: NA = not applicable. See "Plans Subject to Coverage and Parity Requirements" regarding the plan types listed above.

[a] Specified plans are subject to parity requirements *if* they cover mental health/substance use disorder benefits and medical/surgical benefits.

[b] These plans can request time-limited parity exemptions if implementation would increase their costs, as specified in law. See footnote 49 for details.

[c] Nongroup and small-group plans (i.e., fully insured group plans offered by small employers) include those sold on and off the exchanges.

[d] These plans are subject to parity primarily because of the incorporation of parity into EHB requirements.

As shown above, most types of private health insurance plans are subject to federal parity laws if they cover MH/SUD benefits and unless otherwise exempted. Small, self-insured group plans are exempt from parity requirements.[48] Certain plans also may qualify for an increased cost exemption

---

[48] 42 U.S.C. §300gg-26(c)(1) and 45 C.F.R. §146.136(f).

under parity law (i.e., plans for which implementing parity would result in increased costs above specified thresholds).[49]

Although the parity exemption for small employers initially applied to both self-insured and fully insured plans, plans subject to EHB requirements also are subject to parity requirements, per EHB and parity regulations.[50]

In contrast to the relationship between EHB and parity requirements, the preventive services coverage requirements do not trigger parity requirements. In other words, if the only MH/SUD benefits a plan covers are the MH/SUD preventive services, in compliance with that federal requirement, this does not constitute coverage of MH/SUD benefits that would generally trigger the requirement to comply with federal parity law.[51] By contrast, if state law requires a plan to cover MH/SUD benefits, the plan would then also be subject to federal parity law, unless otherwise exempt.

Certain Other Types of Plans

Certain other types of private health plans, such as grandfathered plans and short-term, limited-duration insurance, do not have to comply with most or all federal health insurance requirements. These and other coverage types are discussed in a separate CRS report.[52]

That report also discusses self-insured, nonfederal governmental plans, which previously could opt out of parity and other specified federal requirements. Per the CAA 2023, these plans can no longer opt out of mental health parity requirements.[53]

---

[49] 42 U.S.C. §300gg-26(c)(2) and 45 C.F.R. §146.136(g). Plans that incur increased "actual total costs" (due to parity requirements, as specified) above 1% in a plan year may claim an exemption from parity law for the following plan year. However, nongroup and small-group plans that must cover the EHB and thus are subject to parity requirements (as discussed in this section) do not appear to be eligible for this exemption, per 45 C.F.R. §146.136(e)(4).

[50] 45 C.F.R. §146.136(e)(4), 45 C.F.R. §156.115(a)(3).

[51] See "Mental Health Parity Requirements."

[52] See CRS Report R46003, *Applicability of Federal Requirements to Selected Health Coverage Arrangements*.

[53] 42 U.S.C. §300gg-21(a)(2)(F).

Appendix. Legislative History Summary Table

Table A-1. Legislative history of mental health parity and selected benefit coverage requirements applicable to private health insurance plans

Public Law	Summary of Relevant Provisions
Mental Health Parity Act of 1996 (MHPA) P.L. 104-204, Title VII (§§701- 703)	Required parity in terms of annual and lifetime limits for MH benefits. Applied parity law to large-employer plans (fully or self-insured) that covered MH and M/S benefits. Provided exemptions for small-employer plans (fully or self-insured) and for plans facing increased costs due to parity implementation. As enacted, set to expire September 30, 2001. (Extended by other laws between 1997 and 2008.)
Paul Wellstone and Pete Domenici Mental Health Parity and Addiction Equity Act of 2008 (MHPAEA) P.L. 110-343, Division C, Title V, Subtitle B (§§511-512)	Expanded scope of parity law to include SUD in addition to MH benefits. Added new parity requirements regarding financial requirements and treatment limitations, benefits furnished by out-of-network providers, and information disclosure. Amended the small-employer and increased-cost exemption provisions. Required biannual DOL reports to Congress on parity compliance, Tri-Agency rulemaking and guidance on parity requirements, and a GAO report on MH/SUD benefit coverage and exclusions. Removed parity law sunset dates.
Patient Protection and Affordable Care Act (ACA, as amended, 2010) P.L. 111-148 (§§1001, 1201, 1302, 1311, 1563)	Required nongroup and small-group plans (i.e., fully insured plans offered by small employers) to cover the EHB, and most plans to cover preventive services without cost sharing. Directly and/or effectively expanded the applicability of parity law to nongroup and small- group plans, as specified.
Helping Families in Mental Health Crisis Reform Act of 2016 (21st Century Cures Act of 2016, Division B) P.L. 114-255, Division B, Title XIII (§§13001-13004, 13007)	Required Tri-Agency reports to Congress on federal parity investigations, annually for five years as specified. Required Tri-Agency "compliance program guidance document" and "additional guidance," other agency activities, and a GAO report to Congress on parity compliance and enforcement. Specified that if the Tri-Agency Secretaries determine a plan has violated parity requirements five times, the Secretaries must audit plan documents in the following plan year. Specified that parity requirements apply to eating disorder benefits, if covered.
SUPPORT for Patients and Communities Act (SUPPORT Act, 2018) P.L. 115-271 (§7182)	Amended Cures Act requirements regarding the content of Tri-Agency reports to Congress on federal parity investigations.
Consolidated Appropriations Act, 2021 (CAA 2021, enacted 2020) P.L. 116-260, Division BB, Title II (§203)	Required plans to perform and document comparative analyses of their NQTLs for MH/SUD and M/S benefits, as specified. Required Tri-Agencies to annually request and review at least 20 NQTL comparative analyses, follow up as specified on noncompliance, and annually report to Congress on these analyses. Amended Cures Act requirements regarding the "compliance program guidance document" and "additional guidance."

Table A-1. (Continued)

Public Law	Summary of Relevant Provisions
Consolidated Appropriations Act, 2023 (CAA 2023, enacted 2022) P.L. 117-328, Division FF, Title I (§§1321, 1331)	Provided that self-insured, nonfederal governmental plans may no longer opt out of mental health parity requirements. Established HHS grants to states "to enforce and ensure compliance with" mental health parity requirements, including the NQTL comparative analyses. Authorized to be appropriated $10 million per year for five fiscal years following enactment for such grants.

Source: CRS analysis of relevant private health insurance provisions in the laws cited. Some of these laws also include parity provisions relevant to public programs (e.g., Medicaid), which are not included in this report.

Notes: MH = mental health; M/S = medical / surgical; SUD = substance use disorder; GAO = Government Accountability Office; Tri-Agency = Department of Health and Human Services (HHS), Department of Labor (DOL), and Department of the Treasury; EHB = essential health benefits; NQTLs = nonquantitative treatment limitations. See "Legislative History" in this report regarding codification of these provisions. See "Plans Subject to Coverage and Parity Requirements" for discussion of plan types. See "Required Federal Reports, Rulemaking, Guidance, and Other Activities" for links to agency reports, guidance, and other resources.

Chapter 3

Strategic Framework for Addressing Youth Mental Health Disparities: Fiscal Years 2022–2031*

National Institute of Mental Health

Foreword

I am pleased to introduce the NIMH Strategic Framework on Youth Mental Health Disparities. Developed in collaboration with the National Institute on Minority Health and Health Disparities, the Eunice Kennedy Shriver National Institute of Child Health and Human Development, and multiple other partners across NIH, HHS, and the federal government, and informed by researchers and care providers across the country, this Framework is a living document that summarizes NIMH's plans and priorities for guiding research to address and reduce mental health disparities among underserved and underrepresented youth (persons aged 24 and under) by 2031.

Our country is in the midst of a youth mental health crisis, including alarming increases in youth suicide in recent years. We also know that youth exposed to racism, discrimination, and other adverse experiences, as well as those from disadvantaged and underserved communities, are disproportionately impacted by mental illnesses, and frequently experience reduced access to high-quality, evidence-based mental health services and receive fewer follow-ups in a variety of provider settings. Addressing these

* This is an edited, reformatted and augmented version of National Institute of Mental Health Publication.

In: Healing Minds
Editor: Wilburn M. Conner
ISBN: 979-8-89530-893-6

challenges will require sustained attention, effort, and resources – all built on a foundation of high-quality research.

As the Director of NIMH's Office for Disparities Research and Workforce Diversity, I am committed to the research mission of informing policies and practices aimed at reducing mental health disparities, promoting equity, and addressing the needs of youth from disadvantaged communities and those who are underrepresented in clinical research, including but not limited to racial and ethnic minoritized youth, and sexual and gender minoritized youth. The Strategic Framework serves as NIMH's blueprint for accomplishing this mission. I invite you to come with us and hold us accountable as we not only implement the Framework, but also continuously refine it to meet evolving challenges and needs, in collaboration with stakeholders such as people with mental illnesses and their families, patient advocates and advocacy groups, health care providers, researchers, and state, local, and federal government partners.

Thank you for your support and attention to this important area of research.

Sincerely,
Christina P.C. Borba, Ph.D., M.P.H.
Director, NIMH Office for Disparities Research and Workforce Diversity

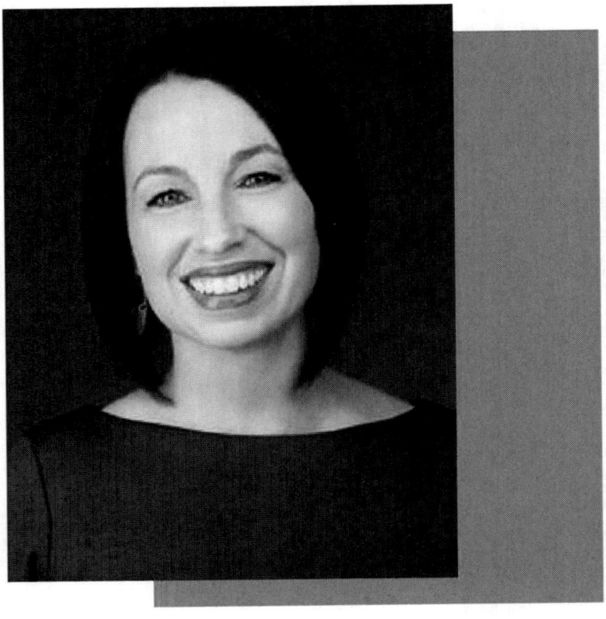

Message from the Nimh Director

As NIMH Director, I am committed to supporting research that addresses mental health disparities – including youth mental health disparities – and informs ways to improve equity in access, utilization, and quality of care for individuals and groups impacted by health disparities. This is a priority that cuts across the whole of NIMH's mission. We need considerably more research focused on innovative solutions for minoritized and underserved youth if we are to truly make a difference.

This Strategic Framework represents a reaffirmation of NIMH's commitment to reducing mental health disparities in youth by 2031 – not only by launching new research programs focused specifically on supporting minoritized youth, but also by integrating this goal more deeply into every aspect of the work that we do across NIMH, ultimately informing mental health policies and practice in real world settings.

In collaboration with our partner agencies and all of you, I fully embrace this opportunity to combat systemic inequities in mental health that impact youth from minoritized groups, and to bring about lasting change for the better in the mental health of all young people.

Sincerely,
Joshua A. Gordon, M.D., Ph.D. Director of NIMH

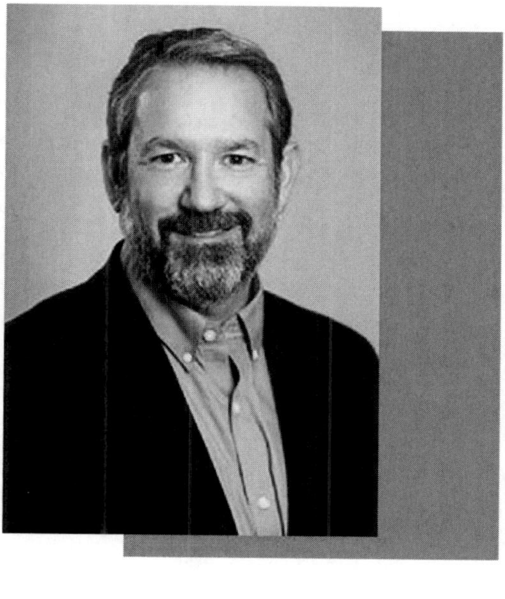

National Institutes of Health

The National Institutes of Health (NIH), within the U.S. Department of Health and Human Services (HHS), is the nation's biomedical research agency – making and supporting vital, lifesaving discoveries and improvements to the health of the nation. The mission of the NIH is to seek fundamental knowledge about the nature and behavior of living systems and apply that knowledge to enhance health, lengthen life, and reduce illness and disability.

National Institute of Mental Health

The National Institute of Mental Health (NIMH) is the lead federal agency for research on mental illnesses. The mission of the NIMH is to transform the understanding and treatment of mental illnesses through basic and clinical research, paving the way for prevention, recovery, and cure. To carry out this mission, NIMH, as established by the Mental Health Act of 1946 and in accordance with Title IV of the Public Health Service Act, conducts and supports biomedical and behavioral research, health services research, research training, and health information dissemination with respect to the causes, diagnosis, treatment, management, and prevention of mental illnesses.

Mental Health Disparities

The NIH National Institute on Minority Health and Health Disparities (NIMHD) defines a health disparity as a health difference, on the basis of one or more health outcomes, that adversely affects disadvantaged populations. U.S. populations negatively impacted by health disparities include Blacks/African Americans, Hispanics/Latinos, American Indians/Alaska Natives (AI/AN), Asian Americans (AA), Native Hawaiians and other Pacific Islanders (NHPI), socioeconomically disadvantaged populations, underserved rural populations, and sexual and gender minorities. Mental health disparities may arise in these populations as a result of differences in the incidence, prevalence, or course of mental illnesses, access to health care, quality of care, experiences of trauma and adversity, and/or inequities in social determinants of health (e.g., education, economic stability, quality of housing, access to health care).

Strategic Framework for Addressing Youth Mental Health Disparities

NIMH initiated the Strategic Framework for Addressing Youth Mental Health Disparities with the overarching goal of advancing scientific knowledge that can be used to inform policies and practices that will reduce mental health disparities in youth by 2031.

This Strategic Framework is structured to align with and supplement the NIMH Strategic Plan for Research and the NIH Minority Health and Health Disparities Strategic Plan. In addition, the Framework complements the priorities of collaborating NIH Institutes, Centers, and Offices (ICOs), including but not limited to NIMHD and the *Eunice Kennedy Shriver* National Institute of Child Health and Human Development (NICHD). The NIMH Office for Disparities Research and Workforce Diversity developed the Strategic Framework, which was refined based on feedback received at the December 2021 conference Identifying Opportunities and Priorities in Youth Mental Health Disparities Research, co-hosted by NIMH, NIMHD, and NICHD. Through 2031, NIMH may periodically update the Framework based on stakeholder feedback, emerging challenges and opportunities, and research advances.

The Strategic Framework encompasses three Components:

- COMPONENT 1: Addressing Knowledge Gaps and Expanding Research Opportunities
- COMPONENT 2: Extending and Supporting Stakeholder Engagement
- COMPONENT 3: Growing the Youth Mental Health Disparities Research Workforce

NIMH seeks to achieve progress in these Components by supporting workforce development and research, and through outreach to and collaboration with a variety of stakeholders. Under each Component, examples of potential actions toward progress as well as examples of potential metrics to assess progress are presented. These examples are not meant to be exhaustive and will be updated and refined as progress is made.

Component 1: Addressing Knowledge Gaps and Expanding Research Opportunities

NIMH will encourage a full and diverse range of research – including basic science, translational science, and services and implementation research – focused on youth mental health disparities through the development of new initiatives and the publication of new Funding Opportunity Announcements (FOAs). These efforts will focus on promoting mental health equity by supporting research on ways to decrease risk, increase resilience and protective factors, improve access to and utilization of quality care, and improve outcomes of treatment and services among populations negatively impacted by mental health disparities.

Examples of potential NIMH actions to address knowledge gaps and expand opportunities for research on youth mental health disparities may include efforts to:

- Support research to elucidate the mechanisms of action of social determinants of mental health, how they can be modified, and how they drive risk of, resilience to, and protection from the development of mental illnesses.
- Support research to identify and understand contextualizing factors, including environmental and historical factors, their impact on biology, emotion, cognition, and behavior, and how they mediate mental health disparities.
- Support research on how local, state, and federal policies, laws, and regulations impact social determinants of mental health, mental health service delivery, and outcomes among youth from populations impacted by mental health disparities.
- Support research on variation in biological and genomic processes within and among diverse populations and settings historically underrepresented in genetics research.
- Support research, including longitudinal studies, to understand and measure how childhood experiences confer resilience to or risk for mental illnesses and suicidal thoughts and behaviors in youth from populations impacted by mental health disparities.
- Support research to improve the specificity of biomarkers and accuracy of culturally appropriate diagnostic assessments (including

risk calculators) for youth from populations impacted by mental health disparities.

- Support the development and validation of culturally appropriate preventive interventions, including systems-level approaches (e.g., in classrooms, schools, communities), for youth and parents from populations impacted by mental health disparities.
- Support the optimization of existing evidence-based approaches to minimize bias in diagnosis and treatment, and to improve continuity of care and mental health outcomes, for youth from populations impacted by mental health disparities.
- Support research to address co-occurring mental illnesses in youth with intellectual and developmental disabilities, including youth with intersectionality with other high-risk groups.
- Support research to improve implementation and availability of mental health prevention and treatment interventions and services, as well as programs to support youth and family functioning, within youth-serving institutions (e.g., educational settings, community based after- school programs, faith-based programs, child welfare programs, juvenile justice settings).
- Support research that uses innovative assessment and analytic methods to examine sub-populations and low base-rate behaviors and to address complex, multi-modal datasets.
- Support translational research on developing, testing, and implementing prevention and treatment interventions that are relevant to communities impacted by health disparities abroad range of ages (e.g., infancy through young adulthood).
- Support research from collaborative teams that include community partners to ensure the outcomes and interpretation of the research reflect the priorities of the population participating in the research.
- Support research to develop targeted interventions by examining risk and resilience within populations impacted by youth mental health disparities.

To estimate progress in addressing knowledge gaps and expanding research opportunities, NIMH could examine:

- Notices of Special Interest (NOSIs) focused on youth mental health disparities.

- FOAs to address youth mental health disparities.
- Grants funded on interventions targeting youth mental health disparities.
- Bibliometrics of NIMH-supported publications (e.g., Relative Citation Ratios).
- Advances related to improving suicide risk prevention and detection among youth from populations impacted by mental health disparities.
- Advances related to improving access, engagement, and effectiveness of evidence-based mental health treatment and services for youth from populations impacted by mental health disparities.
- Advances related to the impact of laws, policies, and structural determinants of health on youth from populations impacted by mental health disparities.

Component 2: Extending and Supporting Stakeholder Engagement

NIMH will engage in outreach, collaboration, and dissemination efforts with youth with mental illnesses and their families, those with interest in or impacted by youth mental health disparities, and those with research expertise. Stakeholders include but are not limited to: patients, families, persons with lived experience, mental health researchers and trainees, other scientists, a range of federal agencies within and outside of HHS, policy makers, non-governmental organizations, educational organizations such as colleges and universities, health care service administrators and payors, clinical care providers, and members of the public. Stakeholder engagement plays an important role in inspiring innovations in science, ensuring the public health relevance of research, encouraging the uptake of evidence-based practices and interventions, decreasing stigma and stereotyping, promoting responsible interpretation and communication of research findings, and increasing overall acceptability of mental health treatments and services, along with public awareness – thus strengthening the public health impact of research.

While NIMH maintains longstanding relationships with numerous stakeholders, additional efforts to include a diversity of perspectives in mental health research will enhance relationships with researchers and populations impacted by health disparities and increase the impact of NIH-supported scientific discoveries. Engagement helps to avoid "othering" and reinforcing stereotypes about youth and families impacted by racial and ethnic health disparities.

Examples of NIMH actions to extend and support stakeholder engagement may include efforts to:

- Seek sustained engagement with stakeholders to inform NIMH's strategies for supporting research that addresses youth mental health disparities.
- Disseminate information about NIMH-supported advances in research on reducing youth mental health disparities.
- Facilitate outreach through professional society and advocacy group meetings to build networking opportunities, connect scientists and community members, and exchange information about the needs of individuals and communities, obstacles to research, and emerging research opportunities related to youth mental health disparities.
- Publish via the NIMH website and social media channels educational materials tailored for families and youth from groups with mental health disparities.
- Encourage NIMH-supported researchers to partner with communities in the development of their research projects, including but not limited to community-based participatory research.
- Promote collaborations across NIH ICOs (e.g., NICHD, NIMHD, the Office of Behavioral and Social Sciences Research (OBSSR)) and with other HHS agencies (e.g., Centers for Medicare and Medicaid Services (CMS), Substance Abuse and Mental Health Services Administration (SAMHSA), Indian Health Service (IHS)) to understand where the gaps in knowledge exist, and how to widely implement evidence-based practices.

To estimate progress in stakeholder engagement, NIMH could examine:

- NIMH-initiated public meetings and outreach activities (e.g., number, reach, impact) about strategies for reducing youth mental health disparities.
- NIMH staff attendance at scientific meetings that cover topics related to youth mental health disparities.
- NIMH data reports related to youth mental health disparities in response to requests from public policy makers.

- Stakeholder engagement with public-facing NIMH messages and educational resources related to youth mental health disparities.
- Investigator-initiated applications incorporating community engagement.
- Collaborations addressing youth mental health disparities across NIHICOs (e.g., NICHD, NIMHD, OBSSR) and with other HHS agencies (e.g., CMS, SAMHSA, IHS).

Component 3: Growing the Youth Mental Health Disparities Research Workforce

NIMH will promote and support the growth and retention of a diverse research workforce, including those well-trained in youth mental health disparities research. To achieve this, NIMH will support a range of research training and career development programs and funding opportunities to build, enhance, and sustain pathways to independent research careers for youth mental health disparities researchers.

Examples of NIMH actions to grow the youth mental health disparities research workforce may include efforts to:

- Promote the training, retention, mentoring, and career transition of investigators in the youth mental health disparities research workforce.
- Participate in cross-NIH programs that promote diversity and inclusivity of the workforce in biomedical research.
- Raise awareness among early-career investigators about the variety of positions that may be involved in youth mental health disparities research.
- Support training for investigators on minimizing bias and other research equity issues.
- Enhance technical assistance, outreach, and capacity-building support to Historically Black Colleges and Universities and other Minority Serving Institutions on applying for research funding, including but not limited to research focused on youth mental health disparities.
- Support the inclusion of diverse perspectives on peer review panels to better appreciate youth mental health disparities research topics.

- Support mechanisms that encourage institutions to diversify their student and faculty populations to enhance the participation and inclusion of individuals from groups that are impacted by mental health disparities.

To estimate progress in growing the youth mental health disparities research workforce, NIMH could examine:

- Grants from Early-Stage Investigators (ESIs) on topics related to youth mental health disparities.
- Individuals supported by NIMH research training and career development mechanisms studying topics related to youth mental health disparities.
- NIMH-supported trainees and ESIs studying topics related to youth mental health disparities who successfully complete the career stage being supported (e.g., completion of pre- or post-doctoral training; transition from "K" award to independent research project grant).
- NIMH-supported trainees and ESIs studying topics related to youth mental health disparities who are successfully retained in the youth mental health disparities research workforce 5-10 years after initial NIMH support.
- Dissemination/reach of NIMH-supported technical assistance and research equity training resources to the youth mental health disparities research workforce.

Chapter 4

Children and Mental Health: Is This Just a Stage?*

National Institute of Mental Health

All children are sad, anxious, irritable, or aggressive at times, and many find it occasionally challenging to sit still, pay attention, or interact with others. In most cases, these are just typical developmental phases. However, such behaviors may also indicate a more serious problem in some children.

What Mental Disorders Can Affect Children?

Many mental disorders can begin in childhood. Examples include anxiety disorders, attention-deficit/hyperactivity disorder (ADHD), depression and other mood disorders, eating disorders, and post-traumatic stress disorder (PTSD).

Early treatment can help children manage their symptoms and support their social and emotional well-being. Many adults reflect on how mental disorders affected their childhood and wish they had received help sooner.

What Are the Signs of Mental Health Conditions in Children?

Distinguishing between challenging behaviors and emotions that are a part of normal development and those that may be cause for concern can be hard.

---

* This is an edited, reformatted and augmented version of The National Institute of Mental Health, NIH Publication No. 24-MH-8085, revised 2024.

In: Healing Minds
Editor: Wilburn M. Conner
ISBN: 979-8-89530-893-6

Consider seeking help if your child's behavior or emotions last for weeks or longer, cause distress for your child or your family, or interfere with your child's functioning at school, at home, or with friends. If your child's behavior is unsafe, or if your child talks about wanting to hurt themselves or someone else, seek help immediately. Learn more about warning signs at www.nimh.nih.gov/children.

When Might Children Benefit from an Evaluation?

Younger Children

- Have frequent tantrums or are irritable much of the time
- Often seem fearful or worried
- Complain about frequent stomachaches or headaches with no known medical cause
- Are in constant motion and cannot sit quietly (except when they are engaged in an activity they enjoy, such as watching videos or playing video games)
- Sleep too much or too little, have frequent nightmares, or seem sleepy during the day
- Are not interested in playing with other children or have difficulty making friends
- Struggle academically or have experienced a recent decline in grades
- Repeat actions or check things many times (for example, repeatedly checking to make sure a door is locked) out of fear that something bad may happen

Older Children

- Have lost interest in things that they used to enjoy
- Have low energy
- Sleep too much or too little or seem sleepy throughout the day
- Have periods of highly elevated energy and activity and require much less sleep than usual
- Spend more and more time alone and avoid social activities with friends or family

- Diet or exercise excessively or fear gaining weight
- Engage in self-harm behaviors (such as cutting or burning their skin)
- Smoke, drink, or use drugs
- Engage in risky or destructive behavior alone or with friends
- Have thoughts of suicide
- Say that they think someone is trying to control their mind or that they hear things that other people cannot hear

Get Immediate Help

If you, your child, or someone you know is struggling or having thoughts of suicide, call or text the 988 Suicide & Crisis Lifeline at *988* or chat at *988lifeline.org*. In life-threatening situations, call *911*.

Where Should I Start If I'm Concerned About My Child's Mental Health?

Being proactive and aware of your child's mental health is an important first step.

If you have concerns about your child's mental health, start by talking with others who frequently interact with your child. For example, ask their teacher about your child's behavior in school, at daycare, or on the playground.

You can talk with your child's pediatrician or health care provider and describe your child's behavior and what you have observed and learned from talking with others. You can also ask the health care provider for a referral to a mental health professional with experience and expertise in evaluating and treating children. Get information about finding a health care provider or accessing treatment at www.nimh.nih.gov/findhelp.

How Is Children's Mental Health Assessed?

An evaluation by a mental health professional can help understand and clarify your child's emotions, behavior, and current situation. Based on this information, the mental health professional can decide if your child would benefit from an intervention and what intervention might work best.

A comprehensive evaluation of a child's mental health usually involves:

- A parent interview to discuss the child's developmental history, temperament, relationships with friends and family, medical history, interests, abilities, and any prior treatment
- Information gathering from the child's school, such as standardized test scores and reports on behavior, capabilities, and difficulties
- If needed, an interview with the child for testing and behavioral observations

Asking questions and providing information to your child's health care provider can improve your child's care. Talking with the health care provider builds trust and leads to better results, quality, safety, and satisfaction with care.

Here are some questions you can ask when meeting with prospective treatment providers.

- Do you use treatment approaches that are supported by research?
- Do you involve parents in the treatment? If so, how are parents involved?
- Will there be "homework" between sessions?
- How will progress be evaluated?
- How soon can we expect to see progress?
- How long should treatment last?

For more ideas on how to start a conversation with your child's health care provider, visit www.nimh.nih.gov/talkingtips.

How Are Childhood Mental Health Disorders Treated?

The mental health professional will review the evaluation results to help determine if a child's emotions and behavior are related to changes or stresses at home or school or if they may indicate a disorder for which they would recommend treatment.

There are several treatment options the mental health professional may recommend.

- Psychotherapy (sometimes called talk therapy), which includes many different approaches such as structured psychotherapies directed at specific conditions. For more information about types of psychotherapies, visit www.nimh.nih.gov/psychotherapies. Effective psychotherapy for children often incorporates:
  - Parent involvement in the treatment
  - Teaching the child skills to practice at home or school (between-session "homework assignments")
  - Measures of progress (such as rating scales and improvements on "homework assignments") that are tracked over time
- Medications, which will depend on the diagnosis and may include antidepressants, stimulants, mood stabilizers, or other medications. For information on
- specific classes of medications, visit www.nimh.nih.gov/medications. Medications are often used in combination with psychotherapy. If multiple health care providers or specialists are involved, treatment information should be shared and coordinated between providers to achieve the best results.
- Family counseling, which includes family members to help them understand how a child's challenges may affect relationships with parents and siblings.
- Support for parents, such as individual or group sessions that include training and the opportunity to talk with other parents. Parental support can provide new strategies for helping a child manage difficult emotions and behavior in a positive way. The therapist can also coach parents on how to work with schools to receive classroom accommodations.

For information about treatment options for specific disorders, visit the NIMH website at www.nimh.nih.gov/health.

How Can the School Support My Child's Mental Health?

Children who have behavioral or emotional challenges that interfere with success in school may benefit from plans or accommodations provided under laws that prevent discrimination against children with disabilities. Your child's health care providers can help you communicate with the school.

A first step may be to ask the school whether accommodations such as an individualized education program (IEP) are appropriate for your child. Accommodations might include providing a child with a tape recorder for taking notes, allowing more time for tests, or adjusting seating in the classroom to reduce distraction.

The U.S. Department of Education offers information and resources on what schools can and, in some cases, must provide for children who would benefit from accommodations and how parents can request evaluation and services for their child.

- The Individuals with Disabilities Education Act (https://sites.ed.gov/idea) consolidates information about how states and public agencies provide early intervention, special education, and related services for infants, toddlers, children, and youth with disabilities.
- The Office for Civil Rights (www.ed.gov/OCR) provides information on federal laws that prohibit discrimination based on disability in public programs, such as schools.
- The Center for Parent Information and Resources (www.parentcenterhub.org/find-your-center) lists Parent Training and Information Centers and Community Parent Resource Centers in each state.

Many organizations listed in the "More information and resources" section also offer information on working with schools and more general information on disorders affecting children.

More Information and Resources

Information on specific disorders is available on the NIMH website (www.nimh.nih.gov/health).

Note: This resource list is provided for informational purposes only. It is not comprehensive and does not constitute an endorsement by NIMH.

The following organizations and agencies have information on symptoms, treatments, and support for childhood mental disorders. Some offer guidance for working with schools and finding mental health professionals. Participating in support groups can provide an avenue for connecting with other parents dealing with similar issues.

- American Academy of Child and Adolescent Psychiatry, Families and Youth (www.aacap org/AACAP/Families_Youth/AACAP/Families_and_Youth/Home.aspx)
- Anxiety and Depression Association of America (https://adaa.org)
- Association for Behavioral and Cognitive Therapies (www.abct.org)
- Centers for Disease Control and Prevention, Children's Mental Health (www.cdc.gov/childrensmentalhealth)
- Child Mind Institute (https://childmind.org/topics-a-z)
- Mental Health America (www.mhanational.org)
- National Alliance on Mental Illness (www.nami.org)
- National Federation of Families (www.ffcmh.org)
- Society of Clinical Child and Adolescent Psychology, Effective Child Therapy (https://effectivechildtherapy.org)
- StopBullying.gov (www.stopbullying.gov)

What Research Is Being Done On Disorders Affecting Children?

NIMH conducts and supports research to help find new and improved ways to diagnose and treat mental disorders that occur in childhood. This research includes studies of risk factors—including genetics, experience, and the environment—which may provide clues to how these disorders develop and how to identify them early.

NIMH also supports efforts to develop and test new interventions, including behavioral, psychotherapeutic, and medication treatments, and ways to improve existing treatments and make them more available in communities, doctor's offices, and schools. Researchers are also exploring whether the benefits of treatment in childhood last into adolescence and adulthood.

What Are Clinical Trials and Why Are They Important?

Children are not little adults, yet they are often given medications and treatments that have been tested only in adults. Research shows that, compared to adults, children respond differently to medications and treatments, both physically and mentally. The way to get the best treatments for children is through research designed specifically for them.

Clinical trials are research studies that look at ways to prevent, detect, or treat diseases and conditions. These studies help show whether a treatment is safe and effective in people.

Some people join clinical trials to help doctors and researchers learn more about a disease and improve health care. Other people, such as those with health conditions, join to try treatments that aren't widely available.

NIMH supports clinical trials across the United States. Talk to a health care provider about clinical trials and whether one is right for your child. For more information, visit www.nimh.nih.gov/clinicaltrials.

For More Information

Learn more at www.nimh.nih.gov/ health. For information about various health topics, visit the National Library of Medicine's MedlinePlus resource at https://medlineplus.gov.

National Institute of Mental Health Office of Science Policy, Planning, and Communications

6001 Executive Boulevard, MSC 9663
Bethesda, MD 20892-9663
Phone: 1-866-615-6464
Email: nimhinfo@nih.gov
Website: www.nimh.nih.gov

Reprints

The information in this publication is in the public domain and may be reused or copied without permission. However, you may not reuse or copy images. Please cite the National Institute of Mental Health as a source. Read our copyright policy to learn more about our guidelines for reusing NIMH content at www.nimh.nih.gov/copyright.

Chapter 5

What Is Telemental Health?*

National Institute of Mental Health

Telemental health is the use of telecommunications or videoconferencing technology to provide mental health services. It is sometimes referred to as telepsychiatry or telepsychology. Research suggests that telemental health services can be effective for many people, including, but not limited to those with attention-deficit/hyperactivity disorder (ADHD), post-traumatic stress disorder (PTSD), depression, and anxiety.

As the need for providing virtual mental health care services has increased, providers are finding ways to use phone and videoconferencing technology to bring therapy, evaluations, interventions, and medication management to individuals where they are.

Although the practice has become much more common, especially as a result of the coronavirus (COVID-19) pandemic, more research is needed to understand when and how telemental health services should be used.

Learn about factors to consider when using telemental health.

Potential Benefits

- Convenience: Telemental health appointments don't require travel and often mean less time off work and smoother logistics coordination for things like transportation or childcare. Patients also can schedule appointments with less advance notice and at more flexible hours.

* This is an edited, reformatted and augmented version of The National Institute of Mental Health NIH Publication No. 21-MH-8155.

In: Healing Minds
Editor: Wilburn M. Conner
ISBN: 979-8-89530-893-6

- Broader reach: The technology is available to people who may not have had access to mental health services previously, including those in remote areas and emergency care situations.
- Fewer barriers: For those who may have been hesitant to look for mental health care in the past, telemental health services might be an easier first step than traditional mental health services.
- Advances in technology: As telemental health services have increased, providers have become more familiar with evolving videoconferencing technology, with some switching to entirely virtual practices.

Potential Drawbacks

- Access to technology: Services may be limited by lack of internet connection and devices.
- Quality issues: Varying levels of technological quality can affect how services are provided and received.
- Cost: Evolving technology means updating equipment, platforms, and networks for patients.
- Privacy: Cameras in users' homes and virtual online platforms pose privacy considerations. Individuals also might be more hesitant to share sensitive personal information with a provider in a situation where others might hear.
- Insurance coverage: The rise in telehealth during the COVID-19 pandemic has led to policy changes to make services accessible to more people. However, it is not known how long such flexibilities will stay in place, and understanding what services are available can be complicated. Coverage and provider licensure requirements vary from state to state.

Finding a Telemental Health Services Provider

Many of the same considerations for finding a provider for in-person mental health services apply to finding a telemental health services provider. Considerations specific to telemental health include:

- Security: As videoconferencing platforms continue to evolve, most providers use secure platforms through which recording isn't possible. Industry best practices for videoconferencing for telemental health services providers suggest selecting platforms with appropriate verification, confidentiality, and security features.
- Introductory sessions: Meeting a provider for the first time in a virtual environment may make it more challenging to determine comfort level. Initial free consultations may make it easier to determine if a telemental health services provider feels like a good fit.

Learn more about getting help and finding a health care provider on the National Institute of Mental Health (NIMH) website at www.nimh.nih.gov/findhelp. The Substance Abuse and Mental Health Services Administration (SAMHSA) offers the Behavioral Health Treatment Services Locator at https://findtreatment.samhsa.gov. Use this online tool to help you find mental health services in your area and to learn whether providers offer telemental health services.

If you are in immediate distress or are thinking about hurting yourself, call the National Suicide Prevention Lifeline toll-free at 1-800-273-TALK (8255)

or the toll-free TTY number at

1-800-799-4TTY (4889). You also can text the Crisis Text Line (HELLO to 741741) or go to the National Suicide Prevention Lifeline website at https://suicidepreventionlifeline.org.

More Resources

- MedlinePlus: Telehealth (https://medlineplus.gov/telehealth.html)
- Department of Health and Human Services: Telehealth (https://www.telehealth.hhs.gov)

Chapter 6

Telehealth Enhancement for Mental Health Act of 2024*

Committee on Energy and Commerce

The Committee on Energy and Commerce, to whom was referred the bill (H.R. 7858) to amend title XVIII of the Social Security Act to establish a Medicare incident to modifier for mental health services furnished through telehealth, having considered the same, reports favorably thereon with amendments and recommends that the bill as amended do pass.

The amendments are as follows:

Strike all after the enacting clause and insert the following:

SECTION 1. SHORT TITLE.

This Act may be cited as the ‘‘Telehealth Enhancement for Mental Health Act of 2024’’ or the ‘‘TELEMH Act of 2024’’.

SEC. 2. ESTABLISHMENT OF MEDICARE INCIDENT TO MODIFIER FOR MENTAL HEALTH SERVICES FURNISHED THROUGH TELEHEALTH AND OTHER TELEHEALTH SERVICES.

Section 1834(m) of the Social Security Act (42 U.S.C. 1395m(m)) is amended by adding at the end the following new paragraph:

‘‘(10) REQUIRED USE OF MODIFIERS IN CERTAIN INSTANCES. — Not later than January 1, 2026, the Secretary shall establish requirements to include a code or modifier, as determined appropriate by the Secretary, in the case of claims for telehealth services under this subsection that are billed incident to a physician's or practitioner's professional service.’’.

Amend the title so as to read:

---

* This is an edited, reformatted and augmented version of House of Representatives Report, Publication No. 118–673, dated September 12, 2024.

In: Healing Minds
Editor: Wilburn M. Conner
ISBN: 979-8-89530-893-6

A bill to amend title XVIII of the Social Security Act to establish a Medicare incident to modifier for mental health services furnished through telehealth and other telehealth services.

Purpose and Summary

H.R. 7858 amends title XVIII of the Social Security Act to establish a Medicare incident to modifier for mental health and other services furnished through telehealth.

Background and Need for Legislation

Prior to the COVID–19 public health emergency, Medicare coverage and reimbursement for services furnished via telehealth was limited and subject to a number of restrictions. Generally, Medicare only reimbursed for telehealth services delivered to a beneficiary in a rural area and at an eligible originating site such as a hospital or physician's office. Medicare also limited reimbursement for telehealth services to a specified set of practitioners, and the program reimbursed only certain covered eligible telehealth services. Additionally, Medicare reimbursed only for telehealth visits that had both audio and visual capabilities (i.e., two-way audiovisual).

Congress greatly expanded Medicare's coverage of telehealth during the COVID–19 Public Health Emergency (PHE). As many as 1 in 4 beneficiaries utilized telehealth during the PHE.[1] Congress further extended these telehealth expansions in the Consolidated Appropriations Act of 2022 beyond the PHE through the end of 2024. Use of telehealth services among Medicare beneficiaries has continued to remain high and far above pre-pandemic levels. Evaluation and management (E/M) services have accounted for almost all of telehealth spending in Medicare. As Congress considers continued extensions of telehealth flexibilities, this bill will increase transparency and allow for more detailed data collection on the types of providers performing telehealth services.

---

[1] Koma, Wyatt, Juliette Cubanski, Tricia Neuman, ''Medicare and Telehealth: Coverage and Use During the COVID–19 Pandemic and Options for the Future'', KFF, 2021, https://www.kff.org/medicare/issue-brief/medicare-and-telehealth-coverage-and-use-during-the-covid-19- pandemic-and-options-for-the-future/.

Committee Action

On April 10, 2024, the Subcommittee on Health held a hearing on H.R. 7858. The title of the hearing was ''Legislative Proposals to Support Patient Access to Telehealth Services.'' The Subcommittee received testimony from:

- Jeanette Ashlock, Patient Advocate, National Multiple Sclerosis Society;
- Fred Riccardi, President, Medicare Rights Center;
- Lee Schwamm, MD, Volunteer, American Health Association; Senior Vice President and Chief Digital Health Officer, Yale New Haven Health System;
- Eve Cunningham, MD, MBA, Group Vice President and Chief of Virtual Care and Digital Health, Providence; and,
- Ateev Mehrotra, MD, MPH, Professor of Health Care Policy and Medicine, Harvard Medical School; Hospitalist, Beth Israel Deaconess Medical Center.

On May 16, 2024, the Subcommittee on Health met in open markup session and forwarded H.R. 7858, as amended, to the full Committee by a recorded vote of 22 yeas and 0 nays.

On June 12, 2024, the full Committee on Energy and Commerce met in open markup session and ordered H.R. 7858, as amended, favorably reported to the House by a recorded vote of 40 yeas and 0 nays.

Committee Votes

Clause 3(b) of rule XIII requires the Committee to list the record votes on the motion to report legislation and amendments thereto. The following reflects the record votes taken during the Committee consideration:

COMMITTEE ON ENERGY AND COMMERCE
118TH CONGRESS
ROLL CALL VOTE # 13

BILL: H.R. 7858, Telehealth Enhancement for Mental Health Act of 2024

AMENDMENT: A motion by Chair Rodgers to order H.R. 7858 favorably reported to the House, as amended (Final Passage).

DISPOSITION: AGREED TO, by a recorded vote of 40 Yeas to 0 Nays.

REPRESENTATIVE	YEAS	NAYS	PRESENT	REPRESENTATIVE	YEAS	NAYS	PRESENT
Rep. Rodgers	X			Rep. Pallone	X		
Rep. Burgess				Rep. Eshoo	X		
Rep. Latta	X			Rep. DeGette			
Rep. Guthrie	X			Rep. Schakowsky	X		
Rep. Griffith	X			Rep. Matsui	X		
Rep. Bilirakis				Rep. Castor	X		
Rep. Bucshon	X			Rep. Sarbanes			
Rep. Hudson	X			Rep. Tonko	X		
Rep. Walberg	X			Rep. Clarke			
Rep. Carter	X			Rep. Cárdenas	X		
Rep. Duncan	X			Rep. Ruiz	X		
Rep. Palmer	X			Rep. Peters	X		
Rep. Dunn	X			Rep. Dingell	X		
Rep. Curtis				Rep. Veasey	X		
Rep. Lesko	X			Rep. Kuster	X		
Rep. Pence	X			Rep. Kelly	X		
Rep. Crenshaw	X			Rep. Barragán			
Rep. Joyce	X			Rep. Blunt Rochester			
Rep. Armstrong				Rep. Soto	X		
Rep. Weber	X			Rep. Craig	X		
Rep. Allen	X			Rep. Schrier	X		
Rep. Balderson	X			Rep. Trahan			
Rep. Fulcher	X			Rep. Fletcher	X		
Rep. Pfluger							
Rep. Harshbarger	X						
Rep. Miller-Meeks	X						
Rep. Cammack							
Rep. Obernolte	X						
Rep. James	X						

06/12/2024

Oversight Findings and Recommendations

Pursuant to clause 2(b)(1) of rule X and clause 3(c)(1) of rule XIII, the Committee held a hearing and made findings that are reflected in this report.

New Budget Authority, Entitlement Authority, and Tax Expenditures

Pursuant to clause 3(c)(2) of rule XIII, the Committee finds that H.R. 7858 would result in no new or increased budget authority, entitlement authority, or tax expenditures or revenues.

Congressional Budget Office Estimate

Pursuant to clause 3(c)(3) of rule XIII, at the time this report was filed, the cost estimate prepared by the Director of the Congressional Budget Office pursuant to section 402 of the Congressional Budget Act of 1974 was not available.

Federal Mandates Statement

The Committee adopts as its own the estimate of Federal mandates prepared by the Director of the Congressional Budget Office pursuant to section 423 of the Unfunded Mandates Reform Act.

Statement of General Performance Goals and Objectives

Pursuant to clause 3(c)(4) of rule XIII, the general performance goal or objective of this legislation is to improve Medicare's delivery of telehealth by collecting data on which type of providers are performing each service billed.

Duplication of Federal Programs

Pursuant to clause 3(c)(5) of rule XIII, no provision of H.R. 7858 is known to be duplicative of another Federal program, including any program that was included in a report to Congress pursuant to section 21 of Public Law 111–139 or the most recent Catalog of Federal Domestic Assistance.

Related Committee and Subcommittee Hearings

Pursuant to clause 3(c)(6) of rule XIII, the following related hearing was used to develop or consider H.R. 7858:

- On April 10, 2024, the Subcommittee on Health held a hearing on H.R. 7858. The title of the hearing was ''Legislative Proposals to Support Patient Access to Telehealth Services.'' The Subcommittee received testimony from:
  - ✓ Jeanette Ashlock, Patient Advocate, National Multiple Sclerosis Society;
  - ✓ Fred Riccardi, President, Medicare Rights Center;
  - ✓ Lee Schwamm, MD, Volunteer, American Health Association; Senior Vice President and Chief Digital Health Officer, Yale New Haven Health System;
  - ✓ Eve Cunningham, MD, MBA, Group Vice President and Chief of Virtual Care and Digital Health, Providence; and,
  - ✓ Ateev Mehrotra, MD, MPH, Professor of Health Care Policy and Medicine, Harvard Medical School; Hospitalist, Beth Israel Deaconess Medical Center.

Committee Cost Estimate

Pursuant to clause 3(d)(1) of rule XIII, the Committee adopts as its own the cost estimate prepared by the Director of the Congressional Budget Office pursuant to section 402 of the Congressional Budget Act of 1974. At the time this report was filed, the estimate was not available.

Earmark, Limited Tax Benefits, and Limited Tariff Benefits

Pursuant to clause 9(e), 9(f), and 9(g) of rule XXI, the Committee finds that H.R. 7858 contains no earmarks, limited tax benefits, or limited tariff benefits.

Advisory Committee Statement

No advisory committees within the meaning of section 5(b) of the Federal Advisory Committee Act were created by this legislation.

Applicability to Legislative Branch

The Committee finds that the legislation does not relate to the terms and conditions of employment or access to public services or accommodations within the meaning of section 102(b)(3) of the Congressional Accountability Act.

Section-by-Section Analysis of the Legislation

Section 1. Short title

Section 1 provides a short title of ''Telehealth Enhancement for Mental Health Act of 2024'' or the ''TELEMH Act of 2024''.

Section 2. Establishment of Medicare incident to modifier for mental health services furnished through telehealth and other telehealth services

Section 2 directs the Secretary to establish a code or modifier for services furnished through telehealth furnished by auxiliary personnel and billed incident to a physician or practitioner's professional services.

Changes in Existing Law Made by the Bill, as Reported

In compliance with clause 3(e) of rule XIII of the Rules of the House of Representatives, changes in existing law made by the bill, as reported, are shown as follows (new matter is printed in italics and existing law in which no change is proposed is shown in roman):

SOCIAL SECURITY ACT

* * * * * * *

TITLE XVIII—HEALTH INSURANCE FOR THE AGED AND DISABLED

* * * * * * *

PART B—SUPPLEMENTARY MEDICAL INSURANCE BENEFITS FOR THE AGED AND DISABLED

* * * * * * *

SPECIAL PAYMENT RULES FOR PARTICULAR ITEMS AND SERVICES

SEC. 1834. (a) PAYMENT FOR DURABLE MEDICAL EQUIPMENT.—

(1) General rule for payment.—

(A) IN GENERAL.—With respect to a covered item (as defined in paragraph (13)) for which payment is determined under this subsection, payment shall be made in the frequency specified in paragraphs (2) through (7) and in an amount equal to 80 percent of the payment basis described in subparagraph (B).

(B) PAYMENT BASIS.—Subject to subparagraph (F)(i), the payment basis described in this subparagraph is the lesser of—

(i) the actual charge for the item, or

(ii) the payment amount recognized under paragraphs (2) through (7) of this subsection for the item; except that clause (i) shall not apply if the covered item is furnished by a public home health agency (or by another home health agency which demonstrates to the satisfaction of the Secretary that a significant portion of its patients are low income) free of charge or at nominal charges to the public.

(C) EXCLUSIVE PAYMENT RULE.—Subject to subparagraph (F)(ii), this subsection shall constitute the exclusive provision of this title for payment for covered items under this part or under part A to a home health agency.

(D) Reduction in fee schedules for certain items.—

With respect to a seat-lift chair or transcutaneous electrical nerve stimulator furnished on or after April 1, 1990, the Secretary shall reduce the payment amount applied under subparagraph (B)(ii) for such an item by 15 percent, and, in the case of a transcutaneous electrical nerve stimulator furnished on or after January 1, 1991, the Secretary shall further reduce such payment amount (as previously reduced) by 45 percent.

(E) Clinical conditions for coverage.—

(i) IN GENERAL.—The Secretary shall establish standards for clinical conditions for payment for covered items under this subsection.

(ii) REQUIREMENTS.—The standards established under clause (i) shall include the specification of types or classes of covered items that require, as a condition of payment under this subsection, a face-to-face examination of the individual by a physician (as defined in section 1861(r)), a physician assistant, nurse practitioner, or a clinical nurse specialist (as those terms are defined in section 1861(aa)(5)) and a prescription for the item.

(iii) PRIORITY OF ESTABLISHMENT OF STANDARDS.—In establishing the standards under this subparagraph, the Secretary shall first establish standards for those covered items for which the Secretary determines there has been a proliferation of use, consistent findings of charges for covered items that are not delivered, or consistent findings of falsification of documentation to provide for payment of such covered items under this part.

(iv) STANDARDS FOR POWER WHEELCHAIRS.—Effective on the date of the enactment of this subparagraph, in the case of a covered item consisting of a motorized or power wheelchair for an individual, payment may not be made for such covered item unless a physician (as defined in section 1861(r)(1)), a physician assistant, nurse practitioner, or a clinical nurse specialist (as those terms are defined in section 1861(aa)(5)) has conducted a face-to-face examination of the individual and written a prescription for the item.

(v) LIMITATION ON PAYMENT FOR COVERED ITEMS.—

Payment may not be made for a covered item under this subsection unless the item meets any standards established under this subparagraph for clinical condition of coverage.

(F) APPLICATION OF COMPETITIVE ACQUISITION; LIMITATION OF INHERENT REASONABLENESS AUTHORITY.—In the case of covered items furnished on or after January 1, 2011, subject to subparagraphs (G) and (H), that are included in a competitive acquisition program in a competitive acquisition area under section 1847(a)—

(i) the payment basis under this subsection for such items and services furnished in such area shall be the payment basis determined under such competitive acquisition program;

(ii) the Secretary may (and, in the case of covered items furnished on or after January 1, 2016, subject to clause (iii), shall) use information on the payment determined under such competitive acquisition programs to adjust the payment amount otherwise recognized under subparagraph (B)(ii) for an area that is not a competitive acquisition area under section 1847 and in the case of such adjustment, paragraph (10)(B) shall not be applied; and

(iii) in the case of covered items furnished on or after January 1, 2016, the Secretary shall continue to make such adjustments described in clause (ii) as, under such competitive acquisition programs, additional covered items are phased in or information is updated as contracts under section 1847 are recompeted in accordance with section 1847(b)(3)(B).

(G) Use of information on competitive bid rates.—

The Secretary shall specify by regulation the methodology to be used in applying the provisions of subparagraph (F)(ii) and subsection (h)(1)(H)(ii). In promulgating such regulation, the Secretary shall consider the costs of items and services in areas in which such provisions would be applied compared to the payment rates for such items and services in competitive acquisition areas.In the case of items and services furnished on or after January 1, 2019, in making any adjustments under clause (ii) or (iii) of subparagraph (F), under subsection (h)(1)(H)(ii), or under section 1842(s)(3)(B), the Secretary shall—

(i) solicit and take into account stakeholder input; and

(ii) take into account the highest amount bid by a winning supplier in a competitive acquisition area and a comparison of each of the following with respect to non-competitive acquisition areas and competitive acquisition areas:

(I) The average travel distance and cost associated with furnishing items and services in the area.

(II) The average volume of items and services furnished by suppliers in the area.

(III) The number of suppliers in the area.

(H) Diabetic supplies.—

(i) IN GENERAL.—On or after the date described in clause (ii), the payment amount under this part for diabetic supplies, including testing strips, that are non-mail order items (as defined by the Secretary) shall be equal to the single payment amounts established under the national mail order competition for diabetic supplies under section 1847.

(ii) DATE DESCRIBED.—The date described in this clause is the date of the implementation of the single payment amounts under the national mail order competition for diabetic supplies under section 1847.

(I) TREATMENT OF VACUUM ERECTION SYSTEMS.—Effective for items and services furnished on and after July 1, 2015, vacuum erection systems described as prosthetic devices described in section 1861(s)(8) shall be treated in the same manner as erectile dysfunction drugs are treated for purposes of section 1860D-2(e)(2)(A).

(2) Payment for inexpensive and other routinely purchased durable medical equipment.—

(A) IN GENERAL.—Payment for an item of durable medical equipment (as defined in paragraph (13))—

(i) the purchase price of which does not exceed $150,

(ii) which the Secretary determines is acquired at least 75 percent of the time by purchase,

(iii) which is an accessory used in conjunction with a nebulizer, aspirator, or a ventilator excluded under paragraph (3)(A), or

(iv) in the case of devices furnished on or after October 1, 2015, which serves as a speech generating device or which is an accessory that is needed for the individual to effectively utilize such a device, shall be made on a rental basis or in a lumpsum amount for the purchase of the item. The payment amount recognized for purchase or rental of such equipment is the amount specified in subparagraph (B) for purchase or rental, except that the total amount of payments with respect to an item may not exceed the payment amount specified in subparagraph (B) with respect to the purchase of the item.

(B) PAYMENT AMOUNT.—For purposes of subparagraph (A), the amount specified in this subparagraph, with respect to the purchase or rental of an item furnished in a carrier service area—

(i) in 1989 and in 1990 is the average reasonable charge in the area for the purchase or rental, respectively, of the item for the 12-month period ending on June 30, 1987, increased by the percentage increase in the consumer price index for all urban consumers (U.S. city average) for the 6-month period ending with December 1987;

(ii) in 1991 is the sum of (I) 67 percent of the local payment amount for the item or device computed under subparagraph (C)(i)(I) for 1991, and (II) 33 percent of the national limited payment amount for the item or device computed under subparagraph (C)(ii) for 1991;

(iii) in 1992 is the sum of (I) 33 percent of the local payment amount for the item or device computed under subparagraph (C)(i)(II) for 1992, and (II) 67 percent of the national limited payment amount for the item or device computed under subparagraph (C)(ii) for 1992; and

(iv) in 1993 and each subsequent year is the national limited payment amount for the item or device computed under subparagraph (C)(ii) for that year (reduced by 10 percent, in the case of a blood glucose testing strip furnished after 1997 for an individual with diabetes).

(C) COMPUTATION OF LOCAL PAYMENT AMOUNT AND NATIONAL LIMITED PAYMENT AMOUNT.—For purposes of subparagraph (B)—

(i) the local payment amount for an item or device for a year is equal to—

(I) for 1991, the amount specified in subparagraph (B)(i) for 1990 increased by the covered item update for 1991, and

(II) for 1992, 1993, and 1994 the amount determined under this clause for the preceding year increased by the covered item update for the year; and

(ii) the national limited payment amount for an item or device for a year is equal to—

(I) for 1991, the local payment amount determined under clause (i) for such item or device for that year, except that the national limited payment amount may not exceed 100 percent of the weighted average of all local payment amounts determined under such clause for such item for that year and may not be less than 85 percent of the weighted average of all local payment amounts determined under such clause for such item,

(II) for 1992 and 1993, the amount determined under this clause for the preceding year increased by the covered item update for such subsequent year,

(III) for 1994, the local payment amount determined under clause (i) for such item or device for that year, except that the national limited payment amount may not exceed 100 percent of the median of all local payment amounts determined under such clause for such item for that year and may not be less than 85 percent of the median of all local payment amounts determined under such clause for such item or device for that year, and

(IV) for each subsequent year, the amount determined under this clause for the preceding year increased by the covered item update for such subsequent year.

(3) Payment for items requiring frequent and substantial servicing.—

(A) IN GENERAL.—Payment for a covered item (such as IPPB machines and ventilators, excluding ventilators that are either continuous airway pressure devices or intermittent assist devices with continuous airway pressure devices) for which there must be frequent and substantial servicing in order to avoid risk to the patient's health shall be made on a monthly basis for the rental of the item and the amount recognized is the amount specified in subparagraph (B).

(B) PAYMENT AMOUNT.—For purposes of subparagraph (A), the amount specified in this subparagraph, with respect to an item or device furnished in a carrier service area—

(i) in 1989 and in 1990 is the average reasonable charge in the area for the rental of the item or device for the 12-month period ending with June 1987, increased by the percentage increase in the consumer price index for all urban consumers (U.S. city average) for the 6-month period ending with December 1987;

(ii) in 1991 is the sum of (I) 67 percent of the local payment amount for the item or device computed under subparagraph (C)(i)(I) for 1991, and (II) 33 percent of the national limited payment amount for the item or device computed under subparagraph (C)(ii) for 1991;

(iii) in 1992 is the sum of (I) 33 percent of the local payment amount for the item or device computed under subparagraph (C)(i)(II) for 1992, and (II) 67 percent of the national limited payment amount for the item or device computed under subparagraph (C)(ii) for 1992; and in 1993 and each subsequent year is the national limited payment amount for the item or device computed under subparagraph (C)(ii) for that year.

(C) COMPUTATION OF LOCAL PAYMENT AMOUNT AND NATIONAL LIMITED PAYMENT AMOUNT.—For purposes of subparagraph (B)—

(i) the local payment amount for an item or device for a year is equal to—

(I) for 1991, the amount specified in subparagraph (B)(i) for 1990 increased by the covered item update for 1991, and

(II) for 1992, 1993, and 1994 the amount determined under this clause for the preceding year increased by the covered item update for the year; and

(ii) the national limited payment amount for an item or device for a year is equal to—

(I) for 1991, the local payment amount determined under clause (i) for such item or device for that year, except that the national limited payment amount may not exceed 100 percent of the weighted average of all local payment amounts determined under such clause for such item for that year and may not be less than 85 percent of the weighted average of all local payment amounts determined under such clause for such item,

(II) for 1992 and 1993, the amount determined under this clause for the preceding year increased by the covered item update for such subsequent year,

(III) for 1994, the local payment amount determined under clause (i) for such item or device for that year, except that the national limited payment amount may not exceed 100 percent of the median of all local payment amounts determined under such clause for such item for that year and may not be less than 85 percent of the median of all local payment amounts determined under such clause for such item or device for that year, and

(IV) for each subsequent year, the amount determined under this clause for the preceding year increased by the covered item update for such subsequent year.

(4) PAYMENT FOR CERTAIN CUSTOMIZED ITEMS.—Payment with respect to a covered item that is uniquely constructed or substantially modified to meet the specific needs of an individual patient, and for that reason cannot be grouped with similar items for purposes of payment under this title, shall be made in a lumpsum amount (A) for the purchase of the item in a payment amount based upon the carrier's individual consideration for that item, and (B) for the reasonable and necessary maintenance and servicing for parts and labor not covered by the supplier's or manufacturer's warranty, when necessary during the period of medical need, and the amount recognized for such maintenance and servicing shall be paid on a lump-sum, as needed basis based upon the carrier's individual consideration for that item. In the case of a wheelchair furnished on or after January 1, 1992, the wheelchair shall be treated as a customized item for purposes of this paragraph if the wheelchair has been measured, fitted, or adapted in consideration of the patient's body size, disability, period of need, or intended use, and has been assembled by a supplier or ordered from a manufacturer who makes available customized features, modifications, or components for wheelchairs that are intended for an individual patient's use in accordance with instructions from the patient's physician.

(5) Payment for oxygen and oxygen equipment.—

(A) IN GENERAL.—Payment for oxygen and oxygen equipment shall be made on a monthly basis in the monthly payment amount recognized under paragraph (9) for oxygen and oxygen equipment (other than portable oxygen equipment), subject to subparagraphs (B), (C), (E), and (F).

(B) ADD-ON FOR PORTABLE OXYGEN EQUIPMENT.—When portable oxygen equipment is used, but subject to subparagraph (D), the payment amount recognized under subparagraph (A) shall be increased by the monthly payment amount recognized under paragraph (9) for portable oxygen equipment.

(C) VOLUME ADJUSTMENT.—When the attending physician prescribes an oxygen flow rate—

(i) exceeding 4 liters per minute, the payment amount recognized under subparagraph (A), subject to subparagraph (D), shall be increased by 50 percent, or

(ii) of less than 1 liter per minute, the payment amount recognized under subparagraph (A) shall be decreased by 50 percent.

(D) LIMIT ON ADJUSTMENT.—When portable oxygen equipment is used and the attending physician prescribes an oxygen flow rate exceeding 4 liters per minute, there shall only be an increase under either subparagraph (B) or (C), whichever increase is larger, and not under both such subparagraphs.

(E) Recertification for patients receiving home OXYGEN THERAPY.—In the case of a patient receiving home oxygen therapy services who, at the time such services are initiated, has an initial arterial blood gas value at or above a partial pressure of 56 or an arterial oxygen saturation at or above 89 percent (or such other values, pressures, or criteria as the Secretary may specify) no payment may be made under this part for such services after the expiration of the 90-day period that begins on the date the patient first receives such services unless the patient's attending physician certifies that, on the basis of a follow-up test of the patient's arterial blood gas value or arterial oxygen saturation conducted during the final 30 days of such 90- day period, there is a medical need for the patient to continue to receive such services.

(F) Rental Cap.—

(i) IN GENERAL.—Payment for oxygen equipment (including portable oxygen equipment) under this paragraph may not extend over a period of continuous use (as determined by the Secretary) of longer than 36 months.

(ii) PAYMENTS AND RULES AFTER RENTAL CAP.—After the 36th continuous month during which payment is made for the equipment under this paragraph—

(I) the supplier furnishing such equipment under this subsection shall continue to furnish the equipment during any period of medical need for the remainder of the reasonable useful lifetime of the equipment, as determined by the Secretary;

(II) payments for oxygen shall continue to be made in the amount recognized for oxygen under paragraph (9) for the period of medical need; and

(III) maintenance and servicing payments shall, if the Secretary determines such payments are reasonable and necessary, be made (for parts and labor not covered by the supplier's or manufacturer's warranty, as determined by the Secretary to be appropriate for the equipment), and such payments shall be in an amount determined to be appropriate by the Secretary.

(6) Payment for other covered items (other than DURABLE MEDICAL EQUIPMENT).—Payment for other covered items (other than durable medical equipment and other covered items described in paragraph (3), (4), or (5)) shall be made in a lumpsum amount for the purchase of the item in the amount of the purchase price recognized under paragraph (8).

(7) Payment for other items of durable medical equipment.—

(A) PAYMENT.—In the case of an item of durable medical equipment not described in paragraphs (2) through (6), the following rules shall apply:

(i) RENTAL.—

(I) IN GENERAL.—Except as provided in clause (iii), payment for the item shall be made on a monthly basis for the rental of the item during the period of medical need (but payments under this clause may not extend over a period of continuous use (as determined by the Secretary) of longer than 13 months).

(II) PAYMENT AMOUNT.—Subject to subclause

(III) and subparagraph (B), the amount recognized for the item, for each of the first 3 months of such period, is 10 percent of the purchase price recognized under paragraph (8) with respect to the item, and, for each of the remaining months of such period, is 7.5 percent of such purchase price.

(III) Special rule for power-driven wheelCHAIRS.—For purposes of payment for power-driven wheelchairs, subclause (II) shall be applied by substituting ''15 percent'' and ''6 percent'' for ''10 percent'' and ''7.5 percent'', respectively.

(ii) OWNERSHIP AFTER RENTAL.—On the first day that begins after the 13th continuous month during which payment is made for the rental of an item under clause (i), the supplier of the item shall transfer title to the item to the individual.

(i) PURCHASE AGREEMENT OPTION FOR COMPLEX, REHABILITATIVE POWER-DRIVEN WHEELCHAIRS.—In the case of a complex, rehabilitative power-driven wheelchair, at the time the supplier furnishes the item, the supplier shall offer the individual the option to purchase the item, and payment for such item shall be made on a lump-sum basis if the individual exercises such option.

(ii) MAINTENANCE AND SERVICING.—After the supplier transfers title to the item under clause (ii) or in the case of a power-driven wheelchair for which a purchase agreement has been entered into under clause (iii), maintenance and servicing payments shall, if the Secretary determines such payments are reasonable and necessary, be made (for parts and labor not covered by the supplier's or manufacturer's warranty, as determined by the Secretary to be appropriate for the particular type of durable medical equipment), and such payments shall be in an amount determined to be appropriate by the Secretary.

(B) Range for rental amounts.—

(i) FOR 1989.—For items furnished during 1989, the payment amount recognized under subparagraph (A)(i) shall not be more than 115 percent, and shall not be less than 85 percent, of the prevailing charge established for rental of the item in January 1987, increased by the percentage increase in the consumer price index for all urban consumers (U.S. city average) for the 6-month period ending with December 1987.

(ii) FOR 1990.—For items furnished during 1990, clause (i) shall apply in the same manner as it applies to items furnished during 1989.

(C) Replacement of items.—

(i) ESTABLISHMENT OF REASONABLE USEFUL LIFETIME.—In accordance with clause (iii), the Secretary shall determine and establish a reasonable useful lifetime for items of durable medical equipment for which payment may be made under this paragraph.

(ii) PAYMENT FOR REPLACEMENT ITEMS.—If the reasonable lifetime of such an item, as so established, has been reached during a continuous period of medical need, or the carrier determines that the item is lost or irreparably damaged, the patient may elect to have payment for an item serving as a replacement for such item made—

(I) on a monthly basis for the rental of the replacement item in accordance with subparagraph (A); or

(II) in the case of an item for which a purchase agreement has been entered into under subparagraph (A)(iii), in a lump-sum amount for the purchase of the item.

(iii) LENGTH OF REASONABLE USEFUL LIFETIME.—The reasonable useful lifetime of an item of durable medical equipment under this subparagraph shall be equal to 5 years, except that, if the Secretary determines that, on the basis of prior experience in making payments for such an item under this title, a reasonable useful lifetime of 5 years is not appropriate with respect to a particular item, the Secretary shall establish an alternative reasonable lifetime for such item.

(2) Purchase price recognized for miscellaneous deVICES AND ITEMS.—For purposes of paragraphs (6) and (7), the amount that is recognized under this paragraph as the purchase price for a covered item is the amount described in subparagraph (C) of this paragraph, determined as follows:

(A) COMPUTATION OF LOCAL PURCHASE PRICE.—Each carrier under section 1842 shall compute a base local purchase price for the item as follows:

(i) The carrier shall compute a base local purchase price, for each item described—

(I) in paragraph (6) equal to the average reasonable charge in the locality for the purchase of the item for the 12-month period ending with June 1987, or

(II) in paragraph (7) equal to the average of the purchase prices on the claims submitted on an assignment-related basis for the unused item supplied during the 6-month period ending with December 1986.

(ii) The carrier shall compute a local purchase price, with respect to the furnishing of each particular item—

(I) in 1989 and 1990, equal to the base local purchase price computed under clause (i) increased by the percentage increase in the consumer price index for all urban consumers (U.S. city average) for the 6-month period ending with December 1987,

(II) in 1991, equal to the local purchase price computed under this clause for the previous year, increased by the covered item update for 1991, and decreased by the percentage by which the average of the reasonable charges for claims paid for all items described in paragraph (7) is lower than the average of the purchase prices submitted for such items during the final 9 months of 1988; or

(III) in 1992, 1993, and 1994 equal to the local purchase price computed under this clause for the previous year increased by the covered item update for the year.

(B) Computation of national limited purchase

PRICE.—With respect to the furnishing of a particular item in a year, the Secretary shall compute a national limited purchase price—

(i) for 1991, equal to the local purchase price computed under subparagraph (A)(ii) for the item for the year, except that such national limited purchase price may not exceed 100 percent of the weighted average of all local purchase prices for the item computed under such subparagraph for the year, and may not be less than 85 percent of the weighted average of all local purchase prices for the item computed under such subparagraph for the year;

(ii) for 1992 and 1993, the amount determined under this subparagraph for the preceding year increased by the covered item update for such subsequent year;

(iii) for 1994, the local purchase price computed under subparagraph (A)(ii) for the item for the year, except that such national limited purchase price may not exceed 100 percent of the median of all local purchase prices computed for the item under such subparagraph for the year and may not be less than 85 percent of the median of all local purchase prices computed under such subparagraph for the item for the year; and

(iv) for each subsequent year, equal to the amount determined under this subparagraph for the preceding year increased by the covered item update for such subsequent year.

(C) PURCHASE PRICE RECOGNIZED.—For purposes of paragraphs (6) and (7), the amount that is recognized under this paragraph as the purchase price for each item furnished—

(i) in 1989 or 1990, is 100 percent of the local purchase price computed under subparagraph (A)(ii)(I);

(ii) in 1991, is the sum of (I) 67 percent of the local purchase price computed under subparagraph (A)(ii)(II) for 1991, and (II) 33 percent of the national limited purchase price computed under subparagraph

(B) for 1991;

(iii) in 1992, is the sum of (I) 33 percent of the local purchase price computed under subparagraph (A)(ii)(III) for 1992, and (II) 67 percent of the national limited purchase price computed under subparagraph

(B) for 1992; and

(iv) in 1993 or a subsequent year, is the national limited purchase price computed under subparagraph

(B) for that year.

(3) Monthly payment amount recognized with respect

TO OXYGEN AND OXYGEN EQUIPMENT.—For purposes of paragraph (5), the amount that is recognized under this paragraph for payment for oxygen and oxygen equipment is the monthly payment amount described in subparagraph (C) of this paragraph. Such amount shall be computed separately (i) for all items of oxygen and oxygen equipment (other than portable oxygen equipment) and (ii) for portable oxygen equipment (each such group referred to in this paragraph as an ''item'').

(A) Computation of local monthly payment rate.—

Each carrier under this section shall compute a base local payment rate for each item as follows:

(i) The carrier shall compute a base local average monthly payment rate per beneficiary as an amount equal to (I) the total reasonable charges for the item during the 12-month period ending with December 1986, divided by (II) the total number of months for all beneficiaries receiving the item in the area during the 12-month period for which the carrier made payment for the item under this title.

(ii) The carrier shall compute a local average monthly payment rate for the item applicable—

(I) to 1989 and 1990, equal to 95 percent of the base local average monthly payment rate computed under clause (i) for the item increased by the percentage increase in the consumer price index for all urban consumers (U.S. city average) for the 6-month period ending with December 1987, or

(II) to 1991, 1992, 1993, and 1994 equal to the local average monthly payment rate computed under this clause for the item for the previous year increased by the covered item increase for the year.

(B) COMPUTATION OF NATIONAL LIMITED MONTHLY PAYMENT RATE.—With respect to the furnishing of an item in a year, the Secretary shall compute a national limited monthly payment rate equal to—

(i) for 1991, the local monthly payment rate computed under subparagraph (A)(ii)(II) for the item for the year, except that such national limited monthly payment rate may not exceed 100 percent of the weighted average of all local monthly payment rates computed for the item under such subparagraph for the year, and may not be less than 85 percent of the weighted average of all local monthly payment rates computed for the item under such subparagraph for the year;

(ii) for 1992 and 1993, the amount determined under this subparagraph for the preceding year increased by the covered item update for such subsequent year;

(iii) for 1994, the local monthly payment rate computed under subparagraph (A)(ii) for the item for the year, except that such national limited monthly payment rate may not exceed 100 percent of the median of all local monthly payment rates computed for the item under such subparagraph for the year and may not be less than 85 percent of the median of all local monthly payment rates computed for the item under such subparagraph for the year;

(iv) for 1995, 1996, and 1997, equal to the amount determined under this subparagraph for the preceding year increased by the covered item update for such subsequent year;

(v) for 1998, 75 percent of the amount determined under this subparagraph for 1997; and

(vi) for 1999 and each subsequent year, 70 percent of the amount determined under this subparagraph for 1997.

(C) MONTHLY PAYMENT AMOUNT RECOGNIZED.—For purposes of paragraph (5), the amount that is recognized under this paragraph as the base monthly payment amount for each item furnished—

(i) in 1989 and in 1990, is 100 percent of the local average monthly payment rate computed under subparagraph (A)(ii) for the item;

(ii) in 1991, is the sum of (I) 67 percent of the local average monthly payment rate computed under subparagraph (A)(ii)(II) for the item for 1991, and (II) 33 percent of the national limited monthly payment rate computed under subparagraph (B)(i) for the item for 1991;

(iii) in 1992, is the sum of (I) 33 percent of the local average monthly payment rate computed under subparagraph (A)(ii)(II) for the item for 1992, and (II) 67 percent of the national limited monthly payment rate computed under subparagraph (B)(ii) for the item for 1992; and

(iv) in a subsequent year, is the national limited monthly payment rate computed under subparagraph

(B) for the item for that year.

(D) Authority to create classes.—

(i) IN GENERAL.—Subject to clause (ii), the Secretary may establish separate classes for any item of oxygen and oxygen equipment and separate national limited monthly payment rates for each of such classes.

(ii) BUDGET NEUTRALITY.—The Secretary may take actions under clause (i) only to the extent such actions do not result in expenditures for any year to be more or less than the expenditures which would have been made if such actions had not been taken. The requirement of the preceding sentence shall not apply beginning with the second calendar quarter beginning on or after the date of the enactment of this sentence.

(4) Exceptions and adjustments.—

(A) AREAS OUTSIDE CONTINENTAL UNITED STATES.—Exceptions to the amounts recognized under the previous provisions of this subsection shall be made to take into account the unique circumstances of covered items furnished in Alaska, Hawaii, or Puerto Rico.

(B) ADJUSTMENT FOR INHERENT REASONABLENESS.—The Secretary is authorized to apply the provisions of paragraphs (8) and (9) of section 1842(b) to covered items and suppliers of such items and payments under this subsection in an area and with respect to covered items and services for which the Secretary does not make a payment amount adjustment under paragraph (1)(F).

(C) Transcutaneous electrical nerve stimulator

(TENS).—In order to permit an attending physician time to determine whether the purchase of a transcutaneous electrical nerve stimulator is medically appropriate for a particular patient, the Secretary may determine an appropriate payment amount for the initial rental of such item for a period of not more than 2 months. If such item is subsequently purchased, the payment amount with respect to such purchase is the payment amount determined under paragraph (2).

(5) Improper billing and requirement of physician order.—

(A) IMPROPER BILLING FOR CERTAIN RENTAL ITEMS.—Notwithstanding any other provision of this title, a supplier of a covered item for which payment is made under this subsection and which is furnished on a rental basis shall continue to supply the item without charge (other than a charge provided under this subsection for the maintenance and servicing of the item) after rental payments may no longer be made under this subsection. If a supplier knowingly and willfully violates the previous sentence, the Secretary may apply sanctions against the supplier under section 1842(j)(2) in the same manner such sanctions may apply with respect to a physician.

(B) Requirement of physician order.—

(i) IN GENERAL.—The Secretary is authorized to require, for specified covered items, that payment may be made under this subsection with respect to the item only if a physician enrolled under section 1866(j) or an eligible professional under section 1848(k)(3)(B) that is enrolled under section 1866(j) has communicated to the supplier, before delivery of the item, a written order for the item.

(ii) REQUIREMENT FOR FACE TO FACE ENCOUNTER.—

The Secretary shall require that such an order be written pursuant to a physician, a physician assistant, a nurse practitioner, or a clinical nurse specialist (as those terms are defined in section 1861(aa)(5)) documenting such physician, physician assistant, practitioner, or specialist has had a face-to-face encounter (including through use of telehealth under subsection

(m) and other than with respect to encounters that are incident to services involved) with the individual involved during the 6-month period preceding such written order, or other reasonable timeframe as determined by the Secretary.

(6) REGIONAL CARRIERS.—The Secretary may designate, by regulation under section 1842, one carrier for one or more entire regions to process all claims within the region for covered items under this section.

(7) COVERED ITEM.—In this subsection, the term ''covered item'' means durable medical equipment (as defined in section 1861(n)), including such equipment described in section 1861(m)(5), but not including implantable items for which payment may be made under section 1833(t).

(8) COVERED ITEM UPDATE.—In this subsection, the term ''covered item update'' means, with respect to a year—

(A) for 1991 and 1992, the percentage increase in the consumer price index for all urban consumers (U.S. city average) for the 12-month period ending with June of the previous year reduced by 1 percentage point;

(B) for 1993, 1994, 1995, 1996, and 1997, the percentage increase in the consumer price index for all urban consumers (U.S. city average) for the 12-month period ending with June of the previous year;

(C) for each of the years 1998 through 2000, 0 percentage points;

(D) for 2001, the percentage increase in the consumer price index for all urban consumers (U.S. city average) for the 12-month period ending with June 2000;

(E) for 2002, 0 percentage points;

(F) for 2003, the percentage increase in the consumer price index for all urban consumers (U.S. urban average) for the 12-month period ending with June of 2002;

(G) for 2004 through 2006—

(i) subject to clause (ii), in the case of class III medical devices described in section 513(a)(1)(C) of the Federal Food, Drug, and Cosmetic Act (21 U.S.C. 360(c)(1)(C)), the percentage increase described in subparagraph (B) for the year involved; and

(ii) in the case of covered items not described in clause (i), 0 percentage points;

(H) for 2007—

(i) subject to clause (ii), in the case of class III medical devices described in section 513(a)(1)(C) of the Federal Food, Drug, and Cosmetic Act (21 U.S.C. 360(c)(1)(C)), the percentage change determined by the Secretary to be appropriate taking into account recommendations contained in the report of the Comptroller General of the United States under section 302(c)(1)(B) of the Medicare Prescription Drug, Improvement, and Modernization Act of 2003; and

(ii) in the case of covered items not described in clause (i), 0 percentage points;

(I) for 2008—

(i) subject to clause (ii), in the case of class III medical devices described in section 513(a)(1)(C) of the Federal Food, Drug, and Cosmetic Act (21 U.S.C. 360(c)(1)(C)), the percentage increase described in subparagraph (B) (as applied to the payment amount for 2007 determined after the application of the percentage change under subparagraph (H)(i)); and

(ii) in the case of covered items not described in clause (i), 0 percentage points;

(J) for 2009—

(i) in the case of items and services furnished in any geographic area, if such items or services were selected for competitive acquisition in any area under the competitive acquisition program under section 1847(a)(1)(B)(i)(I) before July 1, 2008, including related accessories but only if furnished with such items and services selected for such competition and diabetic supplies but only if furnished through mail order, - 9.5 percent; or in the case of other items and services, the percentage increase in the consumer price index for all urban consumers (U.S. urban average) for the 12- month period ending with June 2008;

(K) for 2010, the percentage increase in the consumer price index for all urban consumers (U.S. urban average) for the 12-month period ending with June of the previous year; and

(L) for 2011 and each subsequent year—

(i) the percentage increase in the consumer price index for all urban consumers (United States city average) for the 12-month period ending with June of the previous year, reduced by—

(ii) the productivity adjustment described in section 1886(b)(3)(B)(xi)(II).

The application of subparagraph (L)(ii) may result in the covered item update under this paragraph being less than 0.0 for a year, and may result in payment rates under this subsection for a year being less than such payment rates for the preceding year.

(9) Advance determinations of coverage for certain items.—

(A) Development of lists of items by secretary.—

The Secretary may develop and periodically update a list of items for which payment may be made under this subsection that the Secretary determines, on the basis of prior payment experience, are frequently subject to unnecessary utilization throughout a carrier's entire service area or a portion of such area.

(B) Development of lists of suppliers by secretary.—The Secretary may develop and periodically update a list of suppliers of items for which payment may be made under this subsection with respect to whom—

(i) the Secretary has found that a substantial number of claims for payment under this part for items furnished by the supplier have been denied on the basis of the application of section 1862(a)(1); or

(ii) the Secretary has identified a pattern of over-utilization resulting from the business practice of the supplier.

(C) DETERMINATIONS OF COVERAGE IN ADVANCE.—A carrier shall determine in advance of delivery of an item whether payment for the item may not be made because the item is not covered or because of the application of section 1862(a)(1) if—

(i) the item is included on the list developed by the Secretary under subparagraph (A);

(ii) the item is furnished by a supplier included on the list developed by the Secretary under subparagraph (B); or

(iii) the item is a customized item (other than inexpensive items specified by the Secretary) and the patient to whom the item is to be furnished or the supplier requests that such advance determination be made.

(10) DISCLOSURE OF INFORMATION AND SURETY BOND.—The Secretary shall not provide for the issuance (or renewal) of a provider number for a supplier of durable medical equipment, for purposes of payment under this part for durable medical equipment furnished by the supplier, unless the supplier provides the Secretary on a continuing basis—

(A) with—

(i) full and complete information as to the identity of each person with an ownership or control interest (as defined in section 1124(a)(3)) in the supplier or in any subcontractor (as defined by the Secretary in regulations) in which the supplier directly or indirectly has a 5 percent or more ownership interest; and

(ii) to the extent determined to be feasible under regulations of the Secretary, the name of any disclosing entity (as defined in section 1124(a)(2)) with respect to which a person with such an ownership or control interest in the supplier is a person with such an ownership or control interest in the disclosing entity; and

(B) with a surety bond in a form specified by the Secretary and in an amount that is not less than $50,000 that the Secretary determines is commensurate with the volume of the billing of the supplier.

The Secretary may waive the requirement of a bond under subparagraph (B) in the case of a supplier that provides a comparable surety bond under State law. The Secretary, at the Secretary's discretion, may impose the requirements of the first sentence with respect to some or all providers of items or services under part A or some or all suppliers or other persons (other than physicians or other practitioners, as defined in section 1842(b)(18)(C)) who furnish items or services under this part.

(11) Prohibition against unsolicited telephone contacts by suppliers.—

(A) IN GENERAL.—A supplier of a covered item under this subsection may not contact an individual enrolled under this part by telephone regarding the furnishing of a covered item to the individual unless 1 of the following applies:

(i) The individual has given written permission to the supplier to make contact by telephone regarding the furnishing of a covered item.

(ii) The supplier has furnished a covered item to the individual and the supplier is contacting the individual only regarding the furnishing of such covered item.

(iii) If the contact is regarding the furnishing of a covered item other than a covered item already furnished to the individual, the supplier has furnished at least 1 covered item to the individual during the 15- month period preceding the date on which the supplier makes such contact.

(B) PROHIBITING PAYMENT FOR ITEMS FURNISHED SUBSEQUENT TO UNSOLICITED CONTACTS.—If a supplier knowingly contacts an individual in violation of subparagraph (A), no payment may be made under this part for any item subsequently furnished to the individual by the supplier.

(C) EXCLUSION FROM PROGRAM FOR SUPPLIERS ENGAGING IN PATTERN OF UNSOLICITED CONTACTS.—If a supplier knowingly contacts individuals in violation of subparagraph (A) to such an extent that the supplier's conduct establishes a pattern of contacts in violation of such subparagraph, the Secretary shall exclude the supplier from participation in the programs under this Act, in accordance with the procedures set forth in subsections (c), (f), and (g) of section 1128.

(12) Refund of amounts collected for certain disallowed items.—

(A) IN GENERAL.—If a nonparticipating supplier furnishes to an individual enrolled under this part a covered item for which no payment may be made under this part by reason of paragraph (17)(B), the supplier shall refund on a timely basis to the patient (and shall be liable to the patient for) any amounts collected from the patient for the item, unless—

(i) the supplier establishes that the supplier did not know and could not reasonably have been expected to know that payment may not be made for the item by reason of paragraph (17)(B), or

(ii) before the item was furnished, the patient was informed that payment under this part may not be made for that item and the patient has agreed to pay for that item.

(B) SANCTIONS.—If a supplier knowingly and willfully fails to make refunds in violation of subparagraph (A), the Secretary may apply sanctions against the supplier in accordance with section 1842(j)(2).

(C) NOTICE.—Each carrier with a contract in effect under this part with respect to suppliers of covered items shall send any notice of denial of payment for covered items by reason of paragraph (17)(B) and for which payment is not requested on an assignment-related basis to the supplier and the patient involved.

(D) TIMELY BASIS DEFINED.—A refund under subparagraph (A) is considered to be on a timely basis only if—

(i) in the case of a supplier who does not request reconsideration or seek appeal on a timely basis, the refund is made within 30 days after the date the supplier receives a denial notice under subparagraph (C), or

(ii) in the case in which such a reconsideration or appeal is taken, the refund is made within 15 days after the date the supplier receives notice of an adverse determination on reconsideration or appeal.

(13) Certain upgraded items.—

(A) Individual's right to choose upgraded item.—

Notwithstanding any other provision of this title, the Secretary may issue regulations under which an individual may purchase or rent from a supplier an item of upgraded durable medical equipment for which payment would be made under this subsection if the item were a standard item.

(B) PAYMENTS TO SUPPLIER.—In the case of the purchase or rental of an upgraded item under subparagraph (A)—

(i) the supplier shall receive payment under this subsection with respect to such item as if such item were a standard item; and

(ii) the individual purchasing or renting the item shall pay the supplier an amount equal to the difference between the supplier's charge and the amount under clause (i).

In no event may the supplier's charge for an upgraded item exceed the applicable fee schedule amount (if any) for such item.

(C) CONSUMER PROTECTION SAFEGUARDS.—Any regulations under subparagraph (A) shall provide for consumer protection standards with respect to the furnishing of upgraded equipment under subparagraph (A). Such regulations shall provide for—

(i) determination of fair market prices with respect to an upgraded item;

(ii) full disclosure of the availability and price of standard items and proof of receipt of such disclosure information by the beneficiary before the furnishing of the upgraded item;

(iii) conditions of participation for suppliers in the billing arrangement;

(iv) sanctions of suppliers who are determined to engage in coercive or abusive practices, including exclusion; and

(v) such other safeguards as the Secretary determines are necessary.

(14) Identification of quality standards.—

(A) IN GENERAL.—Subject to subparagraph (C), the Secretary shall establish and implement quality standards for suppliers of items and services described in subparagraph

(D) to be applied by recognized independent accreditation organizations (as designated under subparagraph (B)) and with which such suppliers shall be required to comply in order to—

(i) furnish any such item or service for which payment is made under this part; and

(ii) receive or retain a provider or supplier number used to submit claims for reimbursement for any such item or service for which payment may be made under this title.

(B) DESIGNATION OF INDEPENDENT ACCREDITATION ORGANIZATIONS.—Not later than the date that is 1 year after the date on which the Secretary implements the quality standards under subparagraph (A), notwithstanding section 1865(a), the Secretary shall designate and approve one or more independent accreditation organizations for purposes of such subparagraph.

(C) QUALITY STANDARDS.—The quality standards described in subparagraph (A) may not be less stringent than the quality standards that would otherwise apply if this paragraph did not apply and shall include consumer services standards.

(D) ITEMS AND SERVICES DESCRIBED.—The items and

services described in this subparagraph are the following items and services, as the Secretary determines appropriate:

(i) Covered items (as defined in paragraph (13)) for which payment may otherwise be made under this subsection.

(ii) Prosthetic devices and orthotics and prosthetics described in section 1834(h)(4).

(iii) Items and services described in section 1842(s)(2).

(iv) Lymphedema compression treatment items (as defined in section 1861(mmm)).

(E) IMPLEMENTATION.—The Secretary may establish by program instruction or otherwise the quality standards under this paragraph, including subparagraph (F), after consultation with representatives of relevant parties. Such standards shall be applied prospectively and shall be published on the Internet website of the Centers for Medicare & Medicaid Services.

(F) APPLICATION OF ACCREDITATION REQUIREMENT.—In implementing quality standards under this paragraph—

(i) subject to clause (ii) and subparagraph (G), the Secretary shall require suppliers furnishing items and services described in subparagraph (D) on or after October 1, 2009, directly or as a subcontractor for another entity, to have submitted to the Secretary evidence of accreditation by an accreditation organization designated under subparagraph (B) as meeting applicable quality standards, except that the Secretary shall not require under this clause pharmacies to obtain such accreditation before January 1, 2010, except that the Secretary shall not require a pharmacy to have submitted to the Secretary such evidence of accreditation prior to January 1, 2011; and

(ii) in applying such standards and the accreditation requirement of clause (i) with respect to eligible professionals (as defined in section 1848(k)(3)(B)), and including such other persons, such as orthotists and prosthetists, as specified by the Secretary, furnishing such items and services—

(I) such standards and accreditation requirement shall not apply to such professionals and persons unless the Secretary determines that the standards being applied are designed specifically to be applied to such professionals and persons; and

(II) the Secretary may exempt such professionals and persons from such standards and requirement if the Secretary determines that licensing, accreditation, or other mandatory quality requirements apply to such professionals and persons with respect to the furnishing of such items and services.

(A) Application of accreditation requirement to certain pharmacies.—

(i) IN GENERAL.—With respect to items and services furnished on or after January 1, 2011, in implementing quality standards under this paragraph—

(I) subject to subclause (II), in applying such standards and the accreditation requirement of subparagraph (F)(i) with respect to pharmacies described in clause (ii) furnishing such items and services, such standards and accreditation requirement shall not apply to such pharmacies; and

(II) the Secretary may apply to such pharmacies an alternative accreditation requirement established by the Secretary if the Secretary determines such alternative accreditation requirement is more appropriate for such pharmacies.

(ii) PHARMACIES DESCRIBED.—A pharmacy described in this clause is a pharmacy that meets each of the following criteria:

(I) The total billings by the pharmacy for such items and services under this title are less than 5 percent of total pharmacy sales, as determined based on the average total pharmacy sales for the previous 3 calendar years, 3 fiscal years, or other yearly period specified by the Secretary.

(II) The pharmacy has been enrolled under section 1866(j) as a supplier of durable medical equipment, prosthetics, orthotics, and supplies, has been issued (which may include the renewal of) a provider number for at least 5 years, and for which a final adverse action (as defined in section 424.57(a) of title 42, Code of Federal Regulations) has not been imposed in the past 5 years.

(III) The pharmacy submits to the Secretary an attestation, in a form and manner, and at a time, specified by the Secretary, that the pharmacy meets the criteria described in subclauses (I) and (II). Such attestation shall be subject to section 1001 of title 18, United States Code.

(IV) The pharmacy agrees to submit materials as requested by the Secretary, or during the course of an audit conducted on a random sample of pharmacies selected annually, to verify that the pharmacy meets the criteria described in subclauses (I) and (II). Materials submitted under the preceding sentence shall include a certification by an accountant on behalf of the pharmacy or the submission of tax returns filed by the pharmacy during the relevant periods, as requested by the Secretary.

(2) Special payment rule for specified items and supplies.—

(A) IN GENERAL.—Notwithstanding the preceding provisions of this subsection, for specified items and supplies (described in subparagraph (B)) furnished during 2005, the payment amount otherwise determined under this subsection for such specified items and supplies shall be reduced by the percentage difference between—

(i) the amount of payment otherwise determined for the specified item or supply under this subsection for 2002, and the amount of payment for the specified item or supply under chapter 89 of title 5, United States Code, as identified in the column entitled ''Median FEHP Price'' in the table entitled ''SUMMARY OF MEDICARE PRICES COMPARED TO VA, MEDICAID, RETAIL, AND FEHP PRICES FOR 16 ITEMS'' included in the Testimony of the Inspector General before the Senate Committee on Appropriations, June 12, 2002, or any subsequent report by the Inspector General.

(B) SPECIFIED ITEM OR SUPPLY DESCRIBED.—For purposes of subparagraph (A), a specified item or supply means oxygen and oxygen equipment, standard wheelchairs (including standard power wheelchairs), nebulizers, diabetic supplies consisting of lancets and testing strips, hospital beds, and air mattresses, but only if the HCPCS code for the item or supply is identified in a table referred to in subparagraph (A)(ii).

(C) Application of update to special payment

AMOUNT.—The covered item update under paragraph (14) for specified items and supplies for 2006 and each subsequent year shall be applied to the payment amount under subparagraph (A) unless payment is made for such items and supplies under section 1847.

(3) SPECIAL PAYMENT RULE FOR DIABETIC SUPPLIES.—Notwithstanding the preceding provisions of this subsection, for purposes of determining the payment amount under this subsection for diabetic supplies furnished on or after the first day of the calendar quarter during 2013 that is at least 30 days after the date of the enactment of this paragraph and before the date described in paragraph (1)(H)(ii), the Secretary shall recalculate and apply the covered item update under paragraph (14) as if subparagraph (J)(i) of such paragraph was amended by striking ‘‘but only if furnished through mail order’’.

(B) FEE SCHEDULES FOR RADIOLOGIST SERVICES.—

(1) DEVELOPMENT.—The Secretary shall develop—

(A) a relative value scale to serve as the basis for the payment for radiologist services under this part, and

(B) using such scale and appropriate conversion factors and subject to subsection (c)(1)(A), fee schedules (on a regional, statewide, locality, or carrier service area basis) for payment for radiologist services under this part, to be implemented for such services furnished during 1989.

(2) CONSULTATION.—In carrying out paragraph (1), the Secretary shall regularly consult closely with the Physician Payment Review Commission, the American College of Radiology, and other organizations representing physicians or suppliers who furnish radiologist services and shall share with them the data and data analysis being used to make the determinations under paragraph (1), including data on variations in current medicare payments by geographic area, and by service and physician specialty.

(3) CONSIDERATIONS.—In developing the relative value scale and fee schedules under paragraph (1), the Secretary—

(A) shall take into consideration variations in the cost of furnishing such services among geographic areas and among different sites where services are furnished, and

(B) may also take into consideration such other factors respecting the manner in which physicians in different specialties furnish such services as may be appropriate to assure that payment amounts are equitable and designed to promote effective and efficient provision of radiologist services by physicians in the different specialties.

(4) SAVINGS.—

(A) BUDGET NEUTRAL FEE SCHEDULES.—The Secretary shall develop preliminary fee schedules for 1989, which are designed to result in the same amount of aggregate payments (net of any coinsurance and deductibles under sections 1833(a)(1)(J) and 1833(b)) for radiologist services furnished in 1989 as would have been made if this subsection had not been enacted.

(B) INITIAL SAVINGS.—The fee schedules established for payment purposes under this subsection for services furnished in 1989 shall be 97 percent of the amounts permitted under these preliminary fee schedules developed under subparagraph (A).

(C) 1990 FEE SCHEDULES.—For radiologist services (other than portable X-ray services) furnished under this part during 1990, after March 31 of such year, the conversion factors used under this subsection shall be 96 percent of the conversion factors that applied under this subsection as of December 31, 1989.

(D) 1991 FEE SCHEDULES.—For radiologist services (other than portable X-ray services) furnished under this part during 1991, the conversion factors used in a locality under this subsection shall, subject to clause (vii), be reduced to the adjusted conversion factor for the locality determined as follows:

(i) NATIONAL WEIGHTED AVERAGE CONVERSION FACTOR.—The Secretary shall estimate the national weighted average of the conversion factors used under this subsection for services furnished during 1990 beginning on April 1, using the best available data.

(ii) REDUCED NATIONAL WEIGHTED AVERAGE.—The national weighted average estimated under clause (i) shall be reduced by 13 percent.

(iii) COMPUTATION OF 1990 LOCALITY INDEX RELATIVE TO NATIONAL AVERAGE.—The Secretary shall establish an index which reflects, for each locality, the ratio of the conversion factor used in the locality under this subsection to the national weighted average estimated under clause (i).

(iv) ADJUSTED CONVERSION FACTOR.—The adjusted conversion factor for the professional or technical component of a service in a locality is the sum of 1⁄2 of the locally-adjusted amount determined under clause (v) and 1⁄2 of the GPCI-adjusted amount determined under clause (vi).

(v) LOCALLY-ADJUSTED AMOUNT.—For purposes of clause (iv), the locally adjusted amount determined under this clause is the product of (I) the national weighted average conversion factor computed under clause (ii), and (II) the index value established under clause (iii) for the locality.

(vi) GPCI-ADJUSTED AMOUNT.—For purposes of clause (iv), the GPCI-adjusted amount determined under this clause is the sum of—

(I) the product of (a) the portion of the reduced national weighted average conversion factor computed under clause (ii) which is attributable to physician work and (b) the geographic work index value for the locality (specified in Addendum C to the Model Fee Schedule for Physician Services (published on September 4, 1990, 55 Federal Register pp. 36238–36243)); and

(II) the product of (a) the remaining portion of the reduced national weighted average conversion factor computed under clause (ii), and (b) the geographic practice cost index value specified in section 1842(b)(14)(C)(iv) for the locality.

In applying this clause with respect to the professional component of a service, 80 percent of the conversion factor shall be considered to be attributable to physician work and with respect to the technical component of the service, 0 percent shall be considered to be attributable to physician work.

(vii) LIMITS ON CONVERSION FACTOR.—The conversion factor to be applied to a locality to the professional or technical component of a service shall not be reduced under this subparagraph by more than 9.5 percent below the conversion factor applied in the locality under subparagraph (C) to such component, but in no case shall the conversion factor be less than 60 percent of the national weighted average of the conversion factors (computed under clause (i)).

(E) RULE FOR CERTAIN SCANNING SERVICES.—In the case of the technical components of magnetic resonance imaging (MRI) services and computer assisted tomography (CAT) services furnished after December 31, 1990, the amount otherwise payable shall be reduced by 10 percent.

(F) SUBSEQUENT UPDATING.—For radiologist services furnished in subsequent years, the fee schedules shall be the schedules for the previous year updated by the percentage increase in the MEI (as defined in section 1842(i)(3)) for the year.

(G) Nonparticipating physicians and suppliers.—

Each fee schedule so established shall provide that the payment rate recognized for nonparticipating physicians and suppliers is equal to the appropriate percent (as defined in section 1842(b)(4)(A)(iv)) of the payment rate recognized for participating physicians and suppliers.

(5) Limiting charges of nonparticipating physicians and suppliers.—

(A) IN GENERAL.—In the case of radiologist services furnished after January 1, 1989, for which payment is made under a fee schedule under this subsection, if a nonparticipating physician or supplier furnishes the service to an individual entitled to benefits under this part, the physician or supplier may not charge the individual more than the limiting charge (as defined in subparagraph (B)).

(B) LIMITING CHARGE DEFINED.—In subparagraph (A),

the term ''limiting charge'' means, with respect to a service furnished—

(i) in 1989, 125 percent of the amount specified for the service in the appropriate fee schedule established under paragraph (1),

(ii) in 1990, 120 percent of the amount specified for the service in the appropriate fee schedule established under paragraph (1), and

(iii) after 1990, 115 percent of the amount specified for the service in the appropriate fee schedule established under paragraph (1).

(C) ENFORCEMENT.—If a physician or supplier knowingly and willfully bills in violation of subparagraph (A), the Secretary may apply sanctions against such physician or supplier in accordance with section 1842(j)(2) in the same manner as such sanctions may apply to a physician.

(6) RADIOLOGIST SERVICES DEFINED.—For the purposes of this subsection and section 1833(a)(1)(J), the term ''radiologist services'' only includes radiology services performed by, or under the direction or supervision of, a physician—

(A) who is certified, or eligible to be certified, by the American Board of Radiology, or

(B) for whom radiology services account for at least 50 percent of the total amount of charges made under this part.

(c) PAYMENT AND STANDARDS FOR SCREENING MAMMOGRAPHY.—

(1) IN GENERAL.—With respect to expenses incurred for screening mammography (as defined in section 1861(jj)), payment may be made only—

(A) for screening mammography conducted consistent with the frequency permitted under paragraph (2); and

(B) if the screening mammography is conducted by a facility that has a certificate (or provisional certificate) issued under section 354 of the Public Health Service Act.

(2) Frequency covered.—

(A) IN GENERAL.—Subject to revision by the Secretary under subparagraph (B)—

(i) no payment may be made under this part for screening mammography performed on a woman under 35 years of age;

(ii) payment may be made under this part for only one screening mammography performed on a woman over 34 years of age, but under 40 years of age; and

(iii) in the case of a woman over 39 years of age, payment may not be made under this part for screening mammography performed within 11 months following the month in which a previous screening mammography was performed.

(B) Revision of frequency.—

(i) REVIEW.—The Secretary, in consultation with the Director of the National Cancer Institute, shall review periodically the appropriate frequency for performing screening mammography, based on age and such other factors as the Secretary believes to be pertinent.

(ii) REVISION OF FREQUENCY.—The Secretary, taking into consideration the review made under clause (i), may revise from time to time the frequency with which screening mammography may be paid for under this subsection.

(d) FREQUENCY LIMITS AND PAYMENT FOR COLORECTAL CANCER SCREENING TESTS.—

(1) Screening fecal-occult blood tests.—

(A) PAYMENT AMOUNT.—The payment amount for colorectal cancer screening tests consisting of screening fecal-occult blood tests is equal to the payment amount established for diagnostic fecal-occult blood tests under section 1833(h).

(B) FREQUENCY LIMIT.—No payment may be made under this part for a colorectal cancer screening test consisting of a screening fecal-occult blood test—

(i) if the individual is under 50 years of age; or

(ii) if the test is performed within the 11 months after a previous screening fecal-occult blood test.

(2) Screening flexible sigmoidoscopies.—

(A) FEE SCHEDULE.—With respect to colorectal cancer screening tests consisting of screening flexible sigmoidoscopies, payment under section 1848 shall be consistent with payment under such section for similar or related services.

(B) PAYMENT LIMIT.—In the case of screening flexible sigmoidoscopy services, payment under this part shall not exceed such amount as the

Secretary specifies, based upon the rates recognized for diagnostic flexible sigmoidoscopy services.

(C) Facility payment limit.—

(i) IN GENERAL.—Notwithstanding subsections (i)(2)(A) and (t) of section 1833, in the case of screening flexible sigmoidoscopy services furnished on or after January 1, 1999, that—

(I) in accordance with regulations, may be performed in an ambulatory surgical center and for which the Secretary permits ambulatory surgical center payments under this part, and

(II) are performed in an ambulatory surgical center or hospital outpatient department, payment under this part shall be based on the lesser of the amount under the fee schedule that would apply to such services if they were performed in a hospital outpatient department in an area or the amount under the fee schedule that would apply to such services if they were performed in an ambulatory surgical center in the same area.

(ii) LIMITATION ON COINSURANCE.—Subject to section 1833(a)(1)(Y), but notwithstanding any other provision of this title, in the case of a beneficiary who receives the services described in clause (i)—

(I) in computing the amount of any applicable copayment, the computation of such coinsurance shall be based upon the fee schedule under which payment is made for the services, and

(II) the amount of such coinsurance is equal to 25 percent of the payment amount under the fee schedule described in subclause (I).

(D) SPECIAL RULE FOR DETECTED LESIONS.—Subject to section 1833(a)(1)(Y), if during the course of such screening flexible sigmoidoscopy, a lesion or growth is detected which results in a biopsy or removal of the lesion or growth, payment under this part shall not be made for the screening flexible sigmoidoscopy but shall be made for the procedure classified as a flexible sigmoidoscopy with such biopsy or removal.

(E) FREQUENCY LIMIT.—No payment may be made under this part for a colorectal cancer screening test consisting of a screening flexible sigmoidoscopy—

(i) if the individual is under 50 years of age; or

(ii) if the procedure is performed within the 47 months after a previous screening flexible sigmoidoscopy or, in the case of an individual who is not at high risk for colorectal cancer, if the procedure is performed within the 119 months after a previous screening colonoscopy.

(3) Screening colonoscopy.—

(A) FEE SCHEDULE.—With respect to colorectal cancer screening test consisting of a screening colonoscopy, payment under section 1848 shall be consistent with payment amounts under such section for similar or related services.

(B) PAYMENT LIMIT.—In the case of screening colonoscopy services, payment under this part shall not exceed such amount as the Secretary specifies, based upon the rates recognized for diagnostic colonoscopy services.

(C) Facility payment limit.—

(i) IN GENERAL.—Notwithstanding subsections (i)(2)(A) and (t) of section 1833, in the case of screening colonoscopy services furnished on or after January 1, 1999, that are performed in an ambulatory surgical center or a hospital outpatient department, payment under this part shall be based on the lesser of the amount under the fee schedule that would apply to such services if they were performed in a hospital out-patient department in an area or the amount under the fee schedule that would apply to such services if they were performed in an ambulatory surgical center in the same area.

(ii) LIMITATION ON COINSURANCE.—Subject to section 1833(a)(1)(Y), but notwithstanding any other provision of this title, in the case of a beneficiary who receives the services described in clause (i)—

(I) in computing the amount of any applicable coinsurance, the computation of such coinsurance shall be based upon the fee schedule under which payment is made for the services, and

(II) the amount of such coinsurance is equal to 25 percent of the payment amount under the fee schedule described in subclause (I).

(D) SPECIAL RULE FOR DETECTED LESIONS.—Subject to section 1833(a)(1)(Y), if during the course of such screening colonoscopy, a lesion or growth is detected which results in a biopsy or removal of the lesion or growth, payment under this part shall not be made for the screening colonoscopy but shall be made for the procedure classified as a colonoscopy with such biopsy or removal.

(E) FREQUENCY LIMIT.—No payment may be made under this part for a colorectal cancer screening test consisting of a screening colonoscopy for individuals at high risk for colorectal cancer if the procedure is performed within the 23 months after a previous screening colonoscopy or for other individuals if the procedure is performed within the 119 months after a previous screening colonoscopy or within 47 months after a previous screening flexible sigmoidoscopy.

(e) ACCREDITATION REQUIREMENT FOR ADVANCED DIAGNOSTIC IMAGING Services.—

(1) In general.—

(A) IN GENERAL.—Beginning with January 1, 2012, with respect to the technical component of advanced diagnostic imaging services for which payment is made under the fee schedule established under section 1848(b) and that are furnished by a supplier, payment may only be made if such supplier is accredited by an accreditation organization designated by the Secretary under paragraph (2)(B)(i).

(B) Advanced diagnostic imaging services defined.—

In this subsection, the term ‘‘advanced diagnostic imaging services’’ includes—

(i) diagnostic magnetic resonance imaging, computed tomography, and nuclear medicine (including positron emission tomography); and

(ii) such other diagnostic imaging services, including services described in section 1848(b)(4)(B) (excluding X-ray, ultrasound, and fluoroscopy), as specified by the Secretary in consultation with physician specialty organizations and other stakeholders.

(C) SUPPLIER DEFINED.—In this subsection, the term ‘‘supplier’’ has the meaning given such term in section 1861(d).

(2) Accreditation organizations.—

(A) FACTORS FOR DESIGNATION OF ACCREDITATION ORGANIZATIONS.—The Secretary shall consider the following factors in designating accreditation organizations under subparagraph (B)(i) and in reviewing and modifying the list of accreditation organizations designated pursuant to subparagraph (C):

(i) The ability of the organization to conduct timely reviews of accreditation applications.

(ii) Whether the organization has established a process for the timely integration of new advanced diagnostic imaging services into the organization’s accreditation program.

(iii) Whether the organization uses random site visits, site audits, or other strategies for ensuring accredited suppliers maintain adherence to the criteria described in paragraph (3).

(iv) The ability of the organization to take into account the capacities of suppliers located in a rural area (as defined in section 1886(d)(2)(D)).

(v) Whether the organization has established reasonable fees to be charged to suppliers applying for accreditation.

(vi) Such other factors as the Secretary determines appropriate.

(B) DESIGNATION.—Not later than January 1, 2010, the Secretary shall designate organizations to accredit suppliers furnishing the technical component of advanced diagnostic imaging services. The list of accreditation organizations so designated may be modified pursuant to subparagraph (C).

(C) Review and modification of list of accreditation organizations.—

(i) IN GENERAL.—The Secretary shall review the list of accreditation organizations designated under subparagraph (B) taking into account the factors under subparagraph (A). Taking into account the results of such review, the Secretary may, by regulation, modify the list of accreditation organizations designated under subparagraph (B).

(ii) SPECIAL RULE FOR ACCREDITATIONS DONE PRIOR TO REMOVAL FROM LIST OF DESIGNATED ACCREDITATION ORGANIZATIONS.—In the case where the Secretary removes an organization from the list of accreditation organizations designated under subparagraph (B), any supplier that is accredited by the organization during the period beginning on the date on which the organization is designated as an accreditation organization under subparagraph (B) and ending on the date on which the organization is removed from such list shall be considered to have been accredited by an organization designated by the Secretary under subparagraph (B) for the remaining period such accreditation is in effect.

(3) CRITERIA FOR ACCREDITATION.—The Secretary shall establish procedures to ensure that the criteria used by an accreditation organization designated under paragraph (2)(B) to evaluate a supplier that furnishes the technical component of advanced diagnostic imaging services for the purpose of accreditation of such supplier is specific to each imaging modality. Such criteria shall include—

(A) standards for qualifications of medical personnel who are not physicians and who furnish the technical component of advanced diagnostic imaging services;

(B) standards for qualifications and responsibilities of medical directors and supervising physicians, including standards that recognize the considerations described in paragraph (4);

(C) procedures to ensure that equipment used in furnishing the technical component of advanced diagnostic imaging services meets performance specifications;

(D) standards that require the supplier have procedures in place to ensure the safety of persons who furnish the technical component of advanced diagnostic imaging services and individuals to whom such services are furnished;

(E) standards that require the establishment and maintenance of a quality assurance and quality control program by the supplier that is adequate and appropriate to ensure the reliability, clarity, and accuracy of the technical quality of diagnostic images produced by such supplier; and

(F) any other standards or procedures the Secretary determines appropriate.

(2) RECOGNITION IN STANDARDS FOR THE EVALUATION OF MEDICAL DIRECTORS AND SUPERVISING PHYSICIANS.—The standards described in paragraph (3)(B) shall recognize whether a medical director or supervising physician—

(A) in a particular specialty receives training in advanced diagnostic imaging services in a residency program;

(B) has attained, through experience, the necessary expertise to be a medical director or a supervising physician;

(C) has completed any continuing medical education courses relating to such services; or

(D) has met such other standards as the Secretary determines appropriate.

(3) Rule for accreditations made prior to designaTION.—In the case of a supplier that is accredited before January 1, 2010, by an accreditation organization designated by the Secretary under paragraph (2)(B) as of January 1, 2010, such supplier shall be considered to have been accredited by an organization designated by the Secretary under such paragraph as of January 1, 2012, for the remaining period such accreditation is in effect.

REDUCTION IN PAYMENTS FOR PHYSICIAN PATHOLOGY SERVICES DURING 1991.—

(1) IN GENERAL.—For physician pathology services furnished under this part during 1991, the prevailing charges used in a locality under this part shall be 7 percent below the prevailing charges used in the locality under this part in 1990 after March 31.

(2) LIMITATION.—The prevailing charge for the technical and professional components of an physician pathology service furnished by a physician through an independent laboratory shall not be reduced pursuant to paragraph (1) to the extent that such reduction would reduce such prevailing charge below 115 percent of the prevailing charge for the professional component of such service when furnished by a hospital-based physician in the same locality. For purposes of the preceding sentence, an independent laboratory is a laboratory that is independent of a hospital and separate from the attending or consulting physicians' office.

(d) PAYMENT FOR OUTPATIENT CRITICAL ACCESS HOSPITAL SERVICES.—

(1) IN GENERAL.—The amount of payment for outpatient critical access hospital services of a critical access hospital is equal to 101 percent of the reasonable costs of the hospital in providing such services, unless the hospital makes the election under paragraph (2).

(2) Election of cost-based hospital outpatient service payment plus fee schedule for professional services.—A critical access hospital may elect to be paid for outpatient critical access hospital services amounts equal to the sum of the following, less the amount that such hospital may charge as described in section 1866(a)(2)(A):

(A) FACILITY FEE.—With respect to facility services, not including any services for which payment may be made under subparagraph (B), 101 percent of the reasonable costs of the critical access hospital in providing such services.

(B) FEE SCHEDULE FOR PROFESSIONAL SERVICES.—With respect to professional services otherwise included within outpatient critical access hospital services, 115 percent of such amounts as would otherwise be paid under this part if such services were not included in outpatient critical access hospital services. Subsections (x) and (y) of section 1833 shall not be taken into account in determining the amounts that would otherwise be paid pursuant to the preceding sentence.

The Secretary may not require, as a condition for applying subparagraph (B) with respect to a critical access hospital, that each physician or other practitioner providing professional services in the hospital must assign billing rights with respect to such services, except that such subparagraph shall not apply to those physicians and practitioners who have not assigned such billing rights.

(3) DISREGARDING CHARGES.—The payment amounts under this subsection shall be determined without regard to the amount of the customary or other charge.

(4) TREATMENT OF CLINICAL DIAGNOSTIC LABORATORY SERVICES.—No coinsurance, deductible, copayment, or other cost- sharing otherwise applicable under this part shall apply with respect to clinical diagnostic laboratory services furnished as an outpatient critical access hospital service. Nothing in this title shall be construed as providing for payment for clinical diagnostic laboratory services furnished as part of outpatient critical access hospital services, other than on the basis described in this subsection. For purposes of the preceding sentence and section

1861(mm)(3), clinical diagnostic laboratory services furnished by a critical access hospital shall be treated as being furnished as part of outpatient critical access services without regard to whether the individual with respect to whom such services are furnished is physically present in the critical access hospital, or in a skilled nursing facility or a clinic (including a rural health clinic) that is operated by a critical access hospital, at the time the specimen is collected.

(5) Coverage of costs for certain emergency room on CALL PROVIDERS.—In determining the reasonable costs of out-patient critical access hospital services under paragraphs (1) and (2)(A), the Secretary shall recognize as allowable costs, amounts (as defined by the Secretary) for reasonable compensation and related costs for physicians, physician assistants, nurse practitioners, and clinical nurse specialists who are on-call (as defined by the Secretary) to provide emergency services but who are not present on the premises of the critical access hospital involved, and are not otherwise furnishing services covered under this title and are not on-call at any other provider or facility.

(e) PAYMENT FOR PROSTHETIC DEVICES AND ORTHOTICS AND PROSTHETICS.—

(1) General rule for payment.—

(A) IN GENERAL.—Payment under this subsection for prosthetic devices and orthotics and prosthetics shall be made in a lump-sum amount for the purchase of the item in an amount equal to 80 percent of the payment basis described in subparagraph (B).

(B) PAYMENT BASIS.—Except as provided in subparagraphs (C), (E), and (H)(i), the payment basis described in this subparagraph is the lesser of—

(i) the actual charge for the item; or

(ii) the amount recognized under paragraph (2) as the purchase price for the item.

(C) EXCEPTION FOR CERTAIN PUBLIC HOME HEALTH AGENCIES.—Subparagraph (B)(i) shall not apply to an item furnished by a public home health agency (or by another home health agency which demonstrates to the satisfaction of the Secretary that a significant portion of its patients are low income) free of charge or at nominal charges to the public.

(D) EXCLUSIVE PAYMENT RULE.—Subject to subparagraph (H)(ii), this subsection shall constitute the exclusive provision of this title for payment for prosthetic devices, orthotics, and prosthetics under this part or under part A to a home health agency.

(E) EXCEPTION FOR CERTAIN ITEMS.—Payment for ostomy supplies, tracheostomy supplies, and urologicals shall be made in accordance with subparagraphs (B) and (C) of section 1834(a)(2).

(F) Special payment rules for certain prosthetics and custom-fabricated orthotics.—

(i) IN GENERAL.—No payment shall be made under this subsection for an item of custom-fabricated orthotics described in clause (ii) or for an item of prosthetics unless such item is—

(I) furnished by a qualified practitioner; and

(II) fabricated by a qualified practitioner or a qualified supplier at a facility that meets such criteria as the Secretary determines appropriate.

(ii) DESCRIPTION OF CUSTOM-FABRICATED ITEM.—

(I) IN GENERAL.—An item described in this clause is an item of custom-fabricated orthotics that requires education, training, and experience to custom-fabricate and that is included in a list established by the Secretary in subclause (II). Such an item does not include shoes and shoe inserts.

(II) LIST OF ITEMS.—The Secretary, in consultation with appropriate experts in orthotics (including national organizations representing manufacturers of orthotics), shall establish and update as appropriate a list of items to which this subparagraph applies. No item may be included in such list unless the item is individually fabricated for the patient over a positive model of the patient.

(iii) QUALIFIED PRACTITIONER DEFINED.—In this subparagraph, the term ''qualified practitioner'' means a physician or other individual who—

(I) s a qualified physical therapist or a qualified occupational therapist;

(II) in the case of a State that provides for the licensing of orthotics and prosthetics, is licensed in orthotics or prosthetics by the State in which the item is supplied; or

(III) in the case of a State that does not provide for the licensing of orthotics and prosthetics, is specifically trained and educated to provide or manage the provision of prosthetics and custom-designed or fabricated orthotics, and is certified by the American Board for Certification in Orthotics and Prosthetics, Inc. or by the Board for Orthotist/Prosthetist Certification, or is credentialed and approved by a program that the Secretary determines, in consultation with appropriate experts in orthotics and prosthetics, has training and education standards that are necessary to provide such prosthetics and orthotics.

(iv) QUALIFIED SUPPLIER DEFINED.—In this subparagraph, the term ''qualified supplier'' means any entity that is accredited by the American

Board for Certification in Orthotics and Prosthetics, Inc. or by the Board for Orthotist/Prosthetist Certification, or accredited and approved by a program that the Secretary determines has accreditation and approval standards that are essentially equivalent to those of such Board.

(G) Replacement of prosthetic devices and parts.—

(i) IN GENERAL.—Payment shall be made for the replacement of prosthetic devices which are artificial limbs, or for the replacement of any part of such devices, without regard to continuous use or useful lifetime restrictions if an ordering physician determines that the provision of a replacement device, or a replacement part of such a device, is necessary because of any of the following:

(I) A change in the physiological condition of the patient.

(II) An irreparable change in the condition of the device, or in a part of the device.

(III) The condition of the device, or the part of the device, requires repairs and the cost of such repairs would be more than 60 percent of the cost of a replacement device, or, as the case may be, of the part being replaced.

(ii) CONFIRMATION MAY BE REQUIRED IF DEVICE OR PART BEING REPLACED IS LESS THAN 3 YEARS OLD.—If a physician determines that a replacement device, or a replacement part, is necessary pursuant to clause (i)—

(I) such determination shall be controlling; and

(II) such replacement device or part shall be deemed to be reasonable and necessary for purposes of section 1862(a)(1)(A); except that if the device, or part, being replaced is less than 3 years old (calculated from the date on which the beneficiary began to use the device or part), the Secretary may also require confirmation of necessity of the replacement device or replacement part, as the case may be.

(H) APPLICATION OF COMPETITIVE ACQUISITION TO ORTHOTICS; LIMITATION OF INHERENT REASONABLENESS AUTHORITY.—In the case of orthotics described in paragraph (2)(C) of section 1847(a) furnished on or after January 1, 2011, subject to subsection (a)(1)(G), that are included in a competitive acquisition program in a competitive acquisition area under such section—

(i) the payment basis under this subsection for such orthotics furnished in such area shall be the payment basis determined under such competitive acquisition program; and

(ii) subject to subsection (a)(1)(G), the Secretary may use information on the payment determined under such competitive acquisition programs to adjust the payment amount otherwise recognized under subparagraph (B)(ii) for an area that is not a competitive acquisition area under section 1847, and in the case of such adjustment, paragraphs (8) and (9) of section 1842(b) shall not be applied.

(2) PURCHASE PRICE RECOGNIZED.—For purposes of paragraph (1), the amount that is recognized under this paragraph as the purchase price for prosthetic devices, orthotics, and prosthetics is the amount described in subparagraph (C) of this paragraph, determined as follows:

(A) COMPUTATION OF LOCAL PURCHASE PRICE.—Each carrier under section 1842 shall compute a base local purchase price for the item as follows:

(i) The carrier shall compute a base local purchase price for each item equal to the average reasonable charge in the locality for the purchase of the item for the 12-month period ending with June 1987.

(ii) The carrier shall compute a local purchase price, with respect to the furnishing of each particular item—

(I) in 1989 and 1990, equal to the base local purchase price computed under clause (i) increased by the percentage increase in the consumer price index for all urban consumers (United States city average) for the 6-month period ending with December 1987, or

(II) in 1991, 1992 or 1993, equal to the local purchase price computed under this clause for the previous year increased by the applicable percentage increase for the year.

(B) COMPUTATION OF REGIONAL PURCHASE PRICE.—With respect to the furnishing of a particular item in each region (as defined by the Secretary), the Secretary shall compute a regional purchase price—

(i) for 1992, equal to the average (weighted by relative volume of all claims among carriers) of the local purchase prices for the carriers in the region computed under subparagraph (A)(ii)(II) for the year, and

(ii) for each subsequent year, equal to the regional purchase price computed under this subparagraph for the previous year increased by the applicable percentage increase for the year.

(C) PURCHASE PRICE RECOGNIZED.—For purposes of paragraph (1) and subject to subparagraph (D), the amount that is recognized under this paragraph as the purchase price for each item furnished—

(i) in 1989, 1990, or 1991, is 100 percent of the local purchase price computed under subparagraph (A)(ii);

(ii) in 1992, is the sum of (I) 75 percent of the local purchase price computed under subparagraph (A)(ii)(II) for 1992, and (II) 25 percent of the regional purchase price computed under subparagraph (B) for 1992;

(iii) in 1993, is the sum of (I) 50 percent of the local purchase price computed under subparagraph (A)(ii)(II) for 1993, and (II) 50 percent of the regional purchase price computed under subparagraph (B) for 1993; and in 1994 or a subsequent year, is the regional purchase price computed under subparagraph (B) for that year.

(D) RANGE ON AMOUNT RECOGNIZED.—The amount that is recognized under subparagraph (C) as the purchase price for an item furnished—

(i) in 1992, may not exceed 125 percent, and may not be lower than 85 percent, of the average of the purchase prices recognized under such subparagraph for all the carrier service areas in the United States in that year; and

(ii) in a subsequent year, may not exceed 120 percent, and may not be lower than 90 percent, of the average of the purchase prices recognized under such subparagraph for all the carrier service areas in the United States in that year.

(3) APPLICABILITY OF CERTAIN PROVISIONS RELATING TO DURABLE MEDICAL EQUIPMENT.—Paragraphs (12) and (17) and subparagraphs (A) and (B) of paragraph (10) and paragraph (11) of subsection (a) shall apply to prosthetic devices, orthotics, and prosthetics in the same manner as such provisions apply to covered items under such subsection.

(4) DEFINITIONS.—In this subsection—

(A) the term ''applicable percentage increase'' means—

(i) for 1991, 0 percent;

(ii) for 1992 and 1993, the percentage increase in the consumer price index for all urban consumers (United States city average) for the 12-month period ending with June of the previous year;

(iii) for 1994 and 1995, 0 percent;

(iv) for 1996 and 1997, the percentage increase in the consumer price index for all urban consumers (United States city average) for the 12-month period ending with June of the previous year;

(v) for each of the years 1998 through 2000, 1 percent;

(vi) for 2001, the percentage increase in the consumer price index for all urban consumers (U.S. city average) for the 12-month period ending with June 2000;

(vii) for 2002, 1 percent;

(viii) for 2003, the percentage increase in the consumer price index for all urban consumers (United States city average) for the 12-month period ending with June of the previous year;

(ix) for 2004, 2005, and 2006, 0 percent;

(x) for for each of 2007 through 2010, the percentage increase in the consumer price index for all urban consumers (United States city average) for the 12-month period ending with June of the previous year; and

(xi) for 2011 and each subsequent year—

(I) the percentage increase in the consumer price index for all urban consumers (United States city average) for the 12-month period ending with June of the previous year, reduced by—

(II) the productivity adjustment described in section 1886(b)(3)(B)(xi)(II).

(B) the term ''prosthetic devices'' has the meaning given such term in section 1861(s)(8), except that such term does not include parenteral and enteral nutrition nutrients, supplies, and equipment and does not include an implantable item for which payment may be made under section 1833(t); and

(C) the term ''orthotics and prosthetics'' has the meaning given such term in section 1861(s)(9) (and includes shoes described in section 1861(s)(12)), but does not include intraocular lenses or medical supplies (including catheters, catheter supplies, ostomy bags, and supplies related to ostomy care) furnished by a home health agency under section 1861(m)(5).

The application of subparagraph (A)(xi)(II) may result in the applicable percentage increase under subparagraph (A) being less than 0.0 for a year, and may result in payment rates under this subsection for a year being less than such payment rates for the preceding year.

(5) Documentation created by orthotists and PROSTHETISTS.—For purposes of determining the reasonableness and medical necessity of orthotics and prosthetics, documentation created by an orthotist or prosthetist shall be considered part of the individual's medical record to support documentation created by eligible professionals described in section 1848(k)(3)(B).

(f) PAYMENT FOR SURGICAL DRESSINGS.—

IN GENERAL.—Payment under this subsection for surgical dressings (described in section 1861(s)(5)) shall be made in a lump sum amount for the purchase of the item in an amount equal to 80 percent of the lesser of—

(A) the actual charge for the item; or (B) a payment amount determined in accordance with the methodology described in subparagraphs (B) and (C) of subsection (a)(2) (except that in applying such methodology, the national limited payment amount referred to in such subparagraphs shall be initially computed based on local payment amounts using average reasonable charges for the 12-month period ending December 31, 1992, increased by the covered item updates described in such subsection for 1993 and 1994).

(2) EXCEPTIONS.—Paragraph (1) shall not apply to surgical dressings that are—

(A) furnished as an incident to a physician's professional service; or

(B) furnished by a home health agency.

(g) REQUIREMENTS FOR SUPPLIERS OF MEDICAL EQUIPMENT AND SUPPLIES.—

(I) Issuance and renewal of supplier number.—

(A) PAYMENT.—Except as provided in subparagraph (C), no payment may be made under this part after the date of the enactment of the Social Security Act Amendments of 1994 for items furnished by a supplier of medical equipment and supplies unless such supplier obtains (and renews at such intervals as the Secretary may require) a supplier number.

(B) Standards for possessing a supplier number.—A supplier may not obtain a supplier number unless—

(i) for medical equipment and supplies furnished on or after the date of the enactment of the Social Security Act Amendments of 1994 and before January 1, 1996, the supplier meets standards prescribed by the Secretary in regulations issued on June 18, 1992; and

(ii) for medical equipment and supplies furnished on or after January 1, 1996, the supplier meets revised standards prescribed by the Secretary (in consultation with representatives of suppliers of medical equipment and supplies, carriers, and consumers) that shall include requirements that the supplier—

(I) comply with all applicable State and Federal licensure and regulatory requirements;

(II) maintain a physical facility on an appropriate site;

(III) have proof of appropriate liability insurance; and

(IV) meet such other requirements as the Secretary may specify.

(C) EXCEPTION FOR ITEMS FURNISHED AS INCIDENT TO A PHYSICIAN'S SERVICE.—Subparagraph (A) shall not apply with respect to medical equipment and supplies furnished incident to a physician's service.

(D) PROHIBITION AGAINST MULTIPLE SUPPLIER NUMBERS.—The Secretary may not issue more than one supplier number to any supplier of medical equipment and supplies unless the issuance of more than one number is appropriate to identify subsidiary or regional entities under the supplier's ownership or control.

(E) PROHIBITION AGAINST DELEGATION OF SUPPLIER DETERMINATIONS.—The Secretary may not delegate (other than by contract under section 1842) the responsibility to determine whether suppliers meet the standards necessary to obtain a supplier number.

(2) Certificates of medical necessity.—

(A) Limitation on information provided by suppliers on certificates of medical necessity.—

(i) IN GENERAL.—Effective 60 days after the date of the enactment of the Social Security Act Amendments of 1994, a supplier of medical equipment and supplies may distribute to physicians, or to individuals entitled to benefits under this part, a certificate of medical necessity for commercial purposes which contains no more than the following information completed by the supplier:

(I) An identification of the supplier and the beneficiary to whom such medical equipment and supplies are furnished.

(II) A description of such medical equipment and supplies.

(III) Any product code identifying such medical equipment and supplies.3

(IV) Any other administrative information (other than information relating to the beneficiary's medical condition) identified by the Secretary.

(ii) INFORMATION ON PAYMENT AMOUNT AND CHARGES.—If a supplier distributes a certificate of medical necessity containing any of the information permitted to be supplied under clause (i), the supplier shall also list on the certificate of medical necessity the fee schedule amount and the supplier's charge for the medical equipment or supplies being furnished prior to distribution of such certificate to the physician.

(iii)PENALTY.—Any supplier of medical equipment and supplies who knowingly and willfully distributes a certificate of medical necessity in violation of clause (i) or fails to provide the information required under clause (ii) is subject to a civil money penalty in an amount not to exceed $1,000 for each such certificate of medical necessity so distributed. The provisions of section 1128A (other than subsections (a) and (b)) shall apply to civil money penalties under this subparagraph in the same manner as they apply to a penalty or proceeding under section 1128A(a).

(B) DEFINITION.—For purposes of this paragraph, the term ''certificate of medical necessity'' means a form or other document containing information required by the carrier to be submitted to show that an item is reasonable and necessary for the diagnosis or treatment of illness or injury or to improve the functioning of a malformed body member.

(3) COVERAGE AND REVIEW CRITERIA.—The Secretary shall annually review the coverage and utilization of items of medical equipment and supplies to determine whether such items should be made subject to coverage and utilization review criteria, and if appropriate, shall develop and apply such criteria to such items.

(4) LIMITATION ON PATIENT LIABILITY.—If a supplier of medical equipment and supplies (as defined in paragraph (5))—

(A) furnishes an item or service to a beneficiary for which no payment may be made by reason of paragraph (1);

(B) furnishes an item or service to a beneficiary for which payment is denied in advance under subsection (a)(15); or

(C) furnishes an item or service to a beneficiary for which payment is denied under section 1862(a)(1);

any expenses incurred for items and services furnished to an individual by such a supplier not on an assigned basis shall be the responsibility of such supplier. The individual shall have no financial responsibility for such expenses and the supplier shall refund on a timely basis to the individual (and shall be liable to the individual for) any amounts collected from the individual for such items or services. The provisions of subsection (a)(18) shall apply to refunds required under the previous sentence in the same manner as such provisions apply to refunds under such subsection.

(5) DEFINITION.—The term ''medical equipment and supplies'' means—

(A) durable medical equipment (as defined in section 1861(n));

(B) prosthetic devices (as described in section 1861(s)(8));

(C) orthotics and prosthetics (as described in section 1861(s)(9));

(D) surgical dressings (as described in section 1861(s)(5));

(E) items and services related to the administration of intravenous immune globulin furnished on or after January 1, 2024, as described in section 1861(zz);

(E) lymphedema compression treatment items (as defined in section 1861(mmm));

(F) such other items as the Secretary may determine; and

(G) for purposes of paragraphs (1) and (3)—

(i)home dialysis supplies and equipment (as described in section 1861(s)(2)(F)),

(ii) immunosuppressive drugs (as described in section 1861(s)(2)(J)),

(iii) therapeutic shoes for diabetics (as described in section 1861(s)(12)),

(iv) oral drugs prescribed for use as an anticancer therapeutic agent (as described in section 1861(s)(2)(Q)), and

(v) self-administered erythropoetin (as described in section 1861(s)(2)(P)).

(h) PAYMENT FOR OUTPATIENT THERAPY SERVICES AND COMprehensive Outpatient Rehabilitation Services.—

(1) IN GENERAL.—With respect to services described in section 1833(a)(8) or 1833(a)(9) for which payment is determined under this subsection, the payment basis shall be—

(A) for services furnished during 1998, the amount determined under paragraph (2); or

(B) for services furnished during a subsequent year, 80 percent of the lesser of—

(i) the actual charge for the services, or

(ii) the applicable fee schedule amount (as defined in paragraph (3)) for the services.

(2) PAYMENT IN 1998 BASED UPON ADJUSTED REASONABLE COSTS.—The amount under this paragraph for services is the lesser of—

(A) the charges imposed for the services, or

(B) the adjusted reasonable costs (as defined in paragraph (4)) for the services, less 20 percent of the amount of the charges imposed for such services.

(3) APPLICABLE FEE SCHEDULE AMOUNT.—In this subsection, the term ‘‘applicable fee schedule amount’’ means, with respect to services furnished in a year, the amount determined under the fee schedule established under section 1848 for such services furnished during the year or, if there is no such fee schedule established for such services, the amount determined under the fee schedule established for such comparable services as the Secretary specifies.

(4) ADJUSTED REASONABLE COSTS.—In paragraph (2), the term ‘‘adjusted reasonable costs’’ means, with respect to any services, reasonable costs determined for such services, reduced by 10 percent. The 10-percent reduction shall not apply to services described in section 1833(a)(8)(B) (relating to services provided by hospitals).

(5) UNIFORM CODING.—For claims for services submitted on or after April 1, 1998, for which the amount of payment is determined under this subsection, the claim shall include a code (or codes) under a uniform coding system specified by the Secretary that identifies the services furnished.

(6) RESTRAINT ON BILLING.—The provisions of subparagraphs (A) and (B) of section 1842(b)(18) shall apply to therapy services for which payment is made under this subsection in the same manner as they apply to services provided by a practitioner described in section 1842(b)(18)(C).

(7) ADJUSTMENT IN DISCOUNT FOR CERTAIN MULTIPLE THERAPY SERVICES.—In the case of therapy services furnished on or after April 1, 2013, and for which payment is made under this subsection pursuant to the applicable fee schedule amount (as defined in paragraph (3)), instead of the 25 percent multiple procedure payment reduction specified in the final rule published by the Secretary in the Federal Register on November 29, 2010, the reduction percentage shall be 50 percent.

(b) ESTABLISHMENT OF FEE SCHEDULE FOR AMBULANCE SERVICES.—

(1) IN GENERAL.—The Secretary shall establish a fee schedule for payment for ambulance services whether provided directly by a supplier or provider or under arrangement with a provider under this part through a negotiated rulemaking process described in title 5, United States Code, and in accordance with the requirements of this subsection.

(2) CONSIDERATIONS.—In establishing such fee schedule, the Secretary shall—

(A) establish mechanisms to control increases in expenditures for ambulance services under this part;

(B) establish definitions for ambulance services which link payments to the type of services provided;

(C) consider appropriate regional and operational differences;

(D) consider adjustments to payment rates to account for inflation and other relevant factors; and

(E) phase in the application of the payment rates under the fee schedule in an efficient and fair manner consistent with paragraph (11), except that such phase-in shall provide for full payment of any national mileage rate for ambulance services provided by suppliers that are paid by carriers in any of the 50 States where payment by a carrier for such services for all such suppliers in such State did not, prior to the implementation of the fee schedule, include a separate amount for all mileage within the county from which the beneficiary is transported.

(3) SAVINGS.—In establishing such fee schedule, the Secretary shall—

(A) ensure that the aggregate amount of payments made for ambulance services under this part during 2000 does not exceed the aggregate amount of payments which would have been made for such services under this part during such year if the amendments made by section 4531(a) of the Balanced Budget Act of 1997 continued in effect, except that in making such determination the Secretary shall assume an update in such payments for 2002 equal to percentage increase in the consumer price index for all urban consumers (U.S. city average) for the 12-month period ending with June of the previous year reduced in the case of 2002 by 1.0 percentage points;

(B) set the payment amounts provided under the fee schedule for services furnished in 2001 and each subsequent year at amounts equal to the payment amounts under the fee schedule for services furnished during the previous year, increased, subject to subparagraph (C) and the succeeding sentence of this paragraph, by the percentage increase in the consumer price index for all urban consumers (U.S. city average) for the 12-month period ending with June of the previous year reduced in the case of 2002 by 1.0 percentage points; and

(C) for 2011 and each subsequent year, after determining the percentage increase under subparagraph (B) for the year, reduce such percentage increase by the productivity adjustment described in section 1886(b)(3)(B)(xi)(II).

The application of subparagraph (C) may result in the percentage increase under subparagraph (B) being less than 0.0 for a year, and may result in payment rates under the fee schedule under this subsection for a year being less than such payment rates for the preceding year.

(4) CONSULTATION.—In establishing the fee schedule for ambulance services under this subsection, the Secretary shall consult with various national organizations representing individuals and entities who furnish and regulate ambulance services and share with such organizations relevant data in establishing such schedule.

(5) LIMITATION ON REVIEW.—There shall be no administrative or judicial review under section 1869 or otherwise of the amounts established under the fee schedule for ambulance services under this subsection, including matters described in paragraph (2).

(6) RESTRAINT ON BILLING.—The provisions of subparagraphs (A) and (B) of section 1842(b)(18) shall apply to ambulance services for which payment is made under this subsection in the same manner as they apply to services provided by a practitioner described in section 1842(b)(18)(C).

(7) CODING SYSTEM.—The Secretary may require the claim for any services for which the amount of payment is determined under this subsection to include a code (or codes) under a uniform coding system specified by the Secretary that identifies the services furnished.

(8) Services furnished by critical access hospitals.—

Notwithstanding any other provision of this subsection, the Secretary shall pay 101 percent of the reasonable costs incurred in furnishing ambulance services if such services are furnished—

(A) by a critical access hospital (as defined in section 1861(mm)(1)), or

(B) by an entity that is owned and operated by a critical access hospital,

but only if the critical access hospital or entity is the only provider or supplier of ambulance services that is located within a 35-mile drive of such critical access hospital.

(9) TRANSITIONAL ASSISTANCE FOR RURAL PROVIDERS.—In the case of ground ambulance services furnished on or after July 1, 2001, and before January 1, 2004, for which the transportation originates in a rural area (as defined in section 1886(d)(2)(D)) or in a rural census tract of a metropolitan statistical area (as determined under the most recent modification of the Goldsmith Modification, originally published in the Federal Register on February 27, 1992 (57 Fed. Reg. 6725)), the fee schedule established under this subsection shall provide that, with respect to the payment rate for mileage for a trip above 17 miles, and up to 50 miles, the rate otherwise established shall be increased by not less than 1⁄2 of the additional payment per mile established for the first 17 miles of such a trip originating in a rural area.

(10) Phase-in providing floor using blend of fee schedULE AND REGIONAL FEE SCHEDULES.—In carrying out the phase-in under paragraph (2)(E) for each level of ground service furnished in a year, the portion of the payment amount that is based on the fee schedule shall be the greater of the amount determined under such fee schedule (without regard to this paragraph) or the following blended rate of the fee schedule under paragraph (1) and of a regional fee schedule for the region involved:

(A) For 2004 (for services furnished on or after July 1, 2004), the blended rate shall be based 20 percent on the fee schedule under paragraph (1) and 80 percent on the regional fee schedule.

(B) For 2005, the blended rate shall be based 40 percent on the fee schedule under paragraph (1) and 60 percent on the regional fee schedule.

(C) For 2006, the blended rate shall be based 60 percent on the fee schedule under paragraph (1) and 40 percent on the regional fee schedule.

(D) For 2007, 2008, and 2009, the blended rate shall be based 80 percent on the fee schedule under paragraph (1) and 20 percent on the regional fee schedule.

(E) For 2010 and each succeeding year, the blended rate shall be based 100 percent on the fee schedule under paragraph (1).

For purposes of this paragraph, the Secretary shall establish a regional fee schedule for each of the nine census divisions (referred to in section 1886(d)(2)) using the methodology (used in establishing the fee schedule under paragraph (1)) to calculate a regional conversion factor and a regional mileage payment rate and using the same payment adjustments and the same relative value units as used in the fee schedule under such paragraph.

(11) ADJUSTMENT IN PAYMENT FOR CERTAIN LONG TRIPS.—In the case of ground ambulance services furnished on or after July 1, 2004, and before January 1, 2009, regardless of where the transportation originates, the fee schedule established under this subsection shall provide that, with respect to the payment rate for mileage for a trip above 50 miles the per mile rate otherwise established shall be increased by 1⁄4 of the payment per mile otherwise applicable to miles in excess of 50 miles in such trip.

(12) Assistance for rural providers furnishing services in low population density areas.—

(A) IN GENERAL.—In the case of ground ambulance services furnished on or after July 1, 2004, and before January 1, 2025, for which the transportation originates in a qualified rural area (identified under subparagraph (B)(iii)), the Secretary shall provide for a percent increase in the base rate of the fee schedule for a trip established under this subsection. In establishing such percent increase, the Secretary shall estimate the average cost per trip for such services (not taking into account mileage) in the lowest quartile as compared to the average cost per trip for such services (not taking into account mileage) in the highest quartile of all rural county populations.

(B) Identification of qualified rural areas.—

(i) DETERMINATION OF POPULATION DENSITY IN AREA.—Based upon data from the United States decennial census for the year 2000, the Secretary shall determine, for each rural area, the population density for that area.

(ii) RANKING OF AREAS.—The Secretary shall rank each such area based on such population density.

(iii) IDENTIFICATION OF QUALIFIED RURAL AREAS.—

The Secretary shall identify those areas (in subparagraph (A) referred to as ‘‘qualified rural areas’’) with the lowest population densities that represent, if each such area were weighted by the population of such area (as used in computing such population densities), an aggregate total of 25 percent of the total of the population of all such areas.

(iv) RURAL AREA.—For purposes of this paragraph, the term ‘‘rural area’’ has the meaning given such term in section 1886(d)(2)(D). If feasible, the Secretary shall treat a rural census tract of a metropolitan statistical area (as determined under the most recent modification of the Goldsmith Modification, originally published in the Federal Register on February 27, 1992 (57 Fed. Reg. 6725) as a rural area for purposes of this paragraph.

(v) JUDICIAL REVIEW.—There shall be no administrative or judicial review under section 1869, 1878, or otherwise, respecting the identification of an area under this subparagraph.

(13) Temporary increase for ground ambulance services.—

(A) IN GENERAL.—After computing the rates with respect to ground ambulance services under the other applicable provisions of this subsection, in the case of such services furnished on or after July 1, 2004, and before January 1, 2007, and for such services furnished on or after July 1, 2008, and before January 1, 2025, for which the transportation originates in—

(i) a rural area described in paragraph (9) or in a rural census tract described in such paragraph, the fee schedule established under this section shall provide that the rate for the service otherwise established, after the application of any increase under paragraphs

(11) and (12), shall be increased by 2 percent (or 3 percent if such service is furnished on or after July 1, 2008, and before January 1, 2025); and

(ii) an area not described in clause (i), the fee schedule established under this subsection shall provide that the rate for the service otherwise established, after the application of any increase under paragraph (11), shall be increased by 1 percent (or 2 percent if such service is furnished on or after July 1, 2008, and before January 1, 2025).

(B) APPLICATION OF INCREASED PAYMENTS AFTER APPLICABLE PERIOD.—The increased payments under subparagraph (A) shall not be taken into account in calculating payments for services furnished after the applicable period specified in such subparagraph.

(14) Providing appropriate coverage of rural air ambulance services.—

(A) IN GENERAL.—The regulations described in section 1861(s)(7) shall provide, to the extent that any ambulance services (whether ground or air) may be covered under such section, that a rural air ambulance service (as defined in subparagraph (C)) is reimbursed under this subsection at the air ambulance rate if the air ambulance service—

(i) is reasonable and necessary based on the health condition of the individual being transported at or immediately prior to the time of the transport; and

(ii) complies with equipment and crew requirements established by the Secretary.

(B) SATISFACTION OF REQUIREMENT OF MEDICALLY NECESSARY.—The requirement of subparagraph (A)(i) is deemed to be met for a rural air ambulance service if—

(i) subject to subparagraph (D), such service is requested by a physician or other qualified medical personnel (as specified by the Secretary) who certifies or reasonably determines that the individual's condition is such that the time needed to transport the individual by land or the instability of transportation by land poses a threat to the individual's survival or seriously endangers the individual's health; or

(ii) such service is furnished pursuant to a protocol that is established by a State or regional emergency medical service (EMS) agency and recognized or approved by the Secretary under which the use of an air ambulance is recommended, if such agency does not have an ownership interest in the entity furnishing such service.

(C) RURAL AIR AMBULANCE SERVICE DEFINED.—For purposes of this paragraph, the term ''rural air ambulance service'' means fixed wing and rotary wing air ambulance service in which the point of pick up of the individual occurs in a rural area (as defined in section 1886(d)(2)(D)) or in a rural census tract of a metropolitan statistical area (as determined under the most recent modification of the Goldsmith Modification, originally published in the Federal Register on February 27, 1992 (57 Fed. Reg. 6725)).

(D) Limitation.—

(i) IN GENERAL.

(ii) Subparagraph (B)(i) shall not apply if there is a financial or employment relationship between the person requesting the rural air ambulance service and the entity furnishing the ambulance service, or an entity under common ownership with the entity furnishing the air ambulance service, or a financial relationship between an immediate family member of such requester and such an entity.

(iii) EXCEPTION.—Where a hospital and the entity furnishing rural air ambulance services are under common ownership, clause (i) shall not apply to remuneration (through employment or other relationship) by the hospital of the requester or immediate family member if the remuneration is for provider-based physician services furnished in a hospital (as described in section 1887) which are reimbursed under part A and the amount of the remuneration is unrelated directly or indirectly to the provision of rural air ambulance services.

(15) PAYMENT ADJUSTMENT FOR NON-EMERGENCY AMBULANCE TRANSPORTS FOR ESRD BENEFICIARIES.—The fee schedule amount otherwise applicable under the preceding provisions of this

subsection shall be reduced by 10 percent for ambulance services furnished during the period beginning on October 1, 2013, and ending on September 30, 2018, and by 23 percent for such services furnished on or after October 1, 2018, consisting of non-emergency basic life support services involving transport of an individual with end-stage renal disease for renal dialysis services (as described in section 1881(b)(14)(B)) furnished other than on an emergency basis by a provider of services or a renal dialysis facility.

(16) Prior authorization for repetitive scheduled non- emergent ambulance transports.—

(A) IN GENERAL.—Beginning January 1, 2017, if the expansion to all States of the model of prior authorization described in paragraph (2) of section 515(a) of the Medicare Access and CHIP Reauthorization Act of 2015 meets the requirements described in paragraphs (1) through (3) of section 1115A(c), then the Secretary shall expand such model to all States.

(B) FUNDING.—The Secretary shall use funds made available under section 1893(h)(10) to carry out this paragraph.

(C) Clarification regarding budget neutrality.—

Nothing in this paragraph may be construed to limit or modify the application of section 1115A(b)(3)(B) to models described in such section, including with respect to the model described in subparagraph (A) and expanded beginning on January 1, 2017, under such subparagraph.

(17) Submission of cost and other information.—

(A) DEVELOPMENT OF DATA COLLECTION SYSTEM.—The Secretary shall develop a data collection system (which may include use of a cost survey) to collect cost, revenue, utilization, and other information determined appropriate by the Secretary with respect to providers of services (in this paragraph referred to as ''providers'') and suppliers of ground ambulance services. Such system shall be designed to collect information—

(i) needed to evaluate the extent to which reported costs relate to payment rates under this subsection;

(ii) on the utilization of capital equipment and ambulance capacity, including information consistent with the type of information described in section 1121(a); and

(iii) on different types of ground ambulance services furnished in different geographic locations, including rural areas and low population density areas described in paragraph (12).

(B) Specification of data collection system.—

(i) IN GENERAL.—The Secretary shall—

(I) not later than December 31, 2019, specify the data collection system under subparagraph (A); and

(II) identify the providers and suppliers of ground ambulance services that would be required to submit information under such data collection system, including the representative sample described in clause (ii).

(ii) DETERMINATION OF REPRESENTATIVE SAMPLE.—

(I) IN GENERAL.—Not later than December 31, 2019, with respect to the data collection for the first year under such system, and for each subsequent year through 2024, the Secretary shall determine a representative sample to submit information under the data collection system.

(II) REQUIREMENTS.—The sample under subclause (I) shall be representative of the different types of providers and suppliers of ground ambulance services (such as those providers and suppliers that are part of an emergency service or part of a government organization) and the geographic locations in which ground ambulance services are furnished (such as urban, rural, and low population density areas).

(III) LIMITATION.—The Secretary shall not include an individual provider or supplier of ground ambulance services in the sample under subclause

(I) in 2 consecutive years, to the extent practicable.

(A) REPORTING OF COST INFORMATION.—For each year, a provider or supplier of ground ambulance services identified by the Secretary under subparagraph (B)(i)(II) as being required to submit information under the data collection system with respect to a period for the year shall submit to the Secretary information specified under the system. Such information shall be submitted in a form and manner, and at a time, specified by the Secretary for purposes of this subparagraph.

(B) Payment reduction for failure to report.—

(i) IN GENERAL.—Beginning January 1, 2022, subject to clause (ii), a 10 percent reduction to payments under this subsection shall be made for the applicable period (as defined in clause (ii)) to a provider or supplier of ground ambulance services that—

(I) is required to submit information under the data collection system with respect to a period under subparagraph (C); and

(II) does not sufficiently submit such information, as determined by the Secretary.

(ii) APPLICABLE PERIOD DEFINED.—For purposes of clause (i), the term ''applicable period'' means, with respect to a provider or supplier of ground ambulance services, a year specified by the Secretary not more than 2 years after the end of the period with respect to which the Secretary has made a determination under clause (i)(II) that the provider or supplier of ground ambulance services failed to sufficiently submit information under the data collection system.

(iii) HARDSHIP EXEMPTION.—The Secretary may exempt a provider or supplier from the payment reduction under clause (i) with respect to an applicable period in the event of significant hardship, such as a natural disaster, bankruptcy, or other similar situation that the Secretary determines interfered with the ability of the provider or supplier of ground ambulance services to submit such information in a timely manner for the specified period.

(iv) INFORMAL REVIEW.—The Secretary shall establish a process under which a provider or supplier of ground ambulance services may seek an informal review of a determination that the provider or supplier is subject to the payment reduction under clause (i).

(C) Ongoing data collection.—

(i) REVISION OF DATA COLLECTION SYSTEM.—The Secretary may, as the Secretary determines appropriate and, if available, taking into consideration the report (or reports) under subparagraph (F), revise the data collection system under subparagraph (A).

(ii) SUBSEQUENT DATA COLLECTION.—In order to continue to evaluate the extent to which reported costs relate to payment rates under this subsection and for other purposes the Secretary deems appropriate, the Secretary shall require providers and suppliers of ground ambulance services to submit information for years after 2024 as the Secretary determines appropriate, but in no case less often than once every 3 years.

(D) Ground ambulance data collection system study.—

(i) IN GENERAL.—Not later than the second June 15th following the date on which the Secretary transmits data for the first representative sample of providers and suppliers of ground ambulance services to the Medicare Payment Advisory Commission, and as determined necessary by such Commission thereafter,, such Commission shall assess, and submit to Congress a report on, information submitted by providers and suppliers of ground ambulance services through the data collection system under subparagraph (A), the adequacy of payments for ground ambulance services under this subsection, and geographic variations in the cost of furnishing such services.

(ii) CONTENTS.—A report under clause (i) shall contain the following:

(I) An analysis of information submitted through the data collection system.

(II) An analysis of any burden on providers and suppliers of ground ambulance services associated with the data collection system.

(III) A recommendation as to whether information should continue to be submitted through such data collection system or if such system should be revised under subparagraph (E)(i).

(IV) Other information determined appropriate by the Commission.

(E) PUBLIC AVAILABILITY.—The Secretary shall post information on the results of the data collection under this paragraph on the Internet website of the Centers for Medicare & Medicaid Services, as determined appropriate by the Secretary.

(F) IMPLEMENTATION.—The Secretary shall implement this paragraph through notice and comment rulemaking.

(G) ADMINISTRATION.—Chapter 35 of title 44, United States Code, shall not apply to the collection of information required under this subsection.

(H) LIMITATIONS ON REVIEW.—There shall be no administrative or judicial review under section 1869, section 1878, or otherwise of the data collection system or identification of respondents under this paragraph.

(I) FUNDING FOR IMPLEMENTATION.—For purposes of carrying out subparagraph (A), the Secretary shall provide for the transfer, from the Federal Supplementary Medical Insurance Trust Fund under section 1841, of $15,000,000 to the Centers for Medicare & Medicaid Services Program Management Account for fiscal year 2018. Amounts transferred under this subparagraph shall remain available until expended.

(c) PAYMENT FOR TELEHEALTH SERVICES.—

(1) IN GENERAL.—Subject to paragraphs (8) and (9), the Secretary shall pay for telehealth services that are furnished via a telecommunications system by a physician (as defined in section 1861(r)) or a practitioner (as defined in paragraph (4)(E)) to an eligible telehealth individual enrolled under this part notwithstanding that the individual physician or practitioner providing the telehealth service is not at the same location as the beneficiary. For purposes of the preceding sentence, in the case of any Federal telemedicine demonstration program conducted in Alaska or Hawaii, the term ‘‘telecommunications system’’ includes store-and-forward technologies that provide for the asynchronous transmission of health care information in single or multimedia formats.

(2) Payment amount.—

(A) DISTANT SITE.—Subject to paragraph (8), the Secretary shall pay to a physician or practitioner located at a distant site that furnishes a telehealth service to an eligible telehealth individual an amount equal to the amount that such physician or practitioner would have been paid under this title had such service been furnished without the use of a telecommunications system.

(B) Facility fee for originating site.—

(i) IN GENERAL.—Subject to clauses (ii) and (iii) and paragraph (6)(C), with respect to a telehealth service, subject to section 1833(a)(1)(U), there shall be paid to the originating site a facility fee equal to—

(I) for the period beginning on October 1, 2001, and ending on December 31, 2001, and for 2002, $20; and

(II) for a subsequent year, the facility fee specified in subclause (I) or this subclause for the preceding year increased by the percentage increase in the MEI (as defined in section 1842(i)(3)) for such subsequent year.

(ii) NO FACILITY FEE IF ORIGINATING SITE IS THE HOME.—No facility fee shall be paid under this subparagraph to an originating site described in paragraph (4)(C)(ii)(X).

(iii) NO FACILITY FEE FOR NEW SITES.—In the case that the emergency period described in section 1135(g)(1)(B) ends before December 31, 2024, with respect to telehealth services identified in paragraph (4)(F)(i) as of the date of the enactment of this clause that are furnished during the period beginning on the first day after the end of such emergency period and ending December 31, 2024, a facility fee shall only be paid under this subparagraph to an originating site that is described in paragraph (4)(C)(ii) (other than subclause (X) of such paragraph).

(C) TELEPRESENTER NOT REQUIRED.—Nothing in this subsection shall be construed as requiring an eligible telehealth individual to be presented by a physician or practitioner at the originating site for the furnishing of a service via a telecommunications system, unless it is medically necessary (as determined by the physician or practitioner at the distant site).

(3) Limitation on beneficiary charges.—

(A) PHYSICIAN AND PRACTITIONER.—The provisions of section 1848(g) and subparagraphs (A) and (B) of section 1842(b)(18) shall apply to a physician or practitioner receiving payment under this subsection in the same manner as they apply to physicians or practitioners under such sections.

(B) ORIGINATING SITE.—The provisions of section 1842(b)(18) shall apply to originating sites receiving a facility fee in the same manner as they apply to practitioners under such section.

(4) DEFINITIONS.—For purposes of this subsection:

(A) DISTANT SITE.—Subject to paragraph (8), the term''distant site'' means the site at which the physician or practitioner is located at the time the service is provided via a telecommunications system.

(B) ELIGIBLE TELEHEALTH INDIVIDUAL.—The term ''eligible telehealth individual'' means an individual enrolled under this part who receives a telehealth service furnished at an originating site.

(C) Originating site.—

(i) IN GENERAL.—Except as provided in clause (iii) and paragraphs (5), (6), and (7), the term''originating site'' means only those sites described in clause (ii) at which the eligible telehealth individual is located at the time the service is furnished via a telecommunications system and only if such site is located—

(I) in an area that is designated as a rural health professional shortage area under section 332(a)(1)(A) of the Public Health Service Act (42 U.S.C. 254e(a)(1)(A));

(II) in a county that is not included in a Metropolitan Statistical Area; or

(III) from an entity that participates in a Federal telemedicine demonstration project that has been approved by (or receives funding from) the Secretary of Health and Human Services as of December 31, 2000.

(ii) SITES DESCRIBED.—The sites referred to in clause (i) are the following sites:

(I) The office of a physician or practitioner.

(II) A critical access hospital (as defined in section 1861(mm)(1)).

(III) A rural health clinic (as defined in section 1861(aa)(2)).

(IV) A Federally qualified health center (as defined in section 1861(aa)(4)).

(V) A hospital (as defined in section 1861(e)).

(VI) A hospital-based or critical access hospital-based renal dialysis center (including satellites).

(VII) A skilled nursing facility (as defined in section 1819(a)).

(VIII) A community mental health center (as defined in section 1861(ff)(3)(B)).

(IX) A renal dialysis facility, but only for purposes of section 1881(b)(3)(B).

(X) The home of an individual, but only for purposes of section 1881(b)(3)(B) or telehealth services described in paragraph (7).

(XI) A rural emergency hospital (as defined in section 1861(kkk)(2)).

(iii) EXPANDING ACCESS TO TELEHEALTH SERVICES.—

In the case that the emergency period described in section 1135(g)(1)(B) ends before December 31, 2024, with respect to telehealth services identified in subparagraph (F)(i) as of the date of the enactment of this clause that are furnished during the period beginning on the first day after the end of such emergency period and ending on December 31, 2024, the term ‘‘originating site’’ means any site in the United States at which the eligible telehealth individual is located at the time the service is furnished via a telecommunications system, including the home of an individual.

(D) PHYSICIAN.—The term ‘‘physician’’ has the meaning given that term in section 1861(r).

(E) PRACTITIONER.—The term ‘‘practitioner’’ has the meaning given that term in section 1842(b)(18)(C) and, in the case that the emergency period described in section 1135(g)(1)(B) ends before December 31, 2024, for the period beginning on the first day after the end of such emergency period and ending on December 31, 2024, shall include a qualified occupational therapist (as such term is used in section 1861(g)), a qualified physical therapist (as such term is used in section 1861(p)), a qualified speech-language pathologist (as defined in section 1861(ll)(4)(A)), and a qualified audiologist (as defined in section 1861(ll)(4)(B)).

(F) Telehealth service.—

(i) IN GENERAL.—Subject to paragraph (8), the term‘‘telehealth service’’ means professional consultations, office visits, and office psychiatry services (identified as of July 1, 2000, by HCPCS codes 99241– 99275, 99201–99215, 90804–90809, and 90862 (and as subsequently modified by the Secretary)), and any additional service specified by the Secretary.

(ii) YEARLY UPDATE.—The Secretary shall establish a process that provides, on an annual basis, for the addition or deletion of services (and HCPCS codes), as appropriate, to those specified in clause (i) for authorized payment under paragraph (1).

(5) Treatment of home dialysis monthly ESRD-related VISIT.—The geographic requirements described in paragraph (4)(C)(i) shall not apply with respect to telehealth services furnished on or after January 1, 2019, for purposes of section 1881(b)(3)(B), at an originating site described in subclause (VI), (IX), or (X) of paragraph (4)(C)(ii).

(6) Treatment of stroke telehealth services.—

(A) Non-application of originating site requireMENTS.—The requirements described in paragraph (4)(C) shall not apply with respect to telehealth services furnished on or after January 1, 2019, for purposes of diagnosis, evaluation, or treatment of symptoms of an acute stroke, as determined by the Secretary.

(B) INCLUSION OF CERTAIN SITES.—With respect to telehealth services described in subparagraph (A), the term ''originating site'' shall include any hospital (as defined in section 1861(e)) or critical access hospital (as defined in section 1861(mm)(1)), any mobile stroke unit (as defined by the Secretary), or any other site determined appropriate by the Secretary, at which the eligible telehealth individual is located at the time the service is furnished via a telecommunications system.

(C) No originating site facility fee for new sites.—

No facility fee shall be paid under paragraph (2)(B) to an originating site with respect to a telehealth service described in subparagraph (A) if the originating site does not otherwise meet the requirements for an originating site under paragraph (4)(C).

(7) Treatment of substance use disorder services and mental health services furnished through telehealth.—

(A) IN GENERAL.—The geographic requirements described in paragraph (4)(C)(i) shall not apply with respect to telehealth services furnished on or after July 1, 2019, to an eligible telehealth individual with a substance use disorder diagnosis for purposes of treatment of such disorder or co-occurring mental health disorder, as determined by the Secretary, or, on or after the first day after the end of the emergency period described in section 1135(g)(1)(B), subject to subparagraph (B), to an eligible telehealth individual for purposes of diagnosis, evaluation, or treatment of a mental health disorder, as determined by the Secretary, at an originating site described in paragraph (4)(C)(ii) (other than an originating site described in subclause (IX) of such paragraph) or, for the period for which clause (iii) of paragraph (4)(C) applies, at any site described in such clause.

(B) Requirements for mental health services furnished through telehealth.—

(i) IN GENERAL.—Payment may not be made under this paragraph for telehealth services furnished on or after the day that is the 152nd day after the end of the emergency period described in section 1135(g)(1)(B)) by a physician or practitioner to an eligible telehealth individual for purposes of diagnosis, evaluation, or treatment of a mental health disorder unless such physician or practitioner furnishes an item or service in person, without the use of telehealth, for which payment is made under this title (or would have been made under this title if such individual were entitled to, or enrolled for, benefits under this title at the time such item or service is furnished)—

(I) within the 6-month period prior to the first time such physician or practitioner furnishes such a telehealth service to the eligible telehealth individual; and

(II) during subsequent periods in which such physician or practitioner furnishes such telehealth services to the eligible telehealth individual, at such times as the Secretary determines appropriate.

(ii) CLARIFICATION.—This subparagraph shall not apply if payment would otherwise be allowed—

(I) under this paragraph (with respect to telehealth services furnished to an eligible telehealth individual with a substance use disorder diagnosis for purposes of treatment of such disorder or co-occurring mental health disorder); or

(II) under this subsection without application of this paragraph.

(8) Enhancing telehealth services for federally qualified health centers and rural health clinics.—

(A) IN GENERAL.—During the emergency period described in section 1135(g)(1)(B) and, in the case that such emergency period ends before December 31, 2024, during the period beginning on the first day after the end of such emergency period and ending on December 31, 2024—

(i) the Secretary shall pay for telehealth services that are furnished via a telecommunications system by a Federally qualified health center or a rural health clinic to an eligible telehealth individual enrolled under this part notwithstanding that the Federally qualified health center or rural clinic providing the telehealth service is not at the same location as the beneficiary;

(ii) the amount of payment to a Federally qualified health center or rural health clinic that serves as a distant site for such a telehealth service shall be determined under subparagraph (B); and

(iii) for purposes of this subsection—

(I) the term ''distant site'' includes a Federally qualified health center or rural health clinic that furnishes a telehealth service to an eligible telehealth individual; and

(II) the term ''telehealth services'' includes a rural health clinic service or Federally qualified health center service that is furnished using telehealth to the extent that payment codes corresponding to services identified by the Secretary under clause (i) or (ii) of paragraph (4)(F) are listed on the corresponding claim for such rural health clinic service or Federally qualified health center service.

(B) Special payment rule.—

(i) IN GENERAL.—The Secretary shall develop and implement payment methods that apply under this subsection to a Federally qualified health center or rural health clinic that serves as a distant site that furnishes a telehealth service to an eligible telehealth individual during the periods for which subparagraph

(A) applies. Such payment methods shall be based on payment rates that are similar to the national average payment rates for comparable telehealth services under the physician fee schedule under section 1848. Notwithstanding any other provision of law, the Secretary may implement such payment methods through program instruction or otherwise.

(ii) EXCLUSION FROM FQHC PPS CALCULATION AND RHC AIR CALCULATION.—Costs associated with telehealth services shall not be used to determine the amount of payment for Federally qualified health center services under the prospective payment system under section 1834(o) or for rural health clinic services under the methodology for all-inclusive rates (established by the Secretary) under section 1833(a)(3).

(9) TREATMENT OF TELEHEALTH SERVICES FURNISHED USING AUDIO-ONLY TELECOMMUNICATIONS TECHNOLOGY.—In the case that the emergency period described in section 1135(g)(1)(B) ends before December 31, 2024, the Secretary shall continue to provide coverage and payment under this part for telehealth services identified in paragraph (4)(F)(i) as of the date of the enactment of this paragraph that are furnished via an audio-only communications system during the period beginning on the first day after the end of such emergency period and ending on December 31, 2024. For purposes of the previous sentence, the term ‘‘telehealth service’’ means a telehealth service identified as of the date of the enactment of this paragraph by a HCPCS code (and any succeeding codes) for which the Secretary has not applied the requirements of paragraph (1) and the first sentence of section 410.78(a)(3) of title 42, Code of Federal Regulations, during such emergency period.

(10) Required use of modifiers in certain instances.—

Not later than January 1, 2026, the Secretary shall establish requirements to include a code or modifier, as determined appropriate by the Secretary, in the case of claims for telehealth services under this subsection that are billed incident to a physician’s or practitioner’s professional service.

(d) AUTHORITY TO MODIFY OR ELIMINATE COVERAGE OF CERTAIN PREVENTIVE SERVICES.—Notwithstanding any other provision of this title, effective beginning on January 1, 2010, if the Secretary determines appropriate, the Secretary may—

(1) modify—

(A) the coverage of any preventive service described in subparagraph (A) of section 1861(ddd)(3) to the extent that such modification is consistent with the recommendations of the United States Preventive Services Task Force; and

(B) the services included in the initial preventive physical examination described in subparagraph (B) of such section; and

(2) provide that no payment shall be made under this title for a preventive service described in subparagraph (A) of such section that has not received a grade of A, B, C, or I by such Task Force.

(e) DEVELOPMENT AND IMPLEMENTATION OF PROSPECTIVE PAYment System.—

(1) Development.—

(A) IN GENERAL.—The Secretary shall develop a prospective payment system for payment for Federally qualified health center services furnished by Federally qualified health centers under this title. Such system shall include a process for appropriately describing the services furnished by Federally qualified health centers and shall establish payment rates for specific payment codes based on such appropriate descriptions of services. Such system shall be established to take into account the type, intensity, and duration of services furnished by Federally qualified health centers. Such system may include adjustments, including geographic adjustments, determined appropriate by the Secretary.

(B) COLLECTION OF DATA AND EVALUATION.—By not later than January 1, 2011, the Secretary shall require Federally qualified health centers to submit to the Secretary such information as the Secretary may require in order to develop and implement the prospective payment system under this subsection, including the reporting of services using HCPCS codes.

(2) Implementation.—

(A) IN GENERAL.—Notwithstanding section 1833(a)(3)(A), the Secretary shall provide, for cost reporting periods beginning on or after October 1, 2014, for payments of prospective payment rates for Federally qualified health center services furnished by Federally qualified health centers under this title in accordance with the prospective payment system developed by the Secretary under paragraph (1).

(B) Payments.—

(i) INITIAL PAYMENTS.—The Secretary shall implement such prospective payment system so that the estimated aggregate amount of prospective payment rates (determined prior to the application of section

1833(a)(1)(Z)) under this title for Federally qualified health center services in the first year that such system is implemented is equal to 100 percent of the estimated amount of reasonable costs (determined without the application of a per visit payment limit or productivity screen and prior to the application of section 1866(a)(2)(A)(ii)) that would have occurred for such services under this title in such year if the system had not been implemented.

(ii) PAYMENTS IN SUBSEQUENT YEARS.—Payment

rates in years after the year of implementation of such system shall be the payment rates in the previous year increased—

(I) in the first year after implementation of such system, by the percentage increase in the MEI (as defined in section 1842(i)(3)) for the year involved; and

(I) in subsequent years, by the percentage increase in a market basket of Federally qualified health center goods and services as promulgated through regulations, or if such an index is not available, by the percentage increase in the MEI (as defined in section 1842(i)(3)) for the year involved.

(B) PREPARATION FOR PPS IMPLEMENTATION.—Notwithstanding any other provision of law, the Secretary may establish and implement by program instruction or otherwise the payment codes to be used under the prospective payment system under this section.

(2) Additional payments for certain fqhcs with physicians or other practitioners receiving data 2000 waivers.—

(A) IN GENERAL.—In the case of a Federally qualified health center with respect to which, beginning on or after January 1, 2019, Federally qualified health center services (as defined in section 1861(aa)(3)) are furnished for the treatment of opioid use disorder by a physician or practitioner who meets the requirements described in subparagraph (C), the Secretary shall, subject to availability of funds under subparagraph (D), make a payment (at such time and in such manner as specified by the Secretary) to such Federally qualified health center after receiving and approving an application submitted by such Federally qualified health center under subparagraph (B). Such a payment shall be in an amount determined by the Secretary, based on an estimate of the average costs of training for purposes of receiving a waiver described in subparagraph (C)(ii). Such a payment may be made only one time with respect to each such physician or practitioner.

(B) APPLICATION.—In order to receive a payment described in subparagraph (A), a Federally qualified health center shall submit to the Secretary an application for such a payment at such time, in such manner, and containing such information as specified by the Secretary. A Federally qualified health center may apply for such a payment for each physician or practitioner described in subparagraph (A) furnishing services described in such subparagraph at such center.

(C) REQUIREMENTS.—For purposes of subparagraph (A), the requirements described in this subparagraph, with respect to a physician or practitioner, are the following:

(i) The physician or practitioner is employed by or working under contract with a Federally qualified health center described in subparagraph (A) that submits an application under subparagraph (B).

(ii) The physician or practitioner first receives a waiver under section 303(h) of the Controlled Substances Act on or after January 1, 2019.

(D) FUNDING.—For purposes of making payments under this paragraph, there are appropriated, out of amounts in the Treasury not otherwise appropriated, $6,000,000, which shall remain available until expended.

(3) Payment for certain services furnished by federally qualified health centers.—

(A) Attending physician services for hospice paTIENTS.—In the case of services described in section?1812(d)(2)(A)(ii) furnished on or after January 1, 2022, by an attending physician (as defined in section 1861(dd)(3)(B), other than a physician or practitioner who is employed by a hospice program) who is employed by or working under contract with a Federally qualified health center, a Federally qualified health center shall be paid for such services under the prospective payment system under this subsection.

(B) Mental health visits furnished via teleCOMMUNICATIONS TECHNOLOGY.—In the case of mental health visits furnished via interactive, real-time, audio and video telecommunications technology or audio-only interactions, the in-person mental health visit requirements established under section 405.2463(b)(3) of title 42 of the Code of Federal Regulations (or a successor regulation) shall not apply prior to January 1, 2025 (or, if later, the first day after the end of the emergency period described in section 1135(g)(1)(B)).

(4) Special payment rule for intensive outpatient services.—

(A) IN GENERAL.—In the case of intensive outpatient services furnished by a Federally qualified health center, the payment amount for such services shall be equal to the amount that would have been paid under this title for such services had such services been covered OPD services furnished by a hospital.

(B) EXCLUSION.—Costs associated with intensive outpatient services shall not be used to determine the amount of payment for Federally qualified health center services under the prospective payment system under this subsection.

(C) QUALITY INCENTIVES TO PROMOTE PATIENT SAFETY AND PUBlic Health in Computed Tomography.—

(1) (1) QUALITY INCENTIVES.—In the case of an applicable computed tomography service (as defined in paragraph (2)) for which payment is made under an applicable payment system (as defined in paragraph (3)) and that is furnished on or after January 1, 2016, using equipment that is not consistent with the CT equipment standard (described in paragraph (4)), the payment amount for such service shall be reduced by the applicable percentage (as defined in paragraph (5)).

(2) Applicable computed tomography services defined.—

In this subsection, the term ''applicable computed tomography service'' means a service billed using diagnostic radiological imaging codes for computed tomography (identified as of January 1, 2014, by HCPCS codes 70450–70498, 71250–71275, 72125–72133, 72191–72194, 73200–73206, 73700–73706, 74150–74178, 74261–74263, and 75571–75574 (and any succeeding codes).

(3) APPLICABLE PAYMENT SYSTEM DEFINED.—In this subsection, the term ''applicable payment system'' means the following:

(A) The technical component and the technical component of the global fee under the fee schedule established under section 1848(b).

(B) The prospective payment system for hospital outpatient department services under section 1833(t).

(4) CONSISTENCY WITH CT EQUIPMENT STANDARD.—In this subsection, the term ''not consistent with the CT equipment standard'' means, with respect to an applicable computed tomography service, that the service was furnished using equipment that does not meet each of the attributes of the National Electrical Manufacturers Association (NEMA) Standard XR- 29-2013, entitled ''Standard Attributes on CT Equipment Related to Dose Optimization and Management''. Through rule-making, the Secretary may apply successor standards.

(5) APPLICABLE PERCENTAGE DEFINED.—In this subsection, the term ''applicable percentage'' means—

(A) for 2016, 5 percent; and

(B) for 2017 and subsequent years, 15 percent.

(6) Implementation.—

(A) INFORMATION.—The Secretary shall require that information be provided and attested to by a supplier and a hospital outpatient department that indicates whether an applicable computed tomography service was furnished that was not consistent with the CT equipment standard (described in paragraph (4)). Such information may be included on a claim and may be a modifier. Such information shall be verified, as appropriate, as part of the periodic accreditation of suppliers under section 1834(e) and hospitals under section 1865(a).

(B) ADMINISTRATION.—Chapter 35 of title 44, United States Code, shall not apply to information described in subparagraph (A).

(D) RECOGNIZING APPROPRIATE USE CRITERIA FOR CERTAIN IMAGing Services.—

(1) Program established.—

(A) IN GENERAL.—The Secretary shall establish a program to promote the use of appropriate use criteria (as defined in subparagraph (B)) for applicable imaging services (as defined in subparagraph (C)) furnished in an applicable setting (as defined in subparagraph (D)) by ordering professionals and furnishing professionals (as defined in subparagraphs (E) and (F), respectively).

(B) APPROPRIATE USE CRITERIA DEFINED.—In this subsection, the term ''appropriate use criteria'' means criteria, only developed or endorsed by national professional medical specialty societies or other provider-led entities, to assist ordering professionals and furnishing professionals in making the most appropriate treatment decision for a specific clinical condition for an individual. To the extent feasible, such criteria shall be evidence-based.

APPLICABLE IMAGING SERVICE DEFINED.—In this subsection, the term ''applicable imaging service'' means an advanced diagnostic imaging service (as defined in subsection (e)(1)(B)) for which the Secretary determines—

(i) one or more applicable appropriate use criteria specified under paragraph (2) apply;

(ii) there are one or more qualified clinical decision support mechanisms listed under paragraph (3)(C); and

(iii) one or more of such mechanisms is available free of charge.

(D) APPLICABLE SETTING DEFINED.—In this subsection, the term ''applicable setting'' means a physician's office, a hospital outpatient department (including an emergency department), an ambulatory surgical center, and any other provider-led outpatient setting determined appropriate by the Secretary.

(E) ORDERING PROFESSIONAL DEFINED.—In this subsection, the term ''ordering professional'' means a physician (as defined in section 1861(r)) or a practitioner described in section 1842(b)(18)(C) who orders an applicable imaging service.

(F) FURNISHING PROFESSIONAL DEFINED.—In this subsection, the term ''furnishing professional'' means a physician (as defined in section 1861(r)) or a practitioner described in section 1842(b)(18)(C) who furnishes an applicable imaging service.

(2) Establishment of applicable appropriate use criteria.—

(A) IN GENERAL.—Not later than November 15, 2015, the Secretary shall through rulemaking, and in consultation with physicians, practitioners, and other stakeholders, specify applicable appropriate use criteria for applicable imaging services only from among appropriate use criteria developed or endorsed by national professional medical specialty societies or other provider-led entities.

(B) CONSIDERATIONS.—In specifying applicable appropriate use criteria under subparagraph (A), the Secretary shall take into account whether the criteria—

(i) have stakeholder consensus;

(ii) are scientifically valid and evidence based; and

(iii) are based on studies that are published and reviewable by stakeholders.

(C) REVISIONS.—The Secretary shall review, on an annual basis, the specified applicable appropriate use criteria to determine if there is a need to update or revise (as appropriate) such specification of applicable appropriate use criteria and make such updates or revisions through rule-making.

(D) TREATMENT OF MULTIPLE APPLICABLE APPROPRIATE USE CRITERIA.—In the case where the Secretary determines that more than one appropriate use criterion applies with respect to an applicable imaging service, the Secretary shall apply one or more applicable appropriate use criteria under this paragraph for the service.

(3) Mechanisms for consultation with applicable appropriate use criteria.—

Identification of mechanisms to consult with applicable appropriate use criteria.—

(i) IN GENERAL.—The Secretary shall specify qualified clinical decision support mechanisms that could be used by ordering professionals to consult with applicable appropriate use criteria for applicable imaging services.

(ii) CONSULTATION.—The Secretary shall consult with physicians, practitioners, health care technology experts, and other stakeholders in specifying mechanisms under this paragraph.

INCLUSION OF CERTAIN MECHANISMS.—Mechanisms specified under this paragraph may include any or all of the following that meet the requirements described in subparagraph (B)(ii):

(I) Use of clinical decision support modules in certified EHR technology (as defined in section 1848(o)(4)).

(II) Use of private sector clinical decision support mechanisms that are independent from certified EHR technology, which may include use of clinical decision support mechanisms available from medical specialty organizations.

(III) Use of a clinical decision support mechanism established by the Secretary.

(B) Qualified clinical decision support mechanisms.—

(i) IN GENERAL.—For purposes of this subsection, a qualified clinical decision support mechanism is a mechanism that the Secretary determines meets the requirements described in clause (ii).

(ii) REQUIREMENTS.—The requirements described in this clause are the following:

(I) The mechanism makes available to the ordering professional applicable appropriate use criteria specified under paragraph (2) and the supporting documentation for the applicable imaging service ordered.

(II) In the case where there is more than one applicable appropriate use criterion specified under such paragraph for an applicable imaging service, the mechanism indicates the criteria that it uses for the service.

(III) The mechanism determines the extent to which an applicable imaging service ordered is consistent with the applicable appropriate use criteria so specified.

(IV) The mechanism generates and provides to the ordering professional a certification or docu mentation that documents that the qualified clinical decision support mechanism was consulted by the ordering professional.

(V) The mechanism is updated on a timely basis to reflect revisions to the specification of applicable appropriate use criteria under such paragraph.

(VI) The mechanism meets privacy and security standards under applicable provisions of law.

(VII) The mechanism performs such other functions as specified by the Secretary, which may include a requirement to provide aggregate feedback to the ordering professional.

(C) List of mechanisms for consultation with applicable appropriate use criteria.—

(i) INITIAL LIST.—Not later than April 1, 2016, the Secretary shall publish a list of mechanisms specified under this paragraph.

(ii) PERIODIC UPDATING OF LIST.—The Secretary shall identify on an annual basis the list of qualified clinical decision support mechanisms specified under this paragraph.

(4) Consultation with applicable appropriate use criteria.—

(A) CONSULTATION BY ORDERING PROFESSIONAL.—Beginning with January 1, 2017, subject to subparagraph (C), with respect to an applicable imaging service ordered by an ordering professional that would be furnished in an applicable setting and paid for under an applicable payment system (as defined in subparagraph (D)), an ordering professional shall—

(i) consult with a qualified decision support mechanism listed under paragraph (3)(C); and

(ii) provide to the furnishing professional the information described in clauses (i) through (iii) of subparagraph (B).

(B) REPORTING BY FURNISHING PROFESSIONAL.—Beginning with January 1, 2017, subject to subparagraph (C), with respect to an applicable imaging service furnished in an applicable setting and paid for under an applicable payment system (as defined in subparagraph (D)), payment for such service may only be made if the claim for the service includes the following:

(i) Information about which qualified clinical decision support mechanism was consulted by the ordering professional for the service.

(ii) Information regarding—

(I) whether the service ordered would adhere to the applicable appropriate use criteria specified under paragraph (2);

(II) whether the service ordered would not adhere to such criteria; or

(III) whether such criteria was not applicable to the service ordered.

(iii) The national provider identifier of the ordering professional (if different from the furnishing professional).

(C) EXCEPTIONS.—The provisions of subparagraphs (A) and (B) and paragraph (6)(A) shall not apply to the following:

(i) EMERGENCY SERVICES.—An applicable imaging service ordered for an individual with an emergency medical condition (as defined in section 1867(e)(1)).

(ii) INPATIENT SERVICES.—An applicable imaging service ordered for an inpatient and for which payment is made under part A.

(iii) SIGNIFICANT HARDSHIP.—An applicable imaging service ordered by an ordering professional who the Secretary may, on a case-by-case basis, exempt from the application of such provisions if the Secretary determines, subject to annual renewal, that consultation with applicable appropriate use criteria would result in a significant hardship, such as in the case of a professional who practices in a rural area without sufficient Internet access.

(D) APPLICABLE PAYMENT SYSTEM DEFINED.—In this subsection, the term ''applicable payment system'' means the following:

(i) The physician fee schedule established under section 1848(b).

(ii) The prospective payment system for hospital outpatient department services under section 1833(t).

(iii) The ambulatory surgical center payment systems under section 1833(i).

(5) Identification of outlier ordering professionals.—

(A) IN GENERAL.—With respect to applicable imaging services furnished beginning with 2017, the Secretary shall determine, on an annual basis, no more than five percent of the total number of ordering professionals who are outlier ordering professionals.

(B) OUTLIER ORDERING PROFESSIONALS.—The determination of an outlier ordering professional shall—

(i) be based on low adherence to applicable appropriate use criteria specified under paragraph (2), which may be based on comparison to other ordering professionals; and

(i) include data for ordering professionals for whom prior authorization under paragraph (6)(A) applies.

(B) USE OF TWO YEARS OF DATA.—The Secretary shall use two years of data to identify outlier ordering professionals under this paragraph.

(C) PROCESS.—The Secretary shall establish a process for determining when an outlier ordering professional is no longer an outlier ordering professional.

(D) CONSULTATION WITH STAKEHOLDERS.—The Secretary shall consult with physicians, practitioners and other stakeholders in developing methods to identify outlier ordering professionals under this paragraph.

(2) Prior authorization for ordering professionals who are outliers.—

(A) IN GENERAL.—Beginning January 1, 2020, subject to paragraph (4)(C), with respect to services furnished during a year, the Secretary shall, for a period determined appropriate by the Secretary, apply prior authorization for applicable imaging services that are ordered by an outlier ordering professional identified under paragraph (5).

(B) APPROPRIATE USE CRITERIA IN PRIOR AUTHORIZATION.—In applying prior authorization under subparagraph (A), the Secretary shall utilize only the applicable appropriate use criteria specified under this subsection.

(C) FUNDING.—For purposes of carrying out this paragraph, the Secretary shall provide for the transfer, from the Federal Supplementary Medical Insurance Trust Fund under section 1841, of $5,000,000 to the Centers for Medicare & Medicaid Services Program Management Account for each of fiscal years 2019 through 2021. Amounts transferred under the preceding sentence shall remain available until expended.

(3) CONSTRUCTION.—Nothing in this subsection shall be construed as granting the Secretary the authority to develop or initiate the development of clinical practice guidelines or appropriate use criteria..

c) PAYMENT FOR RENAL DIALYSIS SERVICES FOR INDIVIDUALS WITH ACUTE KIDNEY INJURY.—

(1) PAYMENT RATE.—In the case of renal dialysis services (as defined in subparagraph (B) of section 1881(b)(14)) furnished under this part by a renal dialysis facility or provider of services paid under such section during a year (beginning with 2017) to an individual with acute kidney injury (as defined in paragraph (2)), the amount of payment under this part for such services shall be the base rate for renal dialysis services determined for such year under such section, as adjusted by any applicable geographic adjustment factor applied under subparagraph (D)(iv)(II) of such section and may be adjusted by the Secretary (on a budget neutral basis for payments under this paragraph) by any other adjustment factor under subparagraph (D) of such section.

(2) INDIVIDUAL WITH ACUTE KIDNEY INJURY DEFINED.—In this subsection, the term ''individual with acute kidney injury'' means an individual who has acute loss of renal function and does not receive renal dialysis services for which payment is made under section 1881(b)(14).

PAYMENT FOR APPLICABLE DISPOSABLE DEVICES.—

(1) SEPARATE PAYMENT.—The Secretary shall make a payment (separate from the payments otherwise made under section 1895) in the amount established under paragraph (3) to a home health agency for an applicable disposable device (as defined in paragraph (2)) when furnished on or after January 1, 2017, to an individual who receives home health services for which payment is made under section 1895(b).

(2) APPLICABLE DISPOSABLE DEVICE.—In this subsection, the term applicable disposable device means a disposable device that, as determined by the Secretary, is—

(A) a disposable negative pressure wound therapy device that is an integrated system comprised of a non-manual vacuum pump, a receptacle for collecting exudate, and dressings for the purposes of wound therapy; and

(B) a substitute for, and used in lieu of, a negative pressure wound therapy durable medical equipment item that is an integrated system of a negative pressure vacuum pump, a separate exudate collection canister, and dressings that would otherwise be covered for individuals for such wound therapy.

(3) PAYMENT.—

(A) IN GENERAL.—The separate payment amount established under this paragraph for an applicable disposable device for a year shall be equal to—

(i) for a year before 2024, the amount of the payment that would be made under section 1833(t) (relating to payment for covered OPD services) for the year for the Level I Healthcare Common Procedure Coding System (HCPCS) code for which the description for a professional service includes the furnishing of such device;

(ii) for 2024, the supply price used to determine the relative value for the service under the fee schedule under section 1848 (as of January 1, 2022) for the applicable disposable device, updated by the specified adjustment described in subparagraph (B) for such year; and

(iii) for 2025 and each subsequent year, the payment amount established under this paragraph for such device for the previous year, updated by the specified adjustment described in subparagraph (B) for such year.

(B) Specified adjustment.—

(i) IN GENERAL.—For purposes of subparagraph (A), the specified adjustment described in this subparagraph for a year is equal to—

(I) the percentage increase in the consumer price index for all urban consumers (United States city average) for the 12-month period ending in June of the previous year; minus

(II) the productivity adjustment described in section 1886(b)(3)(B)(xi)(II) for such year.

(ii) CLARIFICATION ON APPLICATION OF THE PRODUCTIVITY ADJUSTMENT.—The application of clause (i)(II) may result in a specified adjustment of less than 0.0 for a year, and may result in the separate payment amount under this subsection for an applicable device for a year being less than such separate payment amount for such device for the preceding year.

(C) Exclusion of nursing and therapy services from SEPARATE PAYMENT.—With respect to applicable devices furnished on or after January 1, 2024, the separate payment amount determined under this paragraph shall not include payment for nursing or therapy services described in section 1861(m). Payment for such nursing or therapy services shall be made under the prospective payment system established under section 1895 and shall not be separately billable.

(4) IMPLEMENTATION.—As part of submitting claims for the separate payment established under this subsection, beginning with 2024, the Secretary shall accept and process claims submitted using the type of bill that is most commonly used by home health agencies to bill services under a home health plan of care.

SITE-OF-SERVICE PRICE TRANSPARENCY.—

(1) IN GENERAL.—In order to facilitate price transparency with respect to items and services for which payment may be made either to a hospital outpatient department or to an ambulatory surgical center under this title, the Secretary shall, for 2018 and each year thereafter, make available to the public via a searchable Internet website, with respect to an appropriate number of such items and services—

(A) the estimated payment amount for the item or service under the outpatient department fee schedule under subsection (t) of section 1833 and the ambulatory surgical center payment system under subsection (i) of such section; and

(B) the estimated amount of beneficiary liability applicable to the item or service.

(2) CALCULATION OF ESTIMATED BENEFICIARY LIABILITY.—For purposes of paragraph (1)(B), the estimated amount of beneficiary liability, with respect to an item or service, is the amount for such item or service for which an individual who does not have coverage under a Medicare supplemental policy certified under section 1882 or any other supplemental insurance coverage is responsible.

(3) IMPLEMENTATION.—In carrying out this subsection, the Secretary—

(A) shall include in the notice described in section 1804(a) a notification of the availability of the estimated amounts made available under paragraph (1); and

(B) may utilize mechanisms in existence on the date of enactment of this subsection, such as the portion of the Internet website of the Centers for Medicare & Medicaid Services on which information comparing physician performance is posted (commonly referred to as the Physician Compare Internet website), to make available such estimated amounts under such paragraph.

(4) FUNDING.—For purposes of implementing this subsection, the Secretary shall provide for the transfer, from the Federal Supplementary Medical Insurance Trust Fund under section 1841 to the Centers for Medicare & Medicaid Services Program Management Account, of $6,000,000 for fiscal year 2017, to remain available until expended.

(f) PAYMENT AND RELATED REQUIREMENTS FOR HOME INFUSION THERAPY.—

(1) PAYMENT.—

Single payment.—

(i) IN GENERAL.—Subject to clause (iii) and subparagraphs (B) and (C), the Secretary shall implement a payment system under which a single payment is made under this title to a qualified home infusion therapy supplier for items and services described in subparagraphs (A) and (B) of section 1861(iii)(2)) furnished by a qualified home infusion therapy supplier (as defined in section 1861(iii)(3)(D)) in coordination with the furnishing of home infusion drugs (as defined in section 1861(iii)(3)(C)) under this part.

(ii) UNIT OF SINGLE PAYMENT.—A unit of single payment under the payment system implemented under this subparagraph is for each infusion drug administration calendar day in the individual's home. The Secretary shall, as appropriate, establish single payment amounts for types of infusion therapy, including to take into account variation in utilization of nursing services by therapy type.

(iii) LIMITATION.—The single payment amount determined under this subparagraph after application of subparagraph (B) and paragraph (3) shall not exceed the amount determined under the fee schedule under section 1848 for infusion therapy services furnished in a calendar day if furnished in a physician office setting, except such single payment shall not reflect more than 5 hours of infusion for a particular therapy in a calendar day.

(B) REQUIRED ADJUSTMENTS.—The Secretary shall adjust the single payment amount determined under subparagraph (A) for home infusion therapy services under section 1861(iii)(1) to reflect other factors such as—

(i) a geographic wage index and other costs that may vary by region; and

(ii) patient acuity and complexity of drug administration.

(C) Discretionary adjustments.—

(i) IN GENERAL.—Subject to clause (ii), the Secretary may adjust the single payment amount determined under subparagraph (A) (after application of subparagraph (B)) to reflect outlier situations and other factors as the Secretary determines appropriate.

(ii) REQUIREMENT OF BUDGET NEUTRALITY.—Any adjustment under this subparagraph shall be made in a budget neutral manner.

(2) CONSIDERATIONS.—In developing the payment system under this subsection, the Secretary may consider the costs of furnishing infusion therapy in the home, consult with home infusion therapy suppliers, consider payment amounts for similar items and services under this part and part A, and consider payment amounts established by Medicare Advantage plans under part C and in the private insurance market for home infusion therapy (including average per treatment day payment amounts by type of home infusion therapy).

Annual updates.—

(A) IN GENERAL.—Subject to subparagraph (B), the Secretary shall update the single payment amount under this subsection from year to year beginning in 2022 by increasing the single payment amount from the prior year by the percentage increase in the Consumer Price Index for all urban consumers (United States city average) for the 12- month period ending with June of the preceding year.

(B) ADJUSTMENT.—For each year, the Secretary shall reduce the percentage increase described in subparagraph

(A) by the productivity adjustment described in section 1886(b)(3)(B)(xi)(II). The application of the preceding sentence may result in a percentage being less than 0.0 for a year, and may result in payment being less than such payment rates for the preceding year.

(4) AUTHORITY TO APPLY PRIOR AUTHORIZATION.—The Secretary may, as determined appropriate by the Secretary, apply prior authorization for home infusion therapy services under section 1861(iii)(1).

(5) Accreditation of qualified home infusion therapy suppliers.—

(A) FACTORS FOR DESIGNATION OF ACCREDITATION ORGANIZATIONS.—The Secretary shall consider the following factors in designating accreditation organizations under subparagraph (B) and in reviewing and modifying the list of accreditation organizations designated pursuant to subparagraph (C):

(i) The ability of the organization to conduct timely reviews of accreditation applications.

(ii) The ability of the organization to take into account the capacities of suppliers located in a rural area (as defined in section 1886(d)(2)(D)).

(iii) Whether the organization has established reasonable fees to be charged to suppliers applying for accreditation.

(iv) Such other factors as the Secretary determines appropriate.

(B) DESIGNATION.—Not later than January 1, 2021, the Secretary shall designate organizations to accredit suppliers furnishing home infusion therapy. The list of accreditation organizations so designated may be modified pursuant to subparagraph (C).

(C) Review and modification of list of accreditation organizations.—

(i) IN GENERAL.—The Secretary shall review the list of accreditation organizations designated under subparagraph (B) taking into account the factors under subparagraph (A). Taking into account the results of such review, the Secretary may, by regulation, modify the list of accreditation organizations designated under subparagraph (B).

(ii) SPECIAL RULE FOR ACCREDITATIONS DONE PRIOR TO REMOVAL FROM LIST OF DESIGNATED ACCREDITATION

ORGANIZATIONS.—In the case where the Secretary removes an organization from the list of accreditation organizations designated under subparagraph (B), any supplier that is accredited by the organization during the period beginning on the date on which the organization is designated as an accreditation organization under subparagraph (B) and ending on the date on which the organization is removed from such list shall be considered to have been accredited by an organization designated by the Secretary under subparagraph

(B) for the remaining period such accreditation is in effect.

(D) Rule for accreditations made prior to designaTION.—In the case of a supplier that is accredited before January 1, 2021, by an accreditation organization designated by the Secretary under subparagraph (B) as of January 1, 2019, such supplier shall be considered to have been accredited by an organization designated by the Secretary under such paragraph as of January 1, 2023, for the remaining period such accreditation is in effect.

(6) NOTIFICATION OF INFUSION THERAPY OPTIONS AVAILABLE PRIOR TO FURNISHING HOME INFUSION THERAPY.—Prior to the furnishing of home infusion therapy to an individual, the physician who establishes the plan described in section 1861(iii)(1) for the individual shall provide notification (in a form, manner, and frequency determined appropriate by the Secretary) of the options available (such as home, physician's office, hospital outpatient department) for the furnishing of infusion therapy under this part.

(7) Home infusion therapy services temporary transitional payment.—

(A) Temporary transitional payment.—

(i) IN GENERAL.—The Secretary shall, in accordance with the payment methodology described in subparagraph (B) and subject to the provisions of this paragraph, provide a home infusion therapy services temporary transitional payment under this part to an eligible home infusion supplier (as defined in subparagraph (F)) for items and services described in subparagraphs (A) and (B) of section 1861(iii)(2)) furnished during the period specified in clause (ii) by such supplier in coordination with the furnishing of transitional home infusion drugs (as defined in clause (iii)).

(ii) PERIOD SPECIFIED.—For purposes of clause (i), the period specified in this clause is the period beginning on January 1, 2019, and ending on the day before the date of the implementation of the payment system under paragraph (1)(A).

(iii) TRANSITIONAL HOME INFUSION DRUG DEFINED.—

For purposes of this paragraph, the term ''transitional home infusion drug'' has the meaning given to the term ''home infusion drug'' under section 1861(iii)(3)(C)), except that clause (ii) of such section shall not apply if a drug described in such clause is identified in clauses (i), (ii), (iii) or (iv) of subparagraph (C) as of the date of the enactment of this paragraph.

(B) PAYMENT METHODOLOGY.—For purposes of this paragraph, the Secretary shall establish a payment methodology, with respect to items and services described in subparagraph (A)(i). Under such payment methodology the Secretary shall—

(i) create the three payment categories described in clauses (i), (ii), and (iii) of subparagraph (C);

(ii) assign drugs to such categories, in accordance with such clauses;

(iii) assign appropriate Healthcare Common Procedure Coding System (HCPCS) codes to each payment category; and

(iv) establish a single payment amount for each such payment category, in accordance with subparagraph (D), for each infusion drug administration calendar day in the individual's home for drugs assigned to such category.

(C) Payment categories.—

(i) PAYMENT CATEGORY 1.—The Secretary shall create a payment category 1 and assign to such category drugs which are covered under the Local Coverage Determination on External Infusion Pumps (LCD number L33794) and billed with the following HCPCS codes (as identified as of January 1, 2018, and as subsequently modified by the Secretary): J0133, J0285, J0287, J0288, J0289, J0895, J1170, J1250, J1265, J1325, J1455, J1457, J1570, J2175, J2260, J2270, J2274, J2278, J3010, or J3285.

(ii) PAYMENT CATEGORY 2.—The Secretary shall create a payment category 2 and assign to such category drugs which are covered under such local coverage determination and billed with the following HCPCS codes (as identified as of January 1, 2018, and as subsequently modified by the Secretary): J1555 JB, J1559 JB, J1561 JB, J1562 JB, J1569 JB, or J1575 JB.

(iii) PAYMENT CATEGORY 3.—The Secretary shall create a payment category 3 and assign to such category drugs which are covered under such local coverage determination and billed with the following HCPCS codes (as identified as of January 1, 2018, and as subsequently modified by the Secretary): J9000, J9039, J9040, J9065, J9100, J9190, J9200, J9360, or J9370.

(iv) INFUSION DRUGS NOT OTHERWISE INCLUDED.—

With respect to drugs that are not included in payment category 1, 2, or 3 under clause (i), (ii), or (iii), respectively, the Secretary shall assign to the most appropriate of such categories, as determined by the Secretary, drugs which are—

(I) covered under such local coverage determination and billed under HCPCS codes J7799 or J7999 (as identified as of July 1, 2017, and as subsequently modified by the Secretary); or

(II) billed under any code that is implemented after the date of the enactment of this paragraph and included in such local coverage determination or included in subregulatory guidance as a home infusion drug described in subparagraph (A)(i).

(D) Payment amounts.—

(i) IN GENERAL.—Under the payment methodology, the Secretary shall pay eligible home infusion suppliers, with respect to items and services described in subparagraph (A)(i) furnished during the period described in subparagraph (A)(ii) by such supplier to an individual, at amounts equal to the amounts determined under the physician fee schedule established under section 1848 for services furnished during the year for codes and units of such codes described in clauses (ii), (iii), and (iv) with respect to drugs included in the payment category under subparagraph (C) specified in the respective clause, determined without application of the geographic adjustment under subsection (e) of such section.

(ii) PAYMENT AMOUNT FOR CATEGORY 1.—For purposes of clause (i), the codes and units described in this clause, with respect to drugs included in payment category 1 described in subparagraph (C)(i), are one unit of HCPCS code 96365 plus three units of HCPCS code 96366 (as identified as of January 1, 2018, and as subsequently modified by the Secretary).

(iii) PAYMENT AMOUNT FOR CATEGORY 2.—For purposes of clause (i), the codes and units described in this clause, with respect to drugs included in payment category 2 described in subparagraph (C)(i), are one unit of HCPCS code 96369 plus three units of HCPCS code 96370 (as identified as of January 1, 2018, and as subsequently modified by the Secretary).

(iv) PAYMENT AMOUNT FOR CATEGORY 3.—For purposes of clause (i), the codes and units described in this clause, with respect to drugs included in payment category 3 described in subparagraph (C)(i), are one unit of HCPCS code 96413 plus three units of HCPCS code 96415 (as identified as of January 1, 2018, and as subsequently modified by the Secretary).

(E) Clarifications.—

(i) INFUSION DRUG ADMINISTRATION DAY.—For purposes of this subsection, with respect to the furnishing of transitional home infusion drugs or home infusion drugs to an individual by an eligible home infusion supplier or a qualified home infusion therapy supplier, a reference to payment to such supplier for an infusion drug administration calendar day in the individual's home shall refer to payment only for the date on which professional services (as described in section 1861(iii)(2)(A)) were furnished to administer such drugs to such individual. For purposes of the previous sentence, an infusion drug administration calendar day shall include all such drugs administered to such individual on such day.

(ii) TREATMENT OF MULTIPLE DRUGS ADMINISTERED ON SAME INFUSION DRUG ADMINISTRATION DAY.—In the case that an eligible home infusion supplier, with respect to an infusion drug administration calendar day in an individual's home, furnishes to such individual transitional home infusion drugs which are not all assigned to the same payment category under subparagraph (C), payment to such supplier for such infusion drug administration calendar day in the individual's home shall be a single payment equal to the amount of payment under this paragraph for the drug, among all such drugs so furnished to such individual during such calendar day, for which the highest payment would be made under this paragraph.

(F) ELIGIBLE HOME INFUSION SUPPLIERS.—In this paragraph, the term ''eligible home infusion supplier'' means a supplier that is enrolled under this part as a pharmacy that provides external infusion pumps and external infusion pump supplies and that maintains all pharmacy licensure requirements in the State in which the applicable infusion drugs are administered.

(G) IMPLEMENTATION.—Notwithstanding any other provision of law, the Secretary may implement this paragraph by program instruction or otherwise.

(g) PAYMENT FOR OUTPATIENT PHYSICAL THERAPY SERVICES AND OUTPATIENT OCCUPATIONAL THERAPY SERVICES FURNISHED BY A THERAPY ASSISTANT.—

(1) IN GENERAL.—In the case of an outpatient physical therapy service or outpatient occupational therapy service furnished on or after January 1, 2022, for which payment is made under section 1848 or subsection (k), that is furnished in whole or in part by a therapy assistant (as defined by the Secretary), the amount of payment for such service shall be an amount equal to 85 percent of the amount of payment otherwise applicable for the service under this part. Nothing in the preceding sentence shall be construed to change applicable requirements with respect to such services.

(2) Use of modifier.—

(A) ESTABLISHMENT.—Not later than January 1, 2019, the Secretary shall establish a modifier to indicate (in a form and manner specified by the Secretary), in the case of an outpatient physical therapy service or outpatient occupational therapy service furnished in whole or in part by a therapy assistant (as so defined), that the service was furnished by a therapy assistant.

(B) REQUIRED USE.—Each request for payment, or bill submitted, for an outpatient physical therapy service or outpatient occupational therapy service furnished in whole or in part by a therapy assistant (as so defined) on or after January 1, 2020, shall include the modifier established under subparagraph (A) for each such service.

(3) IMPLEMENTATION.—The Secretary shall implement this subsection through notice and comment rulemaking.

(h) OPIOID USE DISORDER TREATMENT SERVICES.—

(1) IN GENERAL.—The Secretary shall pay to an opioid treatment program (as defined in paragraph (2) of section 1861(jjj)) an amount that is equal to 100 percent of a bundled payment under this part for opioid use disorder treatment services (as defined in paragraph (1) of such section) that are furnished by such program to an individual during an episode of care (as defined by the Secretary) beginning on or after January 1, 2020. The Secretary shall ensure, as determined appropriate by the Secretary, that no duplicative payments are made under this part or part D for items and services furnished by an opioid treatment program.

(2) CONSIDERATIONS.—The Secretary may implement this subsection through one or more bundles based on the type of medication provided (such

as buprenorphine, methadone, naltrexone, or a new innovative drug), the frequency of services, the scope of services furnished, characteristics of the individuals furnished such services, or other factors as the Secretary determine appropriate. In developing such bundles, the Secretary may consider payment rates paid to opioid treatment programs for comparable services under State plans under title XIX or under the TRICARE program under chapter 55 of title 10 of the United States Code.

(3) ANNUAL UPDATES.—The Secretary shall provide an update each year to the bundled payment amounts under this subsection.

(i) PAYMENT RULES RELATING TO RURAL EMERGENCY HOSPITALS.—

(1) PAYMENT FOR RURAL EMERGENCY HOSPITAL SERVICES.—In the case of rural emergency hospital services (as defined in section 1861(kkk)(1)), furnished by a rural emergency hospital (as defined in section 1861(kkk)(2)) on or after January 1, 2023, the amount of payment for such services shall be equal to the amount of payment that would otherwise apply under section 1833(t) for covered OPD services (as defined in section 1833(t)(1)(B) (other than clause (ii) of such section)), increased by 5 percent to reflect the higher costs incurred by such hospitals, and shall include the application of any copayment amount determined under section 1833(t)(8) as if such increase had not occurred.

(2) Additional facility payment.—

(A) IN GENERAL.—The Secretary shall make monthly payments to a rural emergency hospital in an amount that is equal to 1⁄12 of the annual additional facility payment specified in subparagraph (B).

(B) Annual additional facility payment amount.—

The annual additional facility payment amount specified in this subparagraph is—

(i) for 2023, a Medicare subsidy amount determined under subparagraph (C); and

(ii) for 2024 and each subsequent year, the amount determined under this subparagraph for the preceding year, increased by the hospital market basket percentage increase.

(C) DETERMINATION OF MEDICARE SUBSIDY AMOUNT.—For purposes of subparagraph (B)(i), the Medicare subsidy amount determined under this subparagraph is an amount equal to—

(i) the excess (if any) of—

(I) the total amount that the Secretary determines was paid under this title to all critical access hospitals in 2019; over

(II) the estimated total amount that the Secretary determines would have been paid under this title to such hospitals in 2019 if payment were made for inpatient hospital, outpatient hospital, and skilled nursing facility services under the applicable prospective payment systems for such services during such year; divided by

(ii) the total number of such hospitals in 2019.

(D) REPORTING ON USE OF THE ADDITIONAL FACILITY PAYMENT.—A rural emergency hospital receiving the additional facility payment under this paragraph shall maintain detailed information as specified by the Secretary as to how the facility has used the additional facility payments. Such information shall be made available to the Secretary upon request.

(3) PAYMENT FOR AMBULANCE SERVICES.—For provisions relating to payment for ambulance services furnished by an entity owned and operated by a rural emergency hospital, see section 1834(l).

(4) Payment for post-hospital extended care services.—

For provisions relating to payment for post-hospital extended care services furnished by a rural emergency hospital that has a unit that is a distinct part licensed as a skilled nursing facility, see section 1888(e).

(5) Source of payments.—

(A) IN GENERAL.—Except as provided in subparagraph (B), payments under this subsection shall be made from the Federal Supplementary Medical Insurance Trust Fund under section 1841.

(B) Additional facility payment and post-hospital

EXTENDED CARE SERVICES.—Payments under paragraph (2) shall be made from the Federal Hospital Insurance Trust Fund under section 1817.

(y) PAYMENT FOR CERTAIN SERVICES FURNISHED BY RURAL HEALTH CLINICS.—

(1) Attending physician services for hospice patients.—

In the case of services described in section 1812(d)(2)(A)(ii) furnished on or after January 1, 2022, by an attending physician (as defined in section 1861(dd)(3)(B), other than a physician or practitioner who is employed by a hospice program) who is employed by or working under contract with a rural health clinic, a rural health clinic shall be paid for such services under the methodology for all-inclusive rates (established by the Secretary) under section 1833(a)(3), subject to the limits described in section 1833(f).

(2) MENTAL HEALTH VISITS FURNISHED VIA TELECOMMUNICATIONS TECHNOLOGY.—In the case of mental health visits furnished via interactive, real-time, audio and video telecommunications

technology or audio-only interactions, the in-person mental health visit requirements established under section 405.2463(b)(3) of title 42 of the Code of Federal Regulations (or a successor regulation) shall not apply prior to January 1, 2025 (or, if later, the first day after the end of the emergency period described in section 1135(g)(1)(B)).

(3) Special payment rule for intensive outpatient services.—

(A) IN GENERAL.—In the case of intensive outpatient services furnished by a rural health clinic, the payment amount for such services shall be equal to the amount that would have been paid under this title for such services had such services been covered OPD services furnished by a hospital.

(B) EXCLUSION.—Costs associated with intensive outpatient services shall not be used to determine the amount of payment for rural health clinic services under the methodology for all-inclusive rates (established by the Secretary) under section 1833(a)(3).

(z) PAYMENT FOR LYMPHEDEMA COMPRESSION TREATMENT ITEMS.—

(1) IN GENERAL.—The Secretary shall determine an appropriate payment basis for lymphedema compression treatment items (as defined in section 1861(mmm)). In making such a determination, the Secretary may take into account payment rates for such items under State plans (or waivers of such plans) under title XIX, the Veterans Health Administration, and group health plans and health insurance coverage (as such terms are defined in section 2791 of the Public Health Service Act), and such other information as the Secretary determines appropriate.

(2) FREQUENCY LIMITATION.—No payment may be made under this part for lymphedema compression treatment items furnished other than at such frequency as the Secretary may establish.

(3) APPLICATION OF COMPETITIVE ACQUISITION.—In the case of lymphedema compression treatment items that are included in a competitive acquisition program in a competitive acquisition area under section 1847(a)—

(A) the payment basis under this subsection for such items furnished in such area shall be the payment basis determined under such competitive acquisition program; and

(B) the Secretary may use information on the payment determined under such competitive acquisition programs to adjust the payment amount otherwise determined under this subsection for an area that is not a competitive acquisition area under section 1847, and in the case of such adjustment, paragraphs (8) and (9) of section 1842(b) shall not be applied.

* * * * * * *

EXCHANGE OF LETTERS WITH ADDITIONAL COMMITTEES OF REFERRAL

JASON SMITH
MISSOURI,
CHAIRMAN

MARK ROMAN, STAFF DIRECTOR
(202) 225-3625

RICHARD E. NEAL
MASSACHUSETTS,
RANKING MEMBER

BRANDON CASEY, STAFF DIRECTOR
(202) 225-4021

U.S. House of Representatives
COMMITTEE ON WAYS AND MEANS
1139 LONGWORTH HOUSE OFFICE BUILDING
Washington, DC 20515

September 11, 2024

The Honorable Cathy McMorris Rodgers
Chair
Committee on Energy and Commerce
2125 Rayburn House Office Building
Washington, D.C. 20515

Dear Chair McMorris Rodgers,

Thank you for your letter regarding H.R. 7858, the "TELEMH Act of 2024." As you noted, the Committee on Ways and Means was granted an additional referral on this bill. I agree to forego action on this bill so that it may proceed expeditiously to the House floor for consideration.

The Committee takes this action with our mutual understanding that by foregoing consideration of H.R. 7858 at this time, we do not waive any jurisdiction over subject matter contained in this bill or similar legislation, and that our Committee will be appropriately consulted and involved as the bill or similar legislation moves forward so that we may address any remaining issues in our jurisdiction. Our Committee also reserves the right to seek appointment of an appropriate number of conferees to any House-Senate conference involving this or similar legislation, and asks that you support any such request.

Finally, I would ask that a copy of our exchange of letters on this matter be included in the Congressional Record during floor consideration of H.R. 7858.

Sincerely,

Jason Smith
Chairman

cc: The Honorable Mike Johnson, Speaker, U.S. House of Representatives
The Honorable Richard Neal, Ranking Member, Committee on Ways and Means
The Honorable Frank Pallone, Jr., Committee on Energy and Commerce
Mr. Jason Smith, Parliamentarian, U.S. House of Representatives

CATHY McMORRIS RODGERS, WASHINGTON
CHAIR

FRANK PALLONE, JR., NEW JERSEY
RANKING MEMBER

ONE HUNDRED EIGHTEENTH CONGRESS

Congress of the United States

House of Representatives

COMMITTEE ON ENERGY AND COMMERCE

2125 RAYBURN HOUSE OFFICE BUILDING
WASHINGTON, DC 20515-6115
Majority (202) 225-3641

September 11, 2024

The Honorable Jason Smith
Chair
Committee on Ways and Means
1102 Longworth House Office Building
Washington, DC 20515

Dear Chair Smith:

I write regarding H.R. 7858, the "TELEMH Act of 2024," which was referred in addition to the Committee on Ways and Means.

I ask that the Committee forgo action on the bill so that it may be scheduled for consideration on the House floor. This concession would in no way affect the Committee's jurisdiction over the subject matter of the bill. In addition, should a conference on the bill be necessary, I would support the Committee's request for conferees on the conference committee. Finally, I would be pleased to include this letter and your response in the *Congressional Record* during debate on the bill.

Thank you for your consideration of my request and for the extraordinary cooperation shown by you and your staff over matters of shared jurisdiction. I look forward to further opportunities to work with you this Congress.

Sincerely,

Cathy McMorris Rodgers
Chair

O

Chapter 7

The Restoring Hope for Mental Health and Well-Being Act of 2022 (Division FF, Title I of P.L. 117-328, the Consolidated Appropriations Act, 2023): Section-by-Section Summary*

Johnathan H. Duff

Summary

The Restoring Hope for Mental Health and Well-Being Act was enacted on December 29, 2022, as Division FF, Title I of the Consolidated Appropriations Act, 2023 (P.L. 117-328). The act primarily reauthorized or amended behavioral health (i.e., mental health and substance use) program authorizations expiring in FY2023. The act reauthorized many behavioral health programs established or reauthorized in 2016 by the 21st Century Cures (P.L. 114-255) or the Comprehensive Addiction and Recovery Act (P.L. 114-198). The act also amended or reauthorized federal programs or regulations related to mental health (e.g., mental health crisis response, suicide prevention, children's mental health) and substance use (e.g., alcohol use, opioid use disorder, recovery housing). Most of the amended provisions authorize grant programs administered by the Substance Abuse and Mental Health Services Administration (SAMHSA) within the Department of Health and Human Services (HHS).

---

* This is an edited, reformatted and augmented version of Congressional Research Service Publication No. R47910, dated January 29, 2024.

In: Healing Minds
Editor: Wilburn M. Conner
ISBN: 979-8-89530-893-6

The Restoring Hope for Mental Health and Well-Being Act is organized into five titles. Each title focuses on a different aspect of behavioral health:

- *Subtitle A ("Mental Health and Crisis Care Needs")* focuses on federal mental health program authorizations, including programs supporting specific services (e.g., crisis response, peer support) or targeting certain populations (e.g., pregnant and postpartum women, individuals with eating disorders or serious mental illness). A reauthorization for SAMHSA's mental health block grant is also included.
- *Subtitle B ("Substance Use Disorder Prevention, Treatment, and Recovery Services")* focuses on federal substance use program authorizations, including programs supporting specific services (e.g., medications for opioid use disorder, recovery housing) or targeting certain populations (e.g., homeless individuals, Indian Tribes or tribal organizations). A reauthorization for SAMHSA's substance use block grant is also included.
- *Subtitle C ("Access to Mental Health Care and Coverage")* focuses on federal authorizations related to the mental health care workforce, access to integrated care services, and private health insurance coverage of behavioral health services (i.e., mental health parity).
- *Subtitle D ("Children and Youth")* focuses on federal mental health program authorizations specifically addressing the mental health and well-being of children and youth. These authorizations address support for school- based programming, suicide prevention activities (e.g., Garrett Lee Smith program reauthorizations), and children with serious emotional disturbances, among others.
- *Subtitle E ("Miscellaneous Provisions")* prohibits the HHS Secretary from allocating funding to carry out any program authorized or amended by the Restoring Hope for Mental Health and Well-Being Act without considering the incidence, prevalence, or determinants of behavioral health issues.

This report provides a section-by-section summary of the Restoring Hope for Mental Health and Well-Being Act, organized by subtitle and chapter of the act. It includes relevant background information, followed by a summary of each provision.

Introduction

The Restoring Hope for Mental Health and Well-Being Act was enacted on December 29, 2022, as Division FF, Title I of the Consolidated Appropriations Act, 2023 (P.L. 117-328). The act primarily reauthorized or amended behavioral health (i.e., mental health and substance use) program authorizations expiring in FY2023. The act reauthorized many programs established or reauthorized in 2016 by the 21st Century Cures Act (Cures Act; P.L. 114-255)[1] or the Comprehensive Addiction and Recovery Act (P.L. 114-198).[2] The act amended or reauthorized specific federal programs related to mental health (e.g., mental health crisis response, suicide prevention, children's mental health) and substance use (e.g., alcohol use, opioid use disorder, recovery housing).

Most of the amended provisions authorize grant programs administered by the Substance Abuse and Mental Health Services Administration (SAMHSA) within the Department of Health and Human Services (HHS). SAMHSA is the federal agency primarily responsible for supporting community-based mental health and substance abuse treatment and prevention services.

SAMHSA provides federal funding to states, local communities, and individual organizations through block grants and other formula and discretionary grants. Through such grants, SAMHSA supports activities that include education and training, prevention programs, early intervention activities, treatment services, and technical assistance. SAMHSA does not provide mental health or substance abuse treatment. Rather, the agency supports states' efforts in providing community- based behavioral health services. SAMHSA derives most of its statutory authority from the Public

---

[1] The 21st Century Cures Act (P.L. 114-255) was signed into law on December 13, 2016. Division B, entitled "Helping Families in Mental Health Crisis," established or reauthorized many federal programs—and amended several regulations—related to mental health. For more information on the behavioral health authorizations in the 21st Century Cures Act, see CRS Report R44718, *The Helping Families in Mental Health Crisis Reform Act of 2016 (Division B of P.L. 114-255)*.

[2] In a couple of cases, the act reauthorized programs established or amended by the SUPPORT for Patients and Communities Act (SUPPORT Act; P.L. 115-271). For more information on the behavioral health authorizations in the SUPPORT Act, see CRS Report R45423, *Public Health and Other Related Provisions in P.L. 115-271, the SUPPORT for Patients and Communities Act*.

Health Service Act (PHSA). More specifically, Title V and Title XIX of the PHSA contain most authorities for SAMHSA programs and activities.[3]

The Restoring Hope for Mental Health and Well-Being Act (H.R. 7666) passed the House as a standalone bill in June 2022. After being received in the Senate and referred to the Committee on Health, Education, Labor, and Pensions, the bill was ultimately incorporated into the Consolidated Appropriations Act, 2023, and enacted on December 29, 2022, as Division FF, Title I of P.L. 117-328.

This report provides a section-by-section summary of the Restoring Hope for Mental Health and Well-Being Act, organized by subtitle and chapter of the act. It includes relevant background information, followed by a summary of each provision.

The Restoring Hope for Mental Health and Well- Being Act: At a Glance

In summary, the subtitles of the Restoring Hope for Mental Health and Well-Being Act address the following:

- *Subtitle A ("Mental Health and Crisis Care Needs")* focuses on federal mental health program authorizations, including programs supporting specific services (e.g., crisis response, peer support) or targeting certain populations (e.g., pregnant and postpartum women, individuals with eating disorders or serious mental illness). A reauthorization for SAMHSA's mental health block grant is also included.
- *Subtitle B ("Substance Use Disorder Prevention, Treatment, and Recovery Services")* focuses on federal substance use program authorizations, including programs supporting specific services (e.g., medications for opioid use disorder, recovery housing) or targeting certain populations (e.g., homeless individuals, Indian Tribes or Tribal organizations). A reauthorization for SAMHSA's substance use block grant is also included.
- *Subtitle C ("Access to Mental Health Care and Coverage")* focuses on federal authorizations related to the mental health care workforce,

[3] For more information on SAMHSA, see CRS Report R46426, *Substance Abuse and Mental Health Services Administration (SAMHSA): Overview of the Agency and Major Programs*.

access to integrated care services, and private health insurance coverage of behavioral health services (i.e., mental health parity).

- *Subtitle D ("Children and Youth")* focuses on federal mental health program authorizations specifically addressing the mental health and well-being of children and youth. These authorizations address support for school-based programming, suicide prevention activities (e.g., Garrett Lee Smith program reauthorizations), and children with serious emotional disturbances, among others.
- *Subtitle E ("Miscellaneous Provisions")* prohibits the HHS Secretary from allocating funding to carry out any program authorized or amended by the Restoring Hope for Mental Health and Well-Being Act without considering the incidence, prevalence, or determinants of behavioral health issues.

The Restoring Hope for Mental Health and Well-Being Act is an authorizing law; it does not appropriate any funds. Some of the programs amended or reauthorized by the law have not received explicit appropriations.

In this report, "Secretary" refers to the HHS Secretary unless otherwise noted.[4]

The Restoring Hope for Mental Health and Well- Being Act: Summary of Provisions[5]

Technical Edits in the Restoring Hope for Mental Health and Well-Being Act

Many of the provisions in the Restoring Hope for Mental Health and Well-Being Act make similar amendments to language throughout Title V of the Public Health Service Act (PHSA). For example, several provisions replace the terms "addiction" and "abuse" with "use disorders" to describe substance use. The changes align the legislative language with current clinical and diagnostic terminology related to substance use disorders. The Restoring Hope for Mental Health and Well-Being provisions also capitalize "Tribes" and "Tribal" in places the terms appear in Title V of the PHSA. When *technical edits* are referenced in the current report, it usually describes these changes.

[4] A table of the abbreviations used in this report appears in the **Appendix**.

[5] Section 1001 introduces Title I of Division FF as the "Restoring Hope for Mental Health and Well-Being Act of 2022."

Subtitle A—Mental Health and Crisis Care Needs

Chapter 1—Crisis Care Services and 9-8-8 Implementation
Section 1101. Behavioral Health Crisis Coordinating Office

Background

The Department of Health and Human Services (HHS)—primarily through the Substance Abuse and Mental Health Services Administration (SAMHSA)—supports state and local response efforts to individuals experiencing a mental health crisis. For example, SAMHSA supports the operation of the 988 Suicide & Crisis Lifeline (Lifeline). In July 2022, the Lifeline transitioned from a 10-digit number (1-800-273-TALK) to a three-digit 9-8-8 hotline. In its published 988 appropriations report, SAMHSA articulated a long-term goal of situating the Lifeline in the center of a broader, more robust crisis response system capable of dispatching mobile response services and providing adequate follow-up care.[6] At the direction of Congress via report language accompanying annual appropriations, SAMHSA established the 988 Behavioral Health Crisis Coordinating Office in 2022 through their general authorities derived from Title V of the Public Health Service Act (PHSA).[7] The purpose of the office is to provide leadership and facilitate coordination of behavioral health crisis services across the nation.[8]

Provision

Section 1101 adds a new PHSA Section 501B establishing a behavioral health crisis coordinating office to "coordinate work relating to behavioral health crisis care" across HHS agencies and departments, including SAMHSA, the Centers for Medicare & Medicaid Services (CMS), and the Health Resources and Services Administration (HRSA). Specified duties of the office include (1) convening stakeholders, (2) operating federal workgroups to make best practices recommendations, and (3) supporting technical assistance, data

---

[6] Substance Abuse and Mental Health Services Administration (SAMHSA), *988 Appropriations Report*, Rockville, MD, December 2021, https://www.samhsa.gov/sites/default/files/988-appropriations-report.pdf.

[7] H.Rept. 117-96; see also "Explanatory Statement Submitted by Ms. DeLauro, Chair of the House Committee on Appropriations, Regarding the House Amendment to the Senate Amendment to H.R. 2471, Consolidated Appropriated Act, 2022," *Congressional Record*, vol. 168, part 42, book IV (March 9, 2022), p. H2679.

[8] SAMHSA, *988 & Behavioral Health Crisis Coordinating Office*, https://www.samhsa.gov/about-us/who-we-are/offices-centers/988-behavioral-crisis-coordinating-office.

analysis, and evaluation functions of behavioral health crisis providers, such as the 988 Suicide & Crisis Lifeline, community mental health centers, Certified Community Behavioral Health Clinics (CCBHCs), and other community behavioral health providers. Section 1101 codifies SAMHSA's 988 Behavioral Health Crisis Coordinating Office, initially established in 2022 under SAMHSA's general authorities.[9]

New PHSA Section 501B authorizes $5 million to be appropriated for each of FY2023-FY2027.

Section 1102. Crisis Response Continuum of Care

Background

During the 2022 transition of the National Suicide Prevention Lifeline from the 10-digit number to the new three-digit *988 Suicide & Crisis Lifeline*, the Biden Administration, executive agencies overseeing the Lifeline, and mental health advocacy groups referred to an opportunity to leverage the launch of 988 to enhance the national mental health crisis response system more broadly.[10] In its National Guidelines for Behavioral Health Crisis Care for instance, SAMHSA described an effective mental health crisis system as a continuum of care that includes crisis contact centers ("someone to talk to"), mobile crisis services ("someone to respond"), and crisis stabilization facilities such as psychiatric receiving centers ("a safe place for help").[11] SAMHSA established the 988 Behavioral Health Crisis Coordinating Office in 2022 to

---

[9] Ibid.

[10] See, for example, HHS, "HHS Awards More Than $130 Million in 988 Lifeline Grants From the Bipartisan Safer Communities Act to Address Nation's Ongoing Mental Health and Substance Use Crises," press release, December 16, 2022, https://www.hhs.gov/about/news/2022/12/16/hhs-awards-more-than-130-million-988-lifeline-grants-bipartisan- safer-communities-act-address-nations-ongoing-mental-health-substance-use-crises.html; and National Council for Mental Wellbeing, *Roadmap to the Ideal Crisis System: Essential Elements, Measurable Standards and Best Practices for Behavioral Health Crisis Response*, March 2021, https://www.thenationalcouncil.org/resources/roadmap-to-the-ideal-crisis-system/.

[11] SAMHSA, *National Guidelines for Behavioral Health Crisis Care*, Best Practice Toolkit, Rockville, MD, 2020, https://www.samhsa.gov/sites/default/files/national-guidelines-for-behavioral-health-crisis-care-02242020.pdf. See also, SAMHSA, *988 Appropriations Report*, Rockville, MD, December 2021, https://www.samhsa.gov/sites/default/files/988-appropriations-report.pdf.

provide leadership and technical assistance related to behavioral health crisis services.[12]

Provision

Section 1102 requires the Secretary, acting through the SAMHSA Assistant Secretary, to identify and publish best practices for a behavioral health crisis response continuum of care. These best practices are to consider (1) the range of service providers (i.e., those that do not require prior authorization from insurance, provide services regardless of ability to pay, operate 24/7, provide services through stabilization or transfer to the next level of care, or address psychiatric stabilization), (2) functions of services (i.e., referral and enrollment in behavioral health care, access points to services within the continuum of care, transfer and receipt of individuals throughout the continuum of care, workforce qualifications, and collaboration with community partners), and (3) service capacity and quality (i.e., volume of services to meet population need, timely responsiveness, capacity to serve different patient populations).

The provision requires SAMHSA to publish the best practices no later than one year after enactment (i.e., December 29, 2023). The provision requires GAO to submit an assessment of behavioral health crisis programs to specified congressional committees no later than three years after enactment (i.e., December 29, 2025) to evaluate which programs meet objectives and performance metrics (with potential data metrics specified).

Section 1103. Suicide Prevention Lifeline Improvement

Background

PHSA Section 520E-3 ("The National Suicide Prevention Lifeline Program") authorizes the National Suicide Prevention Lifeline, a national hotline providing crisis counseling and referral services to individuals experiencing suicidal thoughts or other mental distress. The 21st Century Cures Act codified the program in PHSA Section 520E-3 in 2016, though the Lifeline had operated since 2005.[13] The authorization for the Lifeline specifies that

---

[12] SAMHSA, *988 & Behavioral Health Crisis Coordinating Office*, https://www.samhsa.gov/about-us/who-we-are/offices-centers/988-behavioral-crisis-coordinating-office. The authority for this office was codified in Section 1101 of the Restoring Hope for Mental Health and Well-Being Act, as described above.

[13] Cures Act §9005.

SAMHSA coordinate a network of 24-hour crisis centers and maintain the suicide prevention hotline to connect callers with local emergency services. Lifeline services have consisted primarily of immediate crisis counseling through the hotline, along with referrals, as needed, to local follow-up services. In 2022, the Lifeline transitioned from a 10-digit phone number to a three-digit 9-8-8 hotline (and rebranded as the *988 Suicide & Crisis Lifeline*).[14] Many saw the launch of 988 as an opportunity to enhance SAMHSA's role in more broadly building and maintaining the national mental health crisis response system.[15]

Section 520E-3 previously authorized $7.2 million (rounded) to be appropriated for each of FY2018-FY2022.

Provision

Section 1103 amends PHSA Section 520E-3 by adding more requirements to the National Suicide Prevention Lifeline authorization.[16] Specifically, Section 1101 authorizes the Secretary, acting through the SAMHSA Assistant Secretary, to support and coordinate a national network of crisis centers for suicide prevention and "mental health crisis intervention services, including appropriate follow-up services."[17] The provision requires SAMHSA to develop and implement a plan to support crisis centers and maintain the Lifeline. Contents of the plan include (1) program evaluation using performance measures to assess progress and improve responsiveness of the Lifeline; (2) crisis center requirements related to participation, call responsiveness, and best practices; (3) recommendations on implementing evidence-based practices; and (4) criteria for periodic testing of the Lifeline. The provision requires SAMHSA to develop the initial plan no later than one year after enactment (i.e., December 29, 2023).

Section 1103 requires the Secretary to complete a study and issue a report on the implementation of the Lifeline plan (specified above), and options to improve data on the Lifeline, no later than two years after development of the

---

[14] While the Lifeline is now known as the *988 Suicide & Crisis Lifeline*, the authorizing provision in Title V of the PHSA (§520E-3; 42 U S.C. §290bb-36c) maintains the "National Suicide Prevention Lifeline Program" title.

[15] See SAMHSA, *988 Appropriations Report*, Rockville, MD, December 2021, https://www.samhsa.gov/sites/default/files/988-appropriations-report.pdf; and National Council for Mental Wellbeing, *Roadmap to the Ideal Crisis System: Essential Elements, Measurable Standards and Best Practices for Behavioral Health Crisis Response*, March 2021, https://www.thenationalcouncil.org/resources/roadmap-to-the-ideal-crisis-system/.

[16] §520E-3; 42 U.S.C. §290bb-36c.

[17] 42 U.S.C. §290bb-36c.

plan. The provision requires GAO to complete a study and submit a report to Congress with specified information on implementation of the Lifeline plan, recommendations for improving the Lifeline, and specified issues related to access to the Lifeline no later than two years after implementation of the plan begins.

Section 1103 also adds requirements to the Lifeline authorization related to sharing data with the Centers for Disease Control and Prevention (CDC) and state and local agencies. More specifically, the provision requires the Secretary to formalize an arrangement between the Lifeline and CDC related to sharing de-identified epidemiological data. It also requires the Secretary to ensure that aggregated data are available to state and local agencies to inform suicide prevention activities.

The provision authorizes the Secretary to carry out a pilot program to research, analyze, and employ various technologies or communication platforms (e.g., social media, texting, and email) for suicide prevention, in addition to the Lifeline telephone and chat services. The Secretary is required to submit a report with specified information on the pilot program no later than 24 months after the pilot program commences.

Section 1103 reauthorizes the National Suicide Prevention Lifeline. PHSA Section 520E-3(f) now authorizes $101.6 million (rounded) to be appropriated for each of FY2023-FY2027.

Chapter 2—Into the Light for Maternal Mental Health and Substance Use Disorders

Section 1111. Screening and Treatment for Maternal Mental Health and Substance Use Disorders

Background

PHSA Section 317L-1 ("Screening and Treatment for Maternal Depression") authorizes a grant program to states for screening, assessment, and treatment of maternal depression. The Health Resources and Services Administration (HRSA) administers the Screening and Treatment for Maternal Depression and Related Behavioral Disorders grant program. HRSA provides grants to states for programs that expand the capacity to assess, treat, and refer pregnant and postpartum women for services for maternal depression and related behavioral health disorders. In FY2018, for example, HRSA funded seven states for programs training health care providers in assessing and treating maternal mental health conditions.[18]

Section 317L-1(e) previously authorized $5 million to be appropriated for each of FY2018- FY2022.

Provision

Section 1111 amends PHSA Section 317L-1 by changing the title to "Screening and Treatment for Maternal Mental Health and Substance Use Disorders." The provision adds Tribes and Tribal organizations as eligible grant recipients. It also expands the purpose of the grants (from "maternal depression" to "maternal mental health") and amends the definition of the population served. The provision makes similar conforming changes throughout Section 317L-1. It requires the Secretary to prioritize eligible entities providing screening and treatment for maternal behavioral health issues through partnerships with community-based organizations in areas with disproportionate need or in health professional shortage areas.

Section 1111 specifies training requirements and amends the types of professionals served through training and resources. It also expands the eligible uses of funds, adding several activities supported by the grant: (1) screening, brief intervention, and treatment; (2) psychiatric consultation; (3) coordination with maternal and child health programs, including child psychiatric access programs; (4) public outreach and awareness; (5) creation of a multistate consortia; and (6) training primary care providers on trauma-informed care, culturally appropriate services, and other best practices. Section 1111 also requires the Secretary to provide technical assistance to grantees and other states and Tribes, and to disseminate best practices based on program evaluation. The provision further adds a new subsection limiting the federal share of grant-supported activities to 90%.

Section 1111 reauthorizes the (renamed) Screening and Treatment for Maternal Mental Health and Substance Use Disorders grant program. PHSA Section 317L-1 now authorizes $24 million to be appropriated for each of FY2023-FY2027.

[18] HRSA, *Screening and Treatment for Maternal Depression and Related Behavioral Disorders Program (MDRBD)*, https://mchb.hrsa.gov/programs-impact/screening-treatment-maternal-depression-related-behavioral-disorders-program-mdrbd.

Section 1112. Maternal Mental Health Hotline

Background

In May 2022, HRSA launched a new Maternal Mental Health Hotline for expecting and new mothers experiencing mental health challenges.[19] The confidential, toll-free hotline connects callers with counselors available to provide mental health support. Individuals who contact the hotline receive brief interventions from trained counselors, or referrals to community-based and telehealth providers for further services. HRSA originally operated the hotline under its general authorities with an explicit appropriation from Congress.[20] PHSA Title III ("General Powers and Duties of the Public Health Service") contains many of the authorizations for HHS Public Health Service agency programs, including several HRSA maternal and child health initiatives.

Provision

Section 1112 amends PHSA Title III Part P ("Additional Programs") by adding a new Section 399V-7 ("Maternal Mental Health Hotline"), which requires the Secretary to maintain a national maternal mental health hotline. The new authorization requires that the hotline provide emotional support, information, brief intervention, and resources to pregnant and postpartum women with behavioral health needs (and to their families or household members). Section 1112 effectively codifies the Maternal Mental Health Hotline launched by HRSA in 2022.

Section 1112 specifies requirements for the hotline (e.g., hours of operation, staffing, services provided). It also requires the Secretary to conduct a public awareness campaign for the hotline and consult with state and local officials, federal agencies, and other related national hotlines, such as the National Suicide Prevention Lifeline.[21] The provision requires the Secretary

---

[19] U.S. Department of Health and Human Services, "HHS Launches New Maternal Mental Health Hotline," press release, May 6, 2022, https://www.hhs.gov/about/news/2022/05/06/hhs-launches-new-maternal-mental-health- hotline.html.

[20] H.Rept. 116-450 and "Explanatory Statement Submitted by Mrs. Lowey, Chairwoman of the House Committee on Appropriations, Regarding the House Amendment to the Senate Amendment to H.R. 133, Consolidated Appropriations Act, 2021," *Congressional Record*, vol. 166, part 218, book IV (December 21, 2020), p. H8620.

[21] The statutory authorization for the National Suicide Prevention Lifeline uses that title; however, as of 2022, the program is more commonly referred to as the *988 Suicide & Crisis Lifeline*.

to submit an annual report to Congress that includes an evaluation of the effectiveness of the hotline and a directory of referral organizations.

New PHSA Section 399V-7 authorizes $10 million to be appropriated for each of FY2023- FY2027.

Section 1113. Task Force on Maternal Mental Health

Background

HHS—primarily through SAMHSA and HRSA—provides resources and administers grants related to maternal behavioral health. For example, HRSA operates the *Maternal Mental Health Hotline* for expecting and new mothers experiencing mental health challenges.[22] Similarly, SAMHSA offers clinical guidance for practitioners treating pregnant and parenting women,[23] toolkits and technical assistance related to maternal mental health,[24] and grant programs addressing health needs of pregnant women affected by substance use.[25] Prior to enactment of the Restoring Hope for Mental Health and Well-Being Act, no authorization for a maternal mental health task force existed.

Provision

Section 1113 requires the Secretary—no later than 180 days after enactment (i.e., June 30, 2023)—to establish a Task Force on Maternal Mental Health (or incorporate the duties specified in the provision into the responsibilities of an existing federal committee or working group). The provision specifies task force membership, which includes the heads of several HHS agencies and other nonfederal members representing various relevant organizations to be appointed by the Secretary. The provision requires designees to be appointed no later than 90 days after enactment (i.e., March 30, 2023).

---

[22] HRSA, *National Maternal Mental Health Hotline*, May 2023, https://mchb.hrsa.gov/national-maternal-mental- health-hotline.

[23] SAMHSA, *Clinical Guidance for Treatment Pregnant and Parenting Women with Opioid Use Disorder and Their Infants*, SMA18-5054, January 2018, https://store.samhsa.gov/product/Clinical-Guidance-for-Treating-Pregnant-and-Parenting-Women-With-Opioid-Use-Disorder-and-Their-Infants/SMA18-5054.

[24] SAMHSA, *Depression in Mothers: More Than the Blues*, SMA14-4878, March 2016, https://store.samhsa.gov/product/Depression-in-Mothers-More-Than-the-Blues/sma14-4878.

[25] SAMHSA, "HHS Announces New Reports and Grant Programs Addressing the Health Needs of Pregnant Women and Children Affected by Substance Use," press release, February 3, 2022, https://www.samhsa.gov/newsroom/press-announcements/20220203/grants-pregnant-women.

Section 1113 specifies the duties of the task force, which include preparing and updating a report that evaluates federal maternal mental health programs and identifies best practices related to prevention, diagnosis, and treatment; referral to supports; and implementation of community- based or multigenerational support for maternal mental health conditions. The task force must also develop a national strategy for maternal mental health, which is to include how federal agencies coordinate efforts to address maternal mental health conditions. The task force is required to solicit public comments and consider the latest research in preparing the report and national strategy.

The provision requires the task force to meet at least two times each year and convene public meetings, as appropriate. The provision also requires the task force to submit a report to specified entities, including federal agencies and certain congressional committees, no later than one year after the first task force meeting (and an updated report annually thereafter). It requires the task force to submit an initial national strategy no later than two years after the first task force meeting, and an updated national strategy annually thereafter. The provision requires the task force to submit a report to governors of all states describing opportunities for local and state partnerships.

Section 1113 requires the task force to terminate on September 30, 2027, and specifies that the task force may not duplicate others HHS efforts.

Section 1114. Residential Treatment Program for Pregnant and Postpartum Women Pilot Program Reauthorization

Background

PHSA Section 508 ("Residential Treatment Programs for Pregnant and Postpartum Women") authorizes SAMHSA's Pregnant and Postpartum Women (PPW) program, which supports residential substance use disorder treatment and recovery support services to pregnant and postpartum women, their children, and other family members.[26] In 2016, the Comprehensive Addiction and Recovery Act (CARA; P.L. 114-198) added an authorization for a pilot program for state substance abuse agencies to support new models of service delivery, family-based approaches, and activities addressing other gaps in care.[27] The new provision added by CARA included a five-year limit on the pilot program.

---

26 HHS, SAMHSA, Justification of Estimates for Appropriations Committees, FY2024.

27 CARA §501; 42 U.S.C. §290bb-1(r).

In 2018, the SUPPORT Act reauthorized PHSA Section 508, amending the authorization for appropriations to $29.9 million (rounded) for each of FY2019-FY2023.[28]

Provision

Section 1114 amends PHSA Section 508 to remove the five-year limit on the pilot program authorized in subsection (r). Additionally, the provision now requires that the pilot program report be submitted to specified congressional committees no later than September 30, 2026.

Chapter 3—Reaching Improved Mental Health Outcomes for Patients

Section 1121. Innovation for Mental Health

Background

In 2016, the 21st Century Cures Act created several new behavioral health authorizations, including for a new National Mental Health and Substance Use Policy Laboratory within SAMHSA, and an Interdepartmental Serious Mental Illness Coordinating Committee established by the Secretary.

Section 7001 of the Cures Act added a new PHSA Section 501A establishing within SAMHSA the National Mental Health Policy Laboratory. The Laboratory's responsibilities include coordinating the implementation of policy changes to improve certain behavioral health-related outcomes, identifying evidence-based practices, reviewing SAMHSA programs to identify duplicative programs or programs that are not evidence-based, and providing recommendations for improving SAMHSA programs. The provision authorized SAMHSA, via the Laboratory, to award grants for (1) evaluating promising service delivery models and (2) expanding the use of evidence-based programs. In 2018, the SUPPORT Act added another responsibility, requiring the Laboratory to provide information to SAMHSA grant applicants regarding the implementation of evidence-based practices and to provide technical assistance to applicants for funding. SAMHSA appointed its first Director of the National Mental Health and Substance Use Policy

[28] 42 U.S.C. §290bb-1(s).

Laboratory in January 2018.[29] SAMHSA announced its third and most recent director in June 2023.[30]

PHSA Section 501A previously authorized $7 million to be appropriated for the period of FY2018-FY2020 to carry out each of the two grant programs (i.e., $14 million total).

Section 6031 of the Cures Act required the Secretary to establish an Interdepartmental Serious Mental Illness Coordinating Committee. The provision specified committee membership, membership terms, and the frequency of committee meetings. It required the committee to produce a report—no later than one year after enactment (i.e., December 2017) and again five years after enactment (i.e., December 2021)—summarizing advances, evaluating federal programs, and recommending services for individuals with serious mental illness (SMI). The Cures Act provision specified that the committee shall terminate six years after it is established; however, it also required the Secretary, upon submission of the committee's second report, to make a recommendation to Congress as to whether operation of the committee should be extended.

SAMHSA administers numerous grants and activities under authorities commonly known as Programs of Regional and National Significance (PRNS) in three areas: mental health, substance abuse treatment, and substance abuse prevention.[31] The mental health PRNS are authorized under PHSA Section 520A ("Priority Mental Health Needs of Regional and National Significance").

Previously, Section 520A authorized $395.6 million (rounded) to be appropriated for each of FY2018-FY2022 for the mental health PRNS.

Provision

Section 1121 amends PHSA Section 501A to reauthorize the National Mental Health and Substance Use Policy Laboratory. The provision requires GAO to prepare a report no later than 18 months after enactment (i.e., June 29, 2024)

---

[29] SAMHSA, *SAMHSA Blog*, Leadership Announcement, January 9, 2018, https://blog.samhsa.gov/tag/policy.

[30] SAMHSA, *About Us/Who We Are/Leadership/Brian Altman*, June 5, 2023, https://www.samhsa.gov/about-us/who-we-are/leadership/biographies/brian-altman.

[31] Under PHSA Title V Part B, the HHS Secretary is required to "address priority ... needs of regional and national significance" in mental health (PHSA §520A), substance abuse treatment (PHSA §509), and substance abuse prevention (PHSA §516); the HHS Secretary may do so "directly or through grants or cooperative agreements with States, political subdivisions of States, Indian tribes and tribal organizations, other public or private nonprofit entities."

on the work of the Laboratory, including the extent to which it is meeting its statutory responsibilities and any recommendations for improvement. The provision makes other technical edits.

PHSA Section 501A(f) now authorizes $10 million to be appropriated for each of FY2023- FY2027 for all activities authorized under the section.

Section 1121 adds a new PHSA Section 501C codifying in the PHSA an authorization for the Interdepartmental Serious Mental Illness Coordinating Committee (and reauthorizing the committee through 2027). The new PHSA provision specifies committee responsibilities and membership (including term duration). The provision requires the committee to produce reports no later than one year and five years after enactment (i.e., December 29, 2023, and December 29, 2027) summarizing research on the prevention, diagnosis, and treatment of SMI and evaluating federal programs for SMI (with specified information to include in the reports). New Section 501C specifies that the committee shall terminate on September 30, 2027. Section 1121 repeals the previous authorization for the committee included in the Cures Act.

Section 1121 reauthorizes SAMHSA's Priority Mental Health Needs of Regional and National Significance (PRNS). PHSA Section 520A now authorizes $599 million (rounded) to be appropriated for each of FY2023-FY2027.

Section 1122. Crisis Care Coordination

Background

Prior to being amended by the Restoring Hope for Mental Health and Well-Being Act, PHSA Section 520F ("Strengthening Community Crisis Response Systems") required the Secretary to award competitive grants (1) to states, localities, Indian Tribes, and Tribal Organizations to enhance community-based crisis response systems, or (2) to states to develop, maintain, or enhance a database of beds at specified inpatient behavioral health treatment facilities. It specified application procedures, defined the requirements of a database of inpatient beds, and required an evaluation. The provision required applicants to include a community-based crisis response plan (as defined) but did not explicitly require mobile crisis services.

In FY2022, SAMHSA established the Cooperative Agreements for Innovative Community Crisis Response Partnerships program under this authority.[32] The purpose of this program is to create or enhance existing mobile crisis response teams that divert individuals experiencing mental health crises from law enforcement in high-need communities. The program supports mobile crisis team services (including co-responder teams) that offer community-based intervention to individuals in need wherever they are located.[33]

PHSA Section 520F previously authorized $12.5 million to be appropriated for the period of FY2018-FY2022 to carry out the program.

PHSA Section 502J ("Mental Health Awareness Training Grants") authorizes a grant program to train teachers, emergency services personnel, law enforcement, and other individuals to identify and appropriately respond to children and adults with a mental disorder. Grants often support training through Mental Health First Aid, a formal eight-hour course on how to identify, understand, and respond to the signs of a crisis, mental health condition, or substance use issue.

Section 520J previously authorized $14.7 million (rounded) to be appropriated annually for each of FY2018-FY2022.

PHSA Section 520L ("Adult Suicide Prevention") authorizes the National Strategy for Suicide Prevention and the Zero Suicide grant programs. The National Strategy for Suicide Prevention grant program supports states and community partners in implementing the National Strategy for Suicide Prevention—a coordinated guide to the nation's suicide prevention efforts.[34] The Zero Suicide program funds evidence-based suicide prevention interventions in health systems.

Section 520L previously authorized $30 million to be appropriated for the period of FY2018- FY2022.

Provision

Section 1122 replaces PHSA Section 520F with a new provision ("Mental Health Crisis Response Partnership Pilot Program") authorizing a pilot program requiring the Secretary to award grants to establish or enhance mobile crisis response teams. The provision effectively codifies SAMHSA's

---

[32] SAMHSA, Justification of Estimates for Appropriations Committees, FY2024, p. 80.

[33] For more information on co-responder teams, see CRS Report R47285, Issues in Law Enforcement Reform: Responding to Mental Health Crises.

[34] U.S. Surgeon General and the National Action Alliance for Suicide Prevention, *2012 National Strategy for Suicide Prevention: Goals and Objectives for Action*, PEP12=NSSPGOALS, September 2012, https://www.hhs.gov/ surgeongeneral/reports-and-publications/suicide-prevention/index.html.

Cooperative Agreements for Innovative Community Crisis Response Partnerships program.[35]

Mobile crisis response teams are defined as a team of individuals available to respond to people in behavioral health crises and provide immediate stabilization, referrals to service, and triage to a higher level of care, if necessary. The provision requires the Secretary to submit a report to Congress no later than September 30, 2024, on previous steps taken by states and localities to strengthen partnerships among specified members of the behavioral health care community, including first responders, primary care providers, and law enforcement, among others. The provision requires the Secretary to submit annual progress reports with specified information on the grant program, including populations served and related outcomes.

New PHSA Section 520F authorizes $10 million to be appropriated for each of FY2023-FY2027.

Section 1122 amends PHSA Section 502J by making several technical edits. It adds evidence- based training and education on suicide intervention and prevention to the list of allowable uses of funds. It also allows SAMHSA to provide technical assistance to grantees.

Section 1122 reauthorizes the mental health awareness training grant program. PHSA Section 502J now authorizes $25 million (rounded) to be appropriated for each of FY2023-FY2027.

Section 1122 amends PHSA Section 520L by making changes to the purpose of the suicide prevention grant programs. It expands the intended population served to all adults instead of those 25 years of age or older, further emphasizes suicide prevention in the purpose of the grant, and adds suicide prevention resources and the promotion of help seeking for those at risk for suicide as allowable components of activities. The provision adds a third technical assistance requirement, in which the Secretary is to identify best practices for referrals and coordination of follow-up care for individuals in the emergency department who are at risk for suicide, and coordination of care after discharge.

Section 1122 reauthorizes the adult suicide prevention grant programs in PHSA Section 520L. PHSA Section 520L now authorizes $30 million to be appropriated for each of FY2023-FY2027.

---

[35] For more information on some mobile crisis response approaches, see CRS Report R47285, *Issues in Law Enforcement Reform: Responding to Mental Health Crises*.

Section 1123. Treatment of Serious Mental Illness

Background

PHSA Section 520M ("Assertive Community Treatment Grant Program") authorizes SAMHSA's Assertive Community Treatment (ACT) for Individuals with Serious Mental Illness (SMI) grant program.[36] Originally authorized by the Cures Act,[37] the ACT for SMI grant program supports a multidisciplinary intervention designed to reduce rehospitalization and improve outcomes in community settings for individuals with serious mental illness.[38]

PHSA Section 520M previously authorized $5 million to be appropriations for the period of FY2018-FY2022.

The Protecting Access to Medicare Act of 2014 (PAMA; P.L. 113-93) Section 224 ("Assisted Outpatient Treatment Grant Program for Individuals with Serious Mental Illness") authorized a four-year pilot program to award grants for Assisted Outpatient Treatment (AOT) programs for individuals with SMI. It limited grant amounts to not exceed $1 million in each year. It originally authorized $15 million to be appropriated annually for each of FY2015-FY2018. In 2018, the Cures Act extended the program's authorization through FY2022.[39]

The Cures Act amended PAMA Section 224 to authorize $15 million to be appropriated annually for each of FY2015-FY2017, $20 million for FY2018, $19 million annually for each of FY2019- FY2020, and $18 million annually for each of FY2021-FY2022.

Provision

Section 1123 amends PHSA Section 520M. The provision requires the Secretary to provide a report on the grant program to specified congressional committees no later than September 30, 2026.

Section 1123 reauthorizes the ACT for SMI grant program. PHSA Section 520M now authorizes $9 million to be appropriated for each of FY2023-FY2027.

Section 1123 amends PAMA Section 224 to remove the four-year pilot aspect of the program. It makes the annual report biennial, specifies to which

---

[36] 42 U.S.C. §290bb-44.
[37] Cures Act §9015.
[38] SAMHSA, *Justification of Estimates for Appropriations Committees, FY2023.*
[39] Cures Act §9014.

congressional committees the report is due, and adds demographic information of the population served to the reporting requirements.

Section 1123 requires GAO to provide a report to specified congressional committees on the efficacy of the assisted outpatient treatment programs funded under PAMA Section 224.

Section 1123 reauthorizes the AOT grant program. PAMA Section 224 now authorizes $22 million to be appropriated for each of FY2023-2027.[40]

Section 1124. Study on the Costs of Serious Mental Illness

Background

Serious mental illness (SMI) is defined as a mental, behavioral, or emotional disorder that substantially interferes with or limits one or more major life activities.[41] According to SAMHSA's National Survey on Drug Use and Health (NSDUH), an estimated 14 million adults in the United States had a serious mental illness in 2021. SMI causes significant functional impairment, often disrupting an individual's social functioning, capacity to participate in the labor force, and ability to maintain stable housing, among other areas of life. The estimated per individual economic burden from SMI can be substantial—comparable to other major health conditions such as cancer and diabetes.[42]

Provision

Section 1124 requires the Secretary, in consultation with SAMHSA, the HHS Assistant Secretary for Planning and Education (ASPE), the Department of Justice (DOJ), the Department of Labor (DOL), and the Department of Housing and Urban Development (HUD), to conduct a study on the costs of serious mental illness with respect to nongovernmental entities, the federal government, and state, local, and Tribal governments.

---

[40] 42. U.S.C. §290aa-17. (Previously 42 U.S.C. §290aa note.)

[41] Excluding developmental disorders and substance use disorders. Common SMI includes psychoses, major depressive disorder, and bipolar disorder. Substance Abuse and Mental Health Services Administration, *Key Substance Use and Mental Health Indicators in the United States: Results from the 2021 National Survey on Drug Use and Health*, HHS Publication No. PEP22-07-01-005, NSDUH Series H-57, Rockville, MD, December 2022.

[42] Seth A. Seabury, Sarah Axeen, Gwyn Pauley, et al., "Measuring the Lifetime Costs of Serious Mental Illness and the Mitigating Effects of Educational Attainment," *Health Affairs*, vol. 38, no. 4 (April 2019).

The provision specifies considerations for the study, which include costs (1) to the health care system for health services, (2) of homelessness, (3) of residential facilities and other supportive housing, (4) of law enforcement and criminal justice system encounters, (5) of serious mental illness on employment, (6) of caring for individual with SMI by family members and caregivers, and (7) any other relevant costs for programs. The provision specifies disaggregation of the data by costs to governments, types of medical and behavioral health conditions, demographic characteristics, prevalence of serious mental illness, and housing status. The Secretary is required to prepare a report on the study's results no later than two years after enactment of the Restoring Hope for Mental Health and Well-Being Act (i.e., December 29, 2024).

Chapter 4—Anna Westin Legacy

Section 1131. Maintaining Education and Training on Eating Disorders

Background

As part of its mission, SAMHSA supports health practitioners through technical assistance and training. Since 2018, SAMHSA has supported a National Center of Excellence for Eating Disorders (NCEED), located at the University of North Carolina at Chapel Hill.[43] The purpose of the program is to develop and disseminate training and technical assistance for health care practitioners on issues related to addressing eating disorders.[44] This center for excellence facilitates the identification of model programs, develops and updates materials related to eating disorders, and ensures that high-quality training is provided to health professionals.

---

[43] National Center of Excellence for Eating Disorders, *National Center of Excellence for Eating Disorders: Our Mission*, https://www.nceedus.org/about/.

[44] SAMHSA, *National Center of Excellence for Eating Disorders (NCEED)*, November 2, 2022, https://www.samhsa.gov/national-center-excellence-eating-disorders-nceed. See also SAMHSA, "SAMHSA announces up to $3.75 million in funding to enhance training efforts to address eating disorders," press release, July 18, 2018, https://www.samhsa.gov/newsroom/press-announcements/20180718.

Provision

Section 1131 adds a new PHSA 520N entitled "Center for Excellence for Eating Disorders for Education and Training on Eating Disorders." The provision effectively codifies the NCEED program, requiring the Secretary acting through the SAMHSA Assistant Secretary, by grant or contract, to maintain a Center of Excellence for Eating Disorders to improve diagnosis and treatment of eating disorders.

The center's specified activities include (1) training and technical assistance for medical providers in screening and referral for treatment for individuals with eating disorders, and for other paraprofessionals in nonclinical community services; (2) developing and disseminating training materials to health care providers regarding effective treatments for eating disorders; (3) collaborating and coordinating with other SAMHSA entities regarding eating disorders; (4) coordinating with CDC, HRSA, and other federal agencies to disseminate training to primary care and mental health care providers; and (5) conducting other activities as determined by the Secretary. The provision also states that the Secretary may support the integration of eating disorder screening, brief intervention, and referral to treatment (SBIRT) with health information technology systems, provide resources to members of the military and veterans, and consult with DOD and VA on SBIRT for eating disorders.

The new PHSA Section 520N authorizes $1 million to be appropriated for each of FY2023- FY2027.

Chapter 5—Community Mental Health Services Block Grant Reauthorization

Section 1141. Reauthorization of Block Grants for Community Mental Health Services

Background

PHSA Title XIX Subpart I ("Block Grants for Community Mental Health Services") authorizes SAMHSA's Community Mental Health Services Block Grant (MHBG). The MHBG supports state efforts in providing community mental health services for adults with serious mental illness (SMI) and children with serious emotional disturbance (SED).[45] SAMHSA distributes MHBG funds to states (including the District of Columbia and specified territories) according to a formula specified in Title XIX of the PHSA.[46] Each state may distribute MHBG funds to local government entities and nongovernmental organizations to provide community mental health services in accordance with the state's plan. States have flexibility in the use of MHBG funds within the framework of the state plan and federal requirements. The state must designate a Single State Agency responsible for administering the grant and submit the state plan to the Secretary every two years.[47] The statutory authorization for the MHBG contains funding set- asides, such as the requirement that a state must expend 10% of the funds to support early SMI.[48]

Beginning in FY2021, Congress has included a set-aside for "evidence-based crisis systems" in annual appropriations for the MHBG[49] This set-aside reflects Congress's recent intentions to support the development and maintenance of a robust mental health crisis response system.[50] The set-aside is intended to support core elements of crisis care programs, such as mobile crisis units, psychiatric stabilization beds, and crisis call centers.[51]

PHSA Section 1920 previously authorized $532.6 million (rounded) to be appropriated for each of FY2018-FY2022 for the MHBG.

Provision

Section 1141 adds a new subsection to PHSA Section 1920 to codify the 5% set-aside of the MHBG for "Evidence-Based Crisis Care Services."[52] Set-aside funding for crisis care services may be used to support crisis call centers, 24/7 mobile crisis services, or crisis stabilization programs.[53] Section 1141 requires

---

[45] SAMHSA's definitions of adults with SMI and children with SED were provided in a 1993 *Federal Register* notice (May 20, 1993; 58 *Federal Register* 29422).

[46] 42 U.S.C. §300x et seq.

[47] For more information, see CRS Report R46426, *Substance Abuse and Mental Health Services Administration (SAMHSA): Overview of the Agency and Major Programs*.

[48] PHSA §1920(c); 42 U.S.C. §300x-9(c).

[49] Rep. Rosa DeLauro, "Explanatory Statement Submitted by Ms. DeLauro, Chair of the House Committee on Appropriations, Regarding the House Amendment to the Senate Amendment to H.R. 2471, Consolidated Appropriations Act, 2022," Proceedings and Debates of the 117th Congress, Second Session, *Congressional Record*, vol. 168, part No. 42, Book IV (March 9, 2022), pp. H2477-H3215.

[50] See, for example, H.Rept. 117-96 and SAMHSA, *Justification of Estimates for Appropriations Committees, FY2023*.

[51] Ibid.

[52] 42 U.S.C. §300x-9(d).

[53] According to the provision, a state may instead elect to expend not less than 10% of the MHBG funds over two fiscal years.

the Secretary to provide a report to Congress no later than September 20, 2025 (and biennially thereafter), on the crisis care strategies and programs supported by the MHBG set-aside. The report must include a description of crisis care activities, populations served, and outcomes of activities, including the program's effects on hospitalization and hospital stays, onset of serious mental illness, and incidents of suicidal ideation and behaviors.

Section 1141 amends PHSA Section 1920 ("Funding") to reauthorize the Community Mental Health Services Block Grant program. PHSA Section 1920 now authorizes $857.6 million (rounded) to be appropriated for each of FY2023-FY2027.

Chapter 6—Peer-Supported Mental Health Services

Section 1151. Peer-Supported Mental Health Services

Background

Support services provided by individuals with lived experiences with mental health and substance use disorders have been recognized as an essential component of comprehensive behavioral health care.[54] Although SAMHSA supports peer involvement in mental health care through activities such as its Consumer-Supporter Technical Assistance Centers, no explicit SAMHSA authority to fund peer-support services in mental health treatment existed prior to enactment of the Restoring Hope for Mental Health and Well-Being Act.[55]

Provision

Section 1151 adds a new PHSA Section 520H entitled "Peer-Supported Mental Health Services." The provision authorizes SAMHSA to administer a

---

[54] SAMHSA, for example, funds a Peer Support Technical Assistance Center and operates a Recovery Community Services Program to strengthen the infrastructure of recovery communities and provide peer recovery support services for individuals with substance use disorders and co-occurring mental health disorders. See SAMHSA, *Recovery Community Services Program*, 2023 Notice of Funding Opportunity, https://www.samhsa.gov/grants/grant- announcements/ti-23-018. See also SAMHSA, *Peer Support Services in Crisis Care*, SAMHSA Advisory, Rockville, MD, June 2022, https://store.samhsa.gov/sites/default/files/pep22-06-04-001.pdf; and SAMHSA, *Peers Supporting Recovery from Mental Health Conditions*, BRSS TACS Infographic, Rockville, MD, 2017, https://www.samhsa.gov/sites/default/files/programs_campaigns/brss_tacs/peers-supporting-recovery-mental-health-conditions-2017.pdf.

[55] SAMHSA, Justification of Estimates for Appropriations Committees, FY2024.

new grant program to develop, expand, and enhance access to peer-delivered mental health services.

Specified use of funds for the new grant program include (1) initiating workforce development activities to recruit and train peer-workforce providers; (2) building connections between various treatment programs; (3) reducing stigma associated with mental health disorders; (4) expanding virtual peer mental health support services; and (5) researching peer-support and mental illness. Eligible entities include consumer-run nonprofit organizations and Indian Tribes and Tribal organizations.

New PHSA Section 520H authorizes $13 million to be appropriated for each of FY2023-FY2027.

Subtitle B—Substance Use Disorder Prevention, Treatment, and Recovery Services: Chapter 1—Native Behavioral Health Resources

Section 1201. Behavioral Health and Substance Use Disorder Resources for Native Americans

Background

PHSA 506A ("Alcohol and Drug Prevention or Treatment Services for Indians and Native Alaskans") authorized a grant program for Native Alaskan entities and Indian Tribes and Tribal organizations for substance use prevention and treatment services. Originally added by the Children's Health Act of 2000 (P.L. 106-310), the program authorization never received an explicit appropriation. SAMHSA reported in its annual Congressional Budget Justification that the activities authorized in Section 506A may be supported with funding from other Programs of Regional or National Significance (PRNS) or block grants.[56] SAMHSA also noted that the agency has the authority to carry out these programs in their general authorities.[57]

PHSA 506A previously authorized $15 million to be appropriated for FY2001, and such sums as necessary for FY2002 and FY2003.

---

[56] See, for example, SAMHSA, Justification of Estimates for Appropriations Committees, FY2002, pp. 37-39.

[57] See, for example, SAMHSA, Justification of Estimates for Appropriations Committees, FY2005, pp. 27-29.

Provision

Section 1201 replaces PHSA Section 506A with a new provision entitled "Behavioral Health and Substance Use Disorder Resources for Native Americans." The provision authorizes a grant program for services for mental health and substance use disorder prevention and treatment among American Indians, Alaska Natives, and Native Hawaiians.

The provision authorizes the Secretary, acting through the SAMHSA Assistant Secretary in coordination with the Indian Health Service (IHS) as appropriate, to administer grant funds through a contract or compact under Title I or V of the Indian Self-Determination and Education Assistance Act.[58] Award amounts are determined by a formula developed by HHS, with consultation from Indian Tribes and Tribal organizations. Eligible entities are required to apply for awards. The authorization requires the Secretary to provide technical assistance to grantees and to assist with program evaluation data and reporting requirements. The provision requires the Secretary to submit a report describing the services supported by the grant program to specified congressional committees no later than three years after enactment (i.e., December 29, 2025).

PHSA Section 506A now authorizes $80 million to be appropriated for each of FY2023-FY2027 for the grant program.

Chapter 2—Summer Barrow Prevention, Treatment, and Recovery Services

Section 1211. Grants for the Benefit of Homeless Individuals

Background

PHSA Section 506 ("Grants for the Benefit of Homeless Individuals") authorizes SAMHSA's Treatment Systems for Homeless program. Reauthorized in 2016 by the Cures Act,[59] PHSA Section 506 requires the Secretary to award grants, contracts, and cooperative agreements to eligible entities, as specified, to provide mental health and substance abuse services to homeless individuals. The section specifies granting preferences, conditions for services provided under the grant, and terms of awards, among other factors.

---

[58] P.L. 93-638, as amended (25 U.S.C. Chapter 46 et seq.).

[59] Cures Act §9001.

PHSA Section 506 previously authorized $41.3 million (rounded) to be appropriated for each of FY2018-FY2022.

Provision

Section 1211 amends PHSA Section 506 by reauthorizing $41.3 million for each of FY2023- FY2027 for the Treatment Systems for Homeless program.

Section 1212. Priority Substance Use Disorder Treatment Needs of Regional and National Significance

Background

PHSA Section 509 ("Priority Substance Abuse Treatment Needs of Regional and National Significance") provides the authorities for SAMHSA's substance abuse treatment grants and activities commonly known as Programs of Regional and National Significance (PRNS).[60] Reauthorized in 2016 by the Cures Act,[61] the substance abuse treatment PRNS includes grant program authorizations, technical assistance, and other activities supporting treatment for substance use disorders. Some PRNS are explicitly authorized in statute; others are carried out under the general authorities included in PHSA Section 509.

PHSA Section 509 previously authorized $333.8 million (rounded) for each of FY2018-FY2022.

Provision

Section 1212 amends PHSA Section 509 by replacing the term "abuse" with "substance use disorder" wherever it appears.[62] The provision makes other technical edits.

Section 1212 reauthorizes SAMHSA's substance use disorder treatment PRNS. PHSA Section 509 now authorizes $521.5 million (rounded) to be appropriated for each of FY2023-FY2027.

---

[60] Under PHSA Title V Part B, Section 509, the HHS Secretary is required to "address priority substance use disorder treatment needs of regional and national significance"; the Secretary may do so "directly or through grants or cooperative agreements with States, political subdivisions of States, Indian tribes or tribal organizations, … or other public or private nonprofit entities" (42 U.S.C. §290bb-2). PRNS authorizations exist for mental health (PHSA §520A) and substance abuse prevention (PHSA §516) also.

[61] Cures Act §7004.

[62] For example, the provision changes the section title to "Priority Substance Use Disorder Treatment Needs of Regional and National Significance."

Section 1213. Evidence-Based Prescription Opioid and Heroin Treatment and Interventions Demonstration

Background

PHSA Section 514B ("Evidence-Based Prescription Opioid and Heroin Treatment and Interventions Demonstration") authorizes a competitive grant program to expand treatment of substance use disorders in geographic areas with a high rate or rapid increase of heroin and other opioid use.[63] The provision was originally added by CARA in 2016.[64] The program authorized under PHSA 514B has never received an explicit appropriation.[65]

Chapter 2—Summer Barrow Prevention, Treatment, and Recovery Services

Section 1211. Grants for the Benefit of Homeless Individuals

Background

PHSA Section 506 ("Grants for the Benefit of Homeless Individuals") authorizes SAMHSA's Treatment Systems for Homeless program. Reauthorized in 2016 by the Cures Act,59 PHSA Section 506 requires the Secretary to award grants, contracts, and cooperative agreements to eligible entities, as specified, to provide mental health and substance abuse services to homeless individuals. The section specifies granting preferences, conditions for services provided under the grant, and terms of awards, among other factors.

PHSA Section 506 previously authorized $41.3 million (rounded) to be appropriated for each of FY2018-FY2022.

PHSA Section 514B previously authorized $25 million to be appropriated for each of FY2017- FY2021.

Provision

Section 1213 amends PHSA Section 514B by replacing the terms "substance abuse" and "addiction" with "substance use disorder." The provision makes other technical edits.

---

[63] 42 U.S.C. §290bb-10.

[64] CARA §301.

[65] Through FY2023.

Section 1213 amends PHSA Section 514B by reauthorizing $25 million to be appropriated for each of FY2023-FY2027.

Section 1214. Priority Substance Use Disorder Prevention Needs of Regional and National Significance

Background

PHSA Section 516 ("Priority Substance Use Disorder Prevention Needs of Regional and National Significance") provides the authorities for SAMHSA's substance use disorder prevention grants and activities, commonly known as Programs of Regional and National Significance (PRNS).[66] Reauthorized in 2016 by the Cures Act,[67] the substance use disorder treatment PRNS includes grant program authorizations, technical assistance, and other activities supporting prevention of substance use disorders. Some PRNS are explicitly authorized in statute; others are carried out under the general authorities included in PHSA Section 516.

Provision

Section 1214 amends PHSA Section 516 by making technical edits.

Section 1214 reauthorizes SAMHSA's substance use disorder prevention PRNS. PHSA Section 516 now authorizes $218.2 million (rounded) to be appropriated for each of FY2023-FY2027.

Section 1215. Sober Truth on Preventing (STOP) Underage Drinking Authorization

Background

PHSA Section 519B ("Programs to Reduce Underage Drinking") authorizes SAMHSA's Sober Truth on Preventing Underage Drinking Act (STOP Act) programs. Originally added by the STOP Act of 2006 (P.L. 109-422) and

---

[66] Under PHSA Title V Part B, Section 516, the HHS Secretary is required to "address priority substance use disorder prevention needs of regional and national significance"; the Secretary may do so "directly or through grants or cooperative agreements with States, political subdivisions of States, Indian tribes or tribal organizations, … or other public or private nonprofit entities" (42 U.S.C. §290bb-22). PRNS authorizations exist for substance use disorder treatment (PHSA §509) and mental health (PHSA §520A) also.

[67] Cures Act §7005.

reauthorized in 2016 by the Cures Act,[68] PHSA Section 519B authorizes a range of activities aimed at reducing underage drinking. The provision provides separate authorizations of appropriations for each specified activity.

PHSA Section 519B previously authorized the following amounts for each of FY2018-FY2022:

- $1 million to support an Interagency Coordinating Committee on the Prevention of Underage Drinking and an annual report on state underage drinking prevention and enforcement activities;
- $1 million for a national media campaign to prevent underage drinking;
- $5 million for "enhancement grants" aimed at maximizing the effectiveness of community-wide approaches to preventing and reducing underage drinking; and
- $6 million for research on underage drinking.
- There was no explicit authorization of appropriations for grants to pediatric health care providers for screening and brief intervention to reduce underage drinking.

Provision

Section 1215 amends PHSA Section 519B by:

- amending the definitions subsection and removing a reference to a 2003 report by the former Institute of Medicine. The provision now requires the National Academies of Sciences, Engineering, and Medicine (NASEM)[69] to report to Congress with the results of a review on research related to underage alcohol use no later than 12 months after enactment (i.e., December 29, 2023);
- replacing subsection (c) to add a new authorization for the interagency coordinating committee on the prevention of underage drinking and adding specified information to the Secretary's annual report to Congress on state underage drinking prevention and enforcement activities, including certain specified surveillance data.

[68] Cures Act §9016.

[69] The National Academies of Sciences, Engineering, and Medicine (NASEM) is a private, nonprofit organization that provides "independent, objective advice to inform policy with evidence, spark progress and innovation, and confront challenging issues for the benefit of society." For more information, see https://www.nationalacademies.org/about.

New subsection (c) adds further direction for the Secretary's annual collaborative report on each state's performance preventing or reducing underage drinking. The new provision clarifies the contents of the report including performance measures developed by the Secretary and other specified details;

- replacing subsection (d) with a new authority for the national media campaign to prevent underage drinking. The provision requires the Secretary in consultation with the National Highway Traffic Safety Administration to continue a media campaign aimed at adults to reduce underage drinking. The provision specifies the purpose of the campaign, describes campaign components, and requires the Secretary to consult with various specified stakeholders. It requires the Secretary to produce an annual report on the media campaign. The provision also provides the Secretary with the authority, based on the availability of funds, to support research on the potential for a youth-oriented national media campaign, with requirements to share such information with Congress;
- replacing subsection (e) with a new authorization for the community-based coalition enhancement grants to prevent underage drinking. The provision increases the maximum amount of each grant, for example, from $50,000 (the previous amount) to $60,000. It removes the authorization for grants directed at preventing and reducing alcohol abuse at institutions of higher education;
- replacing subsection (f) to include an authorization for grants to pediatric health care providers to reduce underage drinking through screening and brief intervention. The provision amends the previous authorization by narrowing the intended population served to adolescents (removing "children"). The provision adds a definition for the term "screening"; and
- replacing subsection (g) to include the authority to collect data and conduct or support research on underage drinking. The provision amends the specified characteristics of the authorized research and includes (1) evaluation of the effectiveness of community-based programs and statewide systems, (2) the reporting of more precise information on the scope of underage drinking and patterns of underage alcohol consumption, (3) development and identification of evidence-based strategies to reduce underage drinking, and (4)

improvement of public health data collection on alcohol use and alcohol-related conditions.

Section 1215 reauthorizes the STOP Act programs. PHSA Section 519B now authorizes the following amounts to be appropriated for each subsection:

- subsection (c): $1 million for each of FY2023-FY2027 to support the Interagency Coordinating Committee on the Prevention of Underage Drinking and an annual report on state underage drinking prevention and enforcement activities;
- subsection (d): $2.5 million for each of FY2023-FY2027 for a national media campaign to prevent underage drinking;
- subsection (e): $11.5 million for each of FY2023-FY2027 for community-based coalition enhancement grants to prevent underage drinking;
- subsection (f): $3 million for each of FY2023-FY2027 for grants to pediatric health care providers to reduce underage drinking through screening and brief intervention;
- subsection (g): $5 million for each of FY2023-FY2027 for research on underage drinking; and $500,000 for FY2023 to contract with NASEM regarding a report on underage drinking.

Section 1216. Grants for Jail Diversion Programs

Background

PHSA Section 520G ("Grants for Jail Diversion Programs") authorizes SAMHSA's Criminal and Juvenile Justice Programs. Reauthorized in 2016 by the Cures Act,[70]70 PHSA Section 520G requires the Secretary to make grants to states, political subdivisions of states, Indian Tribes, and Tribal organizations, directly or through agreements, for jail diversion programs (i.e., programs to divert individuals with mental illness from the criminal justice system to community-based services).

Section 520G previously authorized $4.3 million (rounded) to be appropriated annually for each of FY2018-FY2022.

---

[70] Cures Act §9002.

Provision

Section 1216 amends PHSA 520G by removing the cap on the number of grants administered, allowing eligible health facilities or nonprofit entities to apply for the grants directly, ensuring peer recovery support services are mentioned in the application, and adding paraprofessional training to the allowable uses of funds. The provision makes other technical edits to the grant authorization.

Section 1216 reauthorizes the Criminal and Juvenile Justice Programs. PHSA Section 520G now authorizes $14 million to be appropriated for each of FY2023-FY2027.

Section 1217. Formula Grants to States

Background

PHSA Section 521 ("Formula Grants to States") authorizes SAMHSA's Projects for Assistance in Transition from Homelessness (PATH) grant program.[71] Reauthorized in 2016 by the Cures Act,[72] the PATH program is a formula grant program that distributes funds to states to support local organizations providing services for people with serious mental illness (including those with co- occurring substance use disorders) who are homeless or at imminent risk of becoming homeless.[73] Up to 20% of the federal payments may be used for housing-related assistance. Other services include (but are not limited to) outreach, mental health and substance use disorder treatment, case management, and job training.[74]

Provision

Section 1217 amends PHSA Section 521 by reauthorizing the PATH formula grant program for FY2023 through FY2027.

---

71 Authorizations for various aspects of the PATH program are included in PHSA Sections 521-535 (42 U.S.C. §290cc- 21 through §290cc-35).

72 Cures Act §9004.

73 The minimum allotment is $300,000 for each of the 50 states, the District of Columbia, and Puerto Rico, and $50,000 for each of Guam, the U.S. Virgin Islands, American Samoa, and the Northern Mariana Islands. Funds are distributed to states in amounts proportional to their populations living in urbanized areas. The formula to determine allotments is included in PHSA Section 524 (42 U.S.C. §290cc-24).

74 For more about PATH, see http://www.samhsa.gov/homelessness-programs-resources/grant-programs-services/path.

Section 1218. Projects for Assistance in Transition from Homelessness

Background

PHSA Section 535 ("Funding") authorizes the appropriations for the PATH program. PHSA Section 535 previously authorized to be appropriated $64.6 million (rounded) for each of FY2018-FY2022 for the PATH program.

Provision

Section 1218 amends PHSA Section 535 by reauthorizing $64.6 million (rounded) to be appropriated for each of FY2023-FY2024.

Section 1219. Grants for Reducing Overdose Deaths

Background

PHSA Section 544 ("Grants for Reducing Overdose Deaths") authorizes SAMHSA's Improving Access to Overdose Treatment grant program. Originally added by CARA in 2016,[75] PHSA Section 544 authorizes a grant program to expand access to FDA-approved drugs for emergency treatment of opioid overdoses. Grants provided a maximum amount of $200,000 per grant year to federally qualified health centers (FQHCs)[76] and federally certified opioid treatment programs (OTPs)[77] for prescribing, purchasing, or training health care providers in the use of FDA- approved overdose reversal medications such as naloxone.[78]

PHSA Section 544 previously authorized $5 million to be appropriated for the period of FY2017- FY2021.

Provision

Section 1219 amends PHSA Section 544 by repealing the $200,000 maximum amount for each grant and changing eligibility for the grant program from FQHCs and OTPs to states, territories, localities, and Tribes. The provision

---

[75] CARA §107 (42 U.S.C. §290dd-3).

[76] For more information on FQHCs, see CRS Report R43937, *Federal Health Centers: An Overview*.

[77] For more information on OTPs, see CRS In Focus IF12348, *Medications for Opioid Use Disorder*.

[78] For more information on naloxone, see CRS In Focus IF12490, *Naloxone for Opioid Overdose: Considerations for Congress*.

adds an authority for grantees to award subgrants to FQHCs, OTPs, and other practitioners using medications for opioid use disorder. The provision adds individuals co-prescribed benzodiazepines to the specified populations served, includes connecting patients to overdose reversal medications in the use of funds, and makes other technical edits. The provision also adds authorities to PHSA Section 544 for the Secretary to provide best practices to specified stakeholders (including prescribers within the VA and DOD) for prescribing FDA-approved drugs for opioid overdoses.

Section 1219 amends PHSA Section 544 to reauthorize $5 million to be appropriated for the period of FY2023-FY2027 for the Improving Access to Overdose program.

Section 1220. Opioid Overdose Reversal Medication Access and Education Grant Programs

Background

PHSA Section 545 ("Opioid Overdose Reversal Medication Access and Education Grant Programs") authorizes a grant program to implement strategies to dispense FDA-approved drugs for emergency treatment of opioid overdose. Originally added by CARA,[79] PHSA Section 545 authorized grants to states to encourage pharmacies to dispense opioid overdose reversal medications, such as naloxone, pursuant to a standing order.[80] The program authorized under PHSA 545 has never received an explicit appropriation as of FY2023.

PHSA Section 545 previously authorized $5 million to be appropriated for the period of FY2017- FY2019.

Provision

Section 1220 amends PHSA Section 545 by amending the title to include "Co-Prescribing" and adding localities and Tribes to the list of eligible grantees.[81] The provision adds co-prescribing FDA-approved medications for opioid

---

[79] CARA §110 "Opioid Overdose Reversal Medication Access and Education Grant Program" (42 U.S.C. §290ee).

[80] For more information on FDA-approved opioid overdose reversal medications and standing orders, see CRS In Focus IF12490, *Naloxone for Opioid Overdose: Considerations for Congress*.

[81] The title for PHSA Section 545 is now "Opioid Overdose Reversal Medication Access, Education, and Co- Prescribing Grant Program."

overdose to the list of required grant activities and removes the specification for pharmacists to be the dispensers of such drugs.[82] The provision also expands the time period for the grant from three years to five years. It amends the limit for using grant funds for public education from 20% to 10% and requires that not less than 20% of the grant be used to offset cost sharing for emergency overdose reversal medications. The provision makes other technical edits regarding language describing FDA approval of opioid overdose reversal medications.

Section 1220 amends PHSA Section 545 to reauthorize $5 million to be appropriated for the period of FY2023-FY2027.

Section 1221. Emergency Department Alternatives to Opioids

Background

SUPPORT for Patients and Communities Act Section 7091 ("Emergency Department Alternatives to Opioids Demonstration Program") authorized SAMHSA's Emergency Department Alternatives to Opioids program. Through this program, SAMHSA provides grants to hospitals and emergency departments to develop, implement, or study alternatives to opioids for pain management in hospital or emergency department settings. The authorizing provision requires SAMHSA to facilitate the development of best practices on opioid alternatives and to provide technical assistance to hospitals and other acute care settings. It also requires the Secretary to submit a report to Congress on the results of the program one year after the completion of the demonstration program.

SUPPORT Act Section 7091 previously authorized $10 million to be appropriated for each of FY2019-FY2021.

Provision

Section 1221 amends SUPPORT Act Section 7091 by removing the demonstration label and making the required report to specified congressional committees annual, due at the end of each year from FY2024 through FY2028.

---

[82] The provision describes "drugs or devices approved, cleared, or otherwise legally marketed under the Federal Food, Drug, and Cosmetic Act for emergency treatment of known or suspected opioid overdose" (42 U.S.C. §290ee). For more information, see CRS Report R41983, *How FDA Approves Drugs and Regulates Their Safety and Effectiveness*.

Section 1221 amends SUPPORT Act Section 7091 by reauthorizing $10 million to be appropriated for each of FY2023-FY2027 for the Emergency Department Alternatives to Opioids program.

Chapter 3—Excellence in Recovery Housing

Background

PHSA Section 550 ("National Recovery Housing Best Practices)" requires the Secretary to develop best practices for operating substance use recovery housing. Originally added by the SUPPORT Act in 2018,[83] PHSA Section 550 defines recovery housing to mean a "shared living environment free from alcohol and illicit drug use and centered on peer support and connection to services that promote sustained recovery from substance use disorders."[84] In identifying these best practices, the Secretary is required to consult with other entities such as SAMHSA, CMS, the HUD Secretary, state health commissioners, health insurers, and individuals with a history of substance use disorder (SUD), among others. The provision requires the Secretary, in consultation with the same specified entities and the Attorney General, to identify common indicators that could be used to identify potentially fraudulent recovery housing operators, as described.

The Secretary is required to disseminate the best practices and common indicators to specified entities, which include state agencies, Tribal organizations, the Attorney General, recovery housing entities, and the public, among others. In carrying out these activities, the Secretary is required to consult with specified entities and to consider how recovery housing supports recovery, prevents relapse and overdose, and improves access to treatment such as medications for opioid use disorder. This provision does not give the Secretary the authority to require states to adhere to minimum standards, though the best practices may include model laws for states to implement suggested minimum standards. SAMHSA published recovery housing best practices in 2019.[85]

---

[83] SUPPORT Act §7031.

[84] 42 U.S.C. §290ee-5.

[85] Substance Abuse and Mental Health Services Administration (SAMHSA), *Recovery Housing: Best Practices and Suggested Guidelines*, 2019. SAMHSA updated these best practices in 2023 subsequent to P.L. 117-328. See SAMHSA, *Best Practices for Recovery Housing*, PEP23-10-00-002, Rockville, MD, 2023, https://www.samhsa.gov/resource/ebp/best-practices-recovery-housing.

PHSA Section 550 previously authorized $3 million to be appropriated for the period of FY2019- FY2021.

PHSA Section 501 ("Substance Abuse and Mental Health Services Administration") provides SAMHSA's general authorities, including those related to the Assistant Secretary and the agency organization.

Section 1231. Clarifying the Role of SAMHSA in Promoting the Availability of High-Quality Recovery Housing

Section 1231 amends PHSA Section 501 by adding a new authority requiring the SAMHSA Assistant Secretary to collaborate with states, federal agencies, and other specified stakeholders with expertise in recovery housing to promote the availability of recovery housing for individuals with substance use disorders.

Section 1232. Developing Guidelines for States to Promote the Availability of High-Quality Recovery Housing

Section 1232 amends PHSA Section 550 by requiring the Secretary to continue to identify, develop, and periodically update best practices for operating recovery housing. The provision adds specifics regarding whom the Secretary must consult with for the best practices. It adds a requirement that the best practices be made publicly available and published on SAMHSA's website. Lastly, it prohibits the Secretary from including best practices for substance use disorder treatment services in the recovery housing best practices.

Section 1233. Coordination of Federal Activities to Promote the Availability of Recovery Housing

Section 1233 amends PHSA Section 550 by adding a new subsection (e) requiring the Secretary, acting through the SAMHSA Assistant Secretary and HUD Secretary, to convene an interagency working group to increase collaboration among federal agencies regarding the promotion of recovery housing for individuals in need.

The new subsection tasks the working group with aligning efforts of federal agencies and avoiding duplication. It also requires the working group to develop a long-term plan for supporting state and local efforts to operate recovery housing consistent with the best practices. The provision specifies the composition of the interagency working group. The working group is required to meet on a quarterly basis and submit a report to specified congressional committees on the work of the group and any recommendations no later than four years after enactment (i.e., December 30, 2026). The provision makes other technical edits.

Section 1234. National Academies of Sciences, Engineering, and Medicine Study and Report

Section 1234 requires the Secretary, acting through the SAMHSA Assistant Secretary, to contract with the National Academies of Sciences, Engineering, and Medicine (NASEM) to study the quality and effectiveness of recovery housing in the United States. The provision tasks NASEM with determining whether the availability of recovery housing meets demand and providing recommendations to promote the availability of recovery housing. It requires the Secretary to contract with NASEM no later than 60 days after enactment (i.e., February 27, 2023) and report to Congress on the results of the review.

Section 1234 authorizes $1.5 million to be appropriated for FY2023.

Section 1235. Grants for States to Promote the Availability of Recovery Housing and Services

Section 1235 amends PHSA Section 550 by authorizing a grant program to support implementation of the national recovery housing best practices.

The provision authorizes the Secretary to award grants to states, Tribes, and territories for technical assistance to implement the national recovery housing best practices and to promote the availability of recovery housing. States receiving such grants are required to submit to SAMHSA, and publish on their state website, a state plan for promotion of recovery housing.

Section 1236. Funding

Section 1235 amends PHSA Section 550 by reauthorizing funding for National Recovery Housing Best Practices activities. PHSA Section 550 now authorizes $5 million to be appropriated for the period of FY2023-FY2027.

Section 1237. Technical Corrections

Section 1237 makes technical corrections to PHSA Title V by redesignating the second PHSA Section 550 (entitled "Sobriety Treatment and Recovery Teams"[86]) as Section 550A and locating it after Section 550.

Chapter 4—Substance Use Prevention, Treatment, and Recovery Services Block Grant

Background

PHSA Title XIX Subpart II ("Block Grants for Prevention and Treatment of Substance Abuse") authorizes SAMHSA's Substance Abuse Prevention and Treatment Block Grant (referred to as the SABG, or sometimes SAPT).[87] The SABG supports state efforts in providing community-based services to prevent and treat substance use disorders. SAMHSA distributes SABG funds to states (including the District of Columbia and specified territories) and one Tribal entity according to a formula specified in Title XIX of the PHSA.[88] Each state may distribute SABG funds to local government entities, administrative service organizations, and prevention and treatment service providers (among others) in accordance with the state's plan.[89] States must designate a Single State Agency responsible for administering the grant and submit an application containing the state plan to the HHS Secretary by the first of October preceding the fiscal year.[90] States have flexibility in the use of SABG funds within the framework of the state plan and federal requirements.

---

[86] The SUPPORT Act Section 8214 inserted a second PHSA Section 550 at the end of title V

[87] PHSA §§1921-1935. Some provisions in PHSA Title XIX, Part B, Subpart III, also apply to the substance use block grant.

[88] 42 U.S.C. §300x et seq.

[89] PHSA §1932(b) (42 U.S.C. §300x-32(b)).

[90] PHSA §1932 (42 U.S.C. §300x-32). Of note, PHSA Section 1958 allows the Assistant Secretary to permit a joint application for the MHBG and SABG.

While the use of funds is generally determined by states, each SABG grantee must expend at least 20% of its SABG allotment on primary prevention strategies.[91]

PHSA Section 1935 authorizes $1.86 billion (rounded) to be appropriated annually for each of FY2018-FY2022 for the SABG.

Section 1241. Eliminating Stigmatizing Language Relating to Substance Use

Section 1241 amends PHSA Title XIX Subpart II (Sections 1921-1935) by replacing the terms "substance abuse" with "substance use disorders." The provision amends the subpart heading to read "Block Grants for Substance Use Prevention, Treatment, and Recovery Services," effectively renaming it the Substance Use Prevention, Treatment, and Recovery Services (SUPTRS) block grant program.[92] It amends PHSA Section 1934 ("Definitions") to define substance use disorder to mean the recurrent use of alcohol or other drugs that causes clinically significant impairment.[93]

Section 1242. Authorizes Activities

Section 1242 amends PHSA Section 1921 ("Formula Grants to States") by adding "recovery support services" to the authorized grant activities stated in subsection (b).

---

91 PHSA §1922(a)(1) (42 U.S.C. §300x-22(a)(1)). Primary prevention strategies refer to interventions designed to avoid manifestations of a disease before the health condition occurs or, in the case of the SABG authorization, "for individuals who do not require treatment for substance abuse." For more information, see CRS Report R46426, *Substance Abuse and Mental Health Services Administration (SAMHSA): Overview of the Agency and Major Programs*.

92 Now referred to by SAMHSA as the SUPTRS block grant, or sometimes SUBG for short. See SAMHSA, *Substance Use Prevention, Treatment, and Recovery Services Block Grant*, updated April, 2023, available at https://www.samhsa.gov/grants/block-grants/subg.

93 42 U.S.C. §300x-34.

Section 1243. State Plan Requirements

Section 1243 amends PHSA Section 1932 ("Application for Grant; Approval of State Plan") by requiring states submitting a plan for the block grants to describe the state's recovery support services and the amount of block grant funds expended for these activities. The provision also makes a conforming edit.

Section 1244. Updating Certain Language Relating to Tribes

Section 1244 amends PHSA Section 1933 ("Determination of Amount of Allotment") by making technical edits, including several related to language pertaining to Tribes.

Section 1245. Block Grants for Substance Use Prevention, Treatment, and Recovery Services

Section 1245 amends PHSA Section 1935 ("Funding") by reauthorizing funding for the substance use block grant. The provision also makes a technical correction.

PHSA Section 1935 now authorizes $1.9 billion (rounded) to be appropriated for each of FY2023-FY2027.

Section 1246. Requirements of Reports and Audits by States

Section 1246 amends PHSA Section 1942 ("Requirement of Reports and Audits by States") by requiring states to include in the report to the Secretary the amount provided to recipients of block grant funds in the state in the previous fiscal year.

Section 1247. Study on Assessment for Use of State Resources

Section 1247 requires the Secretary, acting through the SAMHSA Assistant Secretary and in consultation with states and local service providers, to conduct a study on strategies to assess community needs related to substance use prevention, treatment, and recovery support services. The study is to facilitate state use of the substance use block grant. The provision requires the Secretary to submit results of the study to specified congressional committees no later than two years after enactment (i.e., December 29, 2024).

Chapter 5—Timely Treatment for Opioid Use Disorder

Section 1251. Study on Exemptions for Treatment of Opioid Use Disorder Through Opioid Treatment Programs During the COVID-19 Public Health Emergency

Background

Social distancing measures and temporary stay-at-home orders associated with the COVID-19 pandemic influenced changes in service delivery for substance use treatment. For substance use treatment that uses certain medications for opioid use disorder (MOUD)—specifically opioid agonist treatments such as methadone and buprenorphine—patients are required by law to attend in person for at least the initial visit for buprenorphine, and daily for methadone.[94] Methadone is typically administered on a daily basis onsite at federally certified opioid treatment programs (OTPs, sometimes known as methadone clinics), with some short-term take-home doses allowed for stable patients.[95]

During the pandemic, SAMHSA and DEA allowed stable patients to receive up to 28 days of take-home medication.[96] DEA also allowed alternative methods for the delivery of methadone to patients under stay-at-

[94] See CRS In Focus IF12348, Medications for Opioid Use Disorder.

[95] As outlined in 42 CFR §8.12. See also Drug Enforcement Administration, Use of Telemedicine While Providing Medication Assisted Treatment (MAT), Diversion Control, May 15, 2018, https://www.samhsa.gov/sites/default/files/ programs_campaigns/medication_assisted/telemedicine-dea-guidance.pdf.

[96] Substance Abuse and Mental Health Services Administration, Opioid Treatment Program (OTP) Guidance, Rockville, MD, March 16, 2020, https://www.samhsa.gov/ sites/default/files/otp-guidance-20200316.pdf. See also CRS Report R46831, Behavioral Health During the COVID-19 Pandemic: Overview and Issues for Congress.

home orders,[97] as well as interstate prescribing privileges for providers.[98] Other changes included relaxing privacy requirements mandated by the Health Insurance Portability and Accountability Act (HIPAA) rules and increasing the use of telehealth to deliver substance use treatment services. In addition, some states employed other methods of service delivery (e.g., mobile units) for treatments that cannot be administered via telehealth, such as MOUD.

In addition to these flexibilities allowed by DEA and SAMHSA during the public health emergency, CFR Title 42 Part 8 allows OTPs to apply for exceptions to certain regulations, including during the COVID-19 pandemic.[99] The public health emergency declaration for the COVID-19 pandemic expired on May 11, 2023.[100]

Provision

Section 1251 requires the SAMHSA Assistant Secretary—in consultation with patients and other stakeholders—to conduct a study on activities carried out pursuant to exemptions granted to states or OTPs during the COVID-19 public health emergency. The provision requires SAMHSA to gather feedback from states and OTPs regarding their experiences implementing exemptions. It also requires that SAMHSA publish a report on the results of the study no later than 180 days after the termination of the COVID-19 public health emergency or at the end of calendar year 2022, whichever is sooner.[101]

---

[97] Letter from Thomas Prevoznik, Deputy Assistant Administrator, Drug Enforcement Administration, to Registered Narcotic Treatment Program, April 7, 2020, https://www.deadiversion.usdoj.gov/GDP/(DEA-DC-025)(DEA078)_Off-site_OTP_delivery_method_(Final)+_esign.pdf.

[98] Letter from William McDermott, Assistant Administrator, Drug Enforcement Administration, to DEA Registrants, March 25, 2020, https://www.deadiversion.usdoj.gov/GDP/(DEA-DC-018)(DEA067)%20DEA%20state%20reciprocity%20(final)(Signed).pdf. For more information and resources related to the COVID-19 pandemic from the Drug Enforcement Administration, see "COVID-19 Information Page," https://www.deadiversion.usdoj.gov/coronavirus.html.

[99] 42 C.F.R. §8.11(h).

[100] See CRS Insight IN12088, Effects of Terminating the Coronavirus Disease 2019 (COVID-19) PHE and NEA Declarations; and Press Release, U.S. Department of Health and Human Services, Fact Sheet: COVID-19 Public Health Emergency Transition Roadmap, February 9, 2023, at https://www.hhs.gov/about/news/2023/02/09/fact-sheet- covid-19-public-health-emergency-transition-roadmap.html.

[101] As declared under PHSA §319 (42 U.S.C. §247d). The public health emergency declaration for the COVID-19 pandemic expired on May 11, 2023.

Section 1252. Changes to Federal Opioid Treatment Standards

Background

Section 302 of the Controlled Substance Act (CSA; "Persons Required to Register") requires every person who manufactures or distributes controlled substances to register with the Attorney General (via DEA).[102] Section 302(e) requires a separate DEA registration for each principal place of business or professional practice where the applicant distributes or dispenses controlled substances.

Federally certified opioid treatment programs (OTPs) generally administer methadone (a schedule II controlled substance) to patients on a daily basis, with staff observing as a patient takes an oral dose of liquid methadone. Some OTPs have operated mobile medication units, in which methadone is dispensed at a remote location to individuals receiving treatment from the OTP.[103] DEA has approved mobile medication units in the past, but it ceased registering these mobile units beginning in 2007.[104] DEA announced in 2021 that it would lift the 14-year moratorium on mobile methadone units, removing the requirement that mobile components of OTPs receive a separate registration.[105]

Title 42, Part 8, of the Code of Federal Regulations, which includes most of the regulations for OTPs, specified that patients admitted to OTPs must "be addicted to opioids for at least one year", prohibiting individuals with opioid use disorder for less than a year from receiving treatment at an OTP.[106]

Provision

Section 1252 amends CSA Section 302(e) by making an exception to the separate registration for OTPs operating mobile methadone units, so long as the mobile unit meets such standards as the Attorney General may establish, effectively codifying in statute DEA's 2021 rule.

---

[102] 21 U.S.C. §822(e).

[103] Brian Chan, Kim Hoffman, Christina Bougatsos, et al., "Mobile Methadone Medication Units: A Brief History, Scoping Review, and Research Opportunity," *Journal of Substance Abuse Treatment*, October 2021.

[104] U.S. Department of Justice, Bureau of Justice Assistance, "DEA Expands Access to Mobile Narcotic Treatment Programs," press release, August 2021, https://bja.ojp.gov/library/publi cations/dea-expands-access-mobile-narcotic- treatment-programs.

[105] Drug Enforcement Administration, "Registration Requirements for Narcotic Treatment Programs with Mobile Components," 86 *Federal Register* 33861, June 28, 2021. DEA refers to OTPs as "narcotic treatment programs."

[106] 42 C.F.R. §8.12(e).

Section 1252 also requires the Secretary to revise the Code of Federal Regulations (42 C.F.R. 8.12(e)(1)) to eliminate the requirement that OTPs admit an individual for treatment only if the individual became "addicted to opioids" at least one year before admission for treatment.

Chapter 6—Additional Provisions Relating to Addiction Treatment

Section 1261. Prohibition

Background

The federal government supports certain harm reduction strategies that emphasize prevention of adverse events associated with substance use, such as overdose and disease transmission. For example, the American Rescue Plan Act (P.L. 117-2) appropriated $30 million for grants to support "community-based overdose prevention programs, syringe services programs, and other harm reduction services."[107] The provision required grants be used for preventing and controlling the spread of infectious diseases, distributing opioid overdose reversal medications, connecting individuals with education and services, and encouraging individuals with substance use disorders to reduce the negative health impacts of substance use. SAMHSA announced the grant program in December 2021.[108]

Provision

Section 1261 prohibits funding from any provision in the Restoring Hope for Mental Health and Well-Being Act from being used to purchase or distribute "pipes or cylindrical objects" intended to be used to smoke or inhale illegal drugs.

---

[107] ARPA §2706.

[108] Substance Abuse and Mental Health Services Administration, "SAMHSA Announced Unprecedented $30 Million Harm Reduction Grant Funding Opportunity to Help Address the Nation's Substance Use and Overdose Epidemic," press release, December 8, 2021, https://www.samhsa.gov/newsroom/press-announcements/202112081000. The HHS Secretary and ONDCP Director released a subsequent statement indicating that no federal funding would be used directly to put pipes in safe smoking kits distributed as part of harm reduction efforts. See U.S. Department of Health and Human Services, "Statement by HHS Secretary Xavier Becerra and ONDCP Director Rahul Gupta," press release, February 9, 2022, https://www.hhs.gov/about/news/2022/02/09/statement-hhs-secretary-xavier-becerra-and-ondcp- director-rahul-gupta.html.

Section 1262. Eliminating Additional Requirements for Dispensing Narcotic Drugs in Schedule III, IV, and V for Maintenance or Detoxification Treatment

Background

CSA Section 303 ("Registration Requirements") specifies the requirements for practitioners registering with DEA to dispense (i.e., prescribe or administer) controlled substances.[109]

The Drug Addiction Treatment Act of 2000 (DATA 2000; P.L. 106-310) amended the CSA to allow qualifying practitioners to dispense schedule III-V narcotic drugs for the purposes of maintenance or detoxification treatment for opioid use disorder (i.e., buprenorphine) outside of federally certified OTPs if they obtained a separate waiver from DEA and SAMHSA (known as a DATA waiver or X waiver).[110] Practitioners with DATA waivers treating opioid use disorder using buprenorphine were subject to certain training requirements and limits on the number of patients they could treat at any time. Most requirements for DATA waivers were outlined in regulations pursuant to the Secretary's rulemaking authority. In 2018, the SUPPORT Act amended the CSA, codifying several DATA waiver policies in CSA Section 303(g).[111]

Provision

Section 1262 amends CSA Section 303 by exempting practitioners who dispense schedule III-V narcotic drugs (i.e., buprenorphine) from obtaining a separate DEA registration.[112] Subsequently, it removes the waiver initially

---

[109] 21 U.S.C. §823.

[110] Buprenorphine was (and remains) the only schedule III controlled substance meeting the conditions for the waiver.

[111] SUPPORT Act §§3201-3203. For more information, see CRS Report R45405, The SUPPORT for Patients and Communities Act (P.L. 115-271): Food and Drug Administration and Controlled Substance Provisions.

[112] Section 1262 amends CSA Section 303(g) (21 U.S.C. §823(g)), where the requirements for a separate registration for OTPs and the description of waiver requirements for the use of schedule III-V drugs in the treatment of opioid use disorder (the DATA waiver) had existed. More specifically, the provision removes CSA Section 303(g)(2), which specified the requirements to obtain a waiver. However, Section 103 of P.L. 117-215, enacted on December 2, 2022, several weeks before the Restoring Hope for Mental Health and Well-Being Act was signed into law (but after the bill had initially passed the House), redesignated CSA Section 303 subsection (f) as (g) and subsection (g) as (h). Restoring Hope for Mental Health and Well-Being Act Section 1262 did not reflect these changes. DEA and SAMHSA have interpreted the act to eliminate the DATA waiver requirement. In codifying the amendment, the Office of Law Revision Counsel also executed the

required by the DATA 2000 Act for practitioners using schedule III-IV drugs for maintenance or detoxification treatment for opioid use disorder outside of an OTP, striking all of the specified requirements for obtaining such waiver.

Thus, under current law, any practitioner registered with DEA to dispense (i.e., prescribe or administer) controlled substances is authorized to use buprenorphine to treat OUD outside of an OTP, subject to state laws. Section 1262 makes other technical and conforming edits.

Section 1263. Requiring Prescribers of Controlled Substances to Complete Training

Background

CSA Section 303 ("Registration Requirements") specifies the requirements for practitioners registering with DEA to dispense (i.e., prescribe or administer) controlled substances.[113] Prior to enactment of the Restoring Hope for Mental Health and Well-Being Act, only practitioners who dispensed narcotic drugs to individuals for maintenance or detoxification treatment (e.g., medications for opioid use disorder) had specific qualification or training requirements related to treating individuals with substance use disorders. For instance, one of the conditions for certain physicians included completing an eight-hour training on treatment and management of patients with opioid use disorder (OUD).[114] Section 1262 removed the requirements for practitioners dispensing schedule III-V narcotics in detoxification or maintenance treatment of OUD. The act thus allows any practitioner registered with DEA to treat OUD using buprenorphine, subject to state laws, and removes the previous additional training requirements for treating individuals with OUD.

Provision

Section 1263 amends CSA Section 303 by adding a requirement for practitioners registering with DEA to prescribe controlled substances to complete a one-time training on treatment and management of patients with

---

revisions in the act to Title 21, Section 823(h), of the U.S. Code, noting that this was the "probable intent of Congress."

[113] 21 U.S.C. §823.

[114] Prior to enactment of the Restoring Hope for Mental Health and Well-Being Act, requirements for DATA waivers were outlined in CSA Section 303(g)(2)(G); 21 U.S.C. §823(g)(2)(G). Between enactment of P.L. 117-215 on December 2, 2022 and enactment of P.L. 117-328 on December 29, 2022, DATA waiver requirements were organized under CSA Section 303(h)(2)(G) (21 U.S.C. §823(h)(2)(G)).

opioid or other substance use disorders.[115] The provision specifies time requirements (no less than eight hours) and allowable training providers. The provision exempts physicians and other practitioners who meet certain specified requirements from the training.

Section 1263 requires the Secretary, in consultation with the Attorney General, to submit a report to specified congressional committees on the effects of the elimination of the DATA waiver (from Section 1262) no later than five years after enactment (i.e., December 29, 2027).

Section 1264. Increase in Number of Days Before Which Certain Controlled Substances Must Be Administered

Background

CSA Section 309A ("Delivery of a Controlled Substance by a Pharmacy to an Administering Practitioner") specifies the conditions for which a pharmacy may deliver a controlled substance to a practitioner for administration. Prior to the enactment of the Restoring Hope for Mental Health and Well-Being Act, a controlled substance had to be administered to a patient no later than 14 days after a practitioner had received it.

Provision

Section 1264 amends CSA Section 309A by extending the allowable timeline between delivery of a controlled substance by a pharmacy to a prescribing practitioner and its administration to a patient, from 14 days to 45 days.

Chapter 7—Opioid Crisis Response

Section 1271. Opioid Prescription Verification

Background

SUPPORT Act Section 3212 ("Programs and Materials for Training on Certain Circumstances Under Which a Pharmacist May Decline to Fill a Prescription") required the Secretary, in consultation with the DEA

[115] The safe management of dental pain and screening, brief intervention, and referral for treatment for patients with opioid and other substance use disorders is also included in the training. The provision exempts veterinarians from the training requirement.

Administrator, the FDA Commissioner, the CDC Director, and the SAMHSA Assistant Secretary, and with input from relevant stakeholders, to develop and disseminate materials for pharmacists, health care providers, and patients. The purpose of these materials is to describe (1) the circumstances under which a pharmacist may deny filling a prescription for a controlled substance because the pharmacist suspects the prescription is fraudulent, forged, or suspicious, and (2) other federal requirements pertaining to declining a prescription for a controlled substance. The Secretary is required to include instructions for the pharmacist on how to decline to fill a prescription, as well as information for health care practitioners and the public on the pharmacist's ability to decline to fill a prescription.

PHSA Section 392A authorizes the CDC Director to award grants and provide training and technical assistance to states, localities, and Indian Tribes to carry out and expand evidence-based prevention activities, which may include (1) improving the efficiency and use of a prescription drug monitoring program (PDMP); (2) promoting community or health system interventions; (3) evaluating interventions to prevent controlled substance overdoses; and (4) implementing projects to advance an innovative prevention approach with respect to new and emerging public health crises. Originally added by the SUPPORT Act,[116] PHSA Section 392A also authorizes the CDC Director to conduct controlled substance overdose data collection activities, and to assist states and localities in doing so through grants, training, and technical assistance.

Provision

Section 1271 amends SUPPORT Act Section 3212 by requiring the Secretary—in consultation with specified federal agencies—to update and disseminate the materials for pharmacists, health care providers, and patients related to the circumstances under which a pharmacist may deny filling a prescription for a controlled substance no later than one year after enactment (i.e., December 29, 2023), and periodically thereafter. The provision specifies that this includes updating and disseminating materials with information for pharmacists on how to verify the identity of the patient.

Section 1271 amends PHSA Section 392A by adding a new subsection (c) that allows the CDC Director to prioritize jurisdictions with a disproportionately high rate of drug overdoses or overdose deaths in awarding the opioid overdose prevention and data collection grants authorized in PHSA

[116] SUPPORT Act §7161.

Section 392A subsections (a) and (b). The provision also makes a technical edit.

Section 1272. Synthetic Opioid and Emerging Drug Misuse Danger Awareness

Background

Led by fentanyl, a synthetic opioid 50-100 times more potent than morphine, synthetic opioids emerged as the leading cause of opioid-related overdose deaths in the United States beginning in 2016.[117] Although the Secretary—and SAMHSA Assistant Secretary and CDC Director—can conduct public awareness campaigns on various issues of public health through general and other specific authorities, no explicit authorization to conduct a campaign for synthetic opioids existed prior to enactment of the Restoring Hope for Mental Health and Well-Being Act.

Provision

Section 1272 requires the Secretary to plan and implement a public education campaign to raise awareness of synthetic opioids, such as fentanyl and fentanyl analogues. That campaign must include disseminating information on the potency of fentanyl and on the services provided by SAMHSA and CDC related to opioid misuse. The provision also requires the campaign to include information on nonopioid pain management treatments. The campaign must be carried out no later than one year after enactment (i.e., December 29, 2023) and be updated as needed to address emerging drug misuse issues. The provision requires an independent evaluation and accompanying report to Congress regarding the effectiveness of the campaign beginning two years after enactment (i.e., December 2024) and two years thereafter (i.e., December 2026).

Section 1272 also requires the Secretary, no later than 18 months after enactment (i.e., June 2024), to disseminate information related to synthetic opioids to health care providers participating in federal programs, publish a

---

117 Merianne Rose Spencer, Arialdi M. Minino, and Margaret Warner, *Drug Overdose Deaths in the United States, 2001-2021*, Centers for Disease Control and Prevention, National Center for Health Statistics, NCHS Data Brief No. 457, December 2022, https://www.cdc.gov/nchs/products/databriefs/db457.htm. Fentanyl, heroin, and some prescription pain medications (such as morphine and oxycodone) belong to the class of drugs known as opioids, which act on receptors in the brain that regulate pain and emotion.

training guide for first responders detailing measures to prevent exposure to synthetic opioids, and conduct outreach to first responders about the availability of the training guide.

Section 1273. Grant Program for State and Tribal Response to Opioid Use Disorders

Background

Section 1003 of the 21st Century Cures Act established the "Account for the State Response to the Opioid Abuse Crisis" in the Treasury, to which $500 million was transferred and deposited for each of FY2017 and FY2018. The resulting grant—the State Targeted Response (STR) to the Opioid Crisis grant program—supplemented state activities related to the opioid crisis. The purpose of the grant program was to increase access to treatment, decrease unmet treatment need, and reduce overdose deaths through prevention, treatment, and recovery activities.

In FY2018, Congress provided $1 billion for similar activities through a new State Opioid Response (SOR) grant program. The appropriation, located in the annual Departments of Labor, Health and Human Services, and Education and Related Agencies (Labor-HHS-ED) Appropriations Act, included a $50 million set-aside for Indian Tribes and an additional 15% set-aside for states with the highest opioid-related mortality rates. Program goals were similar to the STR grants with an emphasis on expanding access to medications for opioid use disorder.

The STR grant authorization expired in FY2018, and the program did not receive any further funding. Rather, Congress increased the SOR grant appropriation by $500 million—the same amount as the STR grants—for a total of $1.5 billion for FY2019.[118] Prior to the Restoring Hope for Mental Health and Well-Being Act, the SOR grants did not have a statutory authorization; grants were authorized annually through that Labor-HHS-ED Appropriations Act.[119]

[118] Subsequent annual appropriations for the SOR grants maintained this increase.

[119] For more information on the history of the STR and SOR grants, see CRS In Focus IF12126, *Opioid Block Grants*.

Provision

Section 1273 replaces Section 1003 of the Cures Act with a new provision authorizing the State Opioid Response grants, effectively codifying the SOR grant program and removing the authorization for the STR grants.

Section 1273 authorizes grants to address opioid and stimulant misuse for states and Tribes.[120] Grants are awarded to the Single State Agency responsible for administering SAMHSA's annual substance use block grant.[121] The provision codifies minimum amounts of $4 million for states and $250,000 for territories. It specifies that the Secretary shall develop a formula for funding allocations and submit it to specified congressional committees. The formula methodology must provide preference to states with a higher relative prevalence of opioid use disorders and overdose deaths. It should include performance assessments for continuation awards and avoid "a funding cliff between States with similar overdose mortality rates to prevent funding reductions when compared to prior year allocations."[122] The authorization codifies the 15% set-aside for states with the highest age-adjusted rate of drug overdose deaths. It caps the amount for Tribes at 5%.

The new statutory authorization for the SOR grants provides more specified uses of funds. According to the provision, SOR-supported activities may include the following:

- Implementing substance use disorder prevention activities (including primary prevention).
- Improving prescription drug monitoring programs (PDMPs).
- Training health care practitioners in pain management, best practices for prescribing opioids, identification of SUDs, referral to treatment programs, preventing diversion, and overdose prevention.

---

120 The SOR grant appropriation has included set-aside for Indian Tribes and Tribal organizations—known as the TOR grants. TOR grants are not distributed by a formula. Instead, Tribes and Tribal organizations apply individually, as a consortia, or in partnership with an urban Indian organization. Funds are distributed noncompetitively based on Tribal population. Other grant requirements are similar to the SOR grant program. Section 1273 codifies authority for the TOR grants.

121 Authorized in Title XIX of the PHSA (42 U.S.C. 300x-21 et seq.). Section 1241 of the Restoring Hope for Mental Health and Well-Being Act renamed this grant the Substance Use Prevention, Treatment, and Recovery (SUPTRS) block grant.

122 Report language accompanying appropriations laws authorizing the SOR grant included similar language. Initially, states receiving additional funding through the 15% set-aside for states with the highest overdose mortality could receive significant reductions in funds in subsequent years if they significantly reduced (or slowed) mortality relative to other states.

- Supporting access to SUD services, including those provided at opioid treatment programs (OTPs) or other outpatient or residential facilities providing MOUD,[123] or in integrated care settings.
- Recovery support services, including peer support, mutual aid programs, housing services, and family support.
- Other public health-related activities addressing substance misuse and use disorders.

Section 1273 specifies reporting requirements for grantees and the Secretary. States receiving funds must report a description of the activities supported by the grant and the population served. The Secretary must submit a report to specified congressional committees no later than September 30, 2024, that summarizes the information provided by the states. The authorization also requires the Secretary to provide technical assistance, including regarding grant applications, to grantees. The provision requires GAO to submit a report to specified congressional committees no later than two years after enactment (i.e., December 29, 2024) that assesses funding allocations and use of funds.

Cures Act Section 1003 now authorizes $1.75 billion to be appropriated for each of FY2023- FY2027.

Subtitle C—Access to Mental Health Care and Coverage: Chapter 1—Improving Uptake and Patient Access to Integrated Care Services

Section 1301. Improving Uptake and Patient Access to Integrated Care Services

Background

PHSA Section 520K ("Integration Incentive Grants and Cooperative Agreements") authorizes SAMHSA's Primary and Behavioral Health Care Integration program. Amended in 2016 by the Cures Act,[124] the provision authorizes the Secretary to fund demonstration projects that provide coordinated and integrated mental health and primary care services. The

---

[123] For more information, see CRS In Focus IF12348, *Medications for Opioid Use Disorder*.
[124] Cures Act §9003.

program provides grants to states and community mental health centers to engage in collaboration, expand infrastructure, and increase the availability of primary health care and wellness services for individuals with serious mental illness or co-occurring mental illness and substance use disorders.[125]

PHSA Section 520K previously authorized $51.9 million (rounded) to be appropriated for each of FY2018-FY2022.

Provision

Section 1301 replaces PHSA Section 520K with a new provision authorizing similar activities, entitled "Improving Uptake and Patient Access to Integrated Care Services." The new authorization makes the following changes:

- Expands eligible entities to include rural health clinics, FQHCs, or primary care practices.
- Amends the definition of integrated care to include the psychiatric collaborative care model and other evidence-based or evidence-informed models, and specifies that integrated care includes coordinating and jointly delivering behavioral and physical health services.
- Adds a definition of the psychiatric collaborative care model.
- Adds a definition for bidirectional integrated care, which means integration of behavioral health care and specialty health care, or primary care into specialty behavioral health settings.
- Adds to the definition of "special population" adults with co-occurring mental health and substance use disorders.
- Changes "Purposes" of the program to "Use of Funds" and expands the use of funds beyond primary care and for all special populations (as now defined). It specifies that the grants support evidence-based or evidence-informed activities; adds recovery services; adds bidirectional integrated care services; adds greater specifications for use of funds (hiring staff, formalizing contractual relationships, purchasing software and other resources, etc.).
- Specifies greater detail regarding the application and partnerships with Tribal, rural, or medically underserved communities, and a description of evidence- based integrated care models other than the psychiatric care model.

---

[125] SAMHSA, Justification of Estimates for Appropriations Committees, FY2023.

- Further specifies that awards are for no more than $2 million (as opposed to exactly $2 million previously), with adjustments by the Secretary permitted.
- Broadens the information included in annual grantee reports and removes requirements to report certain specific outcomes.
- Adds training and information on the psychiatric collaborative care model to the technical assistance authorization for grantees.

The new authorization requires a report to specified congressional committees no later than 18 months after enactment (i.e., June 29, 2024), and annually thereafter, summarizing the annual grantee reports and including other specified information on outcomes. The provision specifies no less than 10% of funds are for implementing the psychiatric collaborative care model (provided the annual appropriation is not less than the FY2022 level).

PHSA Section 520K now authorizes $60 million to be appropriated for each of FY2023-FY2027.

Chapter 2—Helping Enable Access to Lifesaving Services

Section 1311. Reauthorization and Provision of Certain Programs to Strengthen the Health Care Workforce

Background

PHSA Section 756 ("Mental and Behavioral Health Education and Training Grants") authorizes the Behavioral Health Workforce Education and Training (BHWET) Program. Administered by HRSA, this program provides grants to support the training of the behavioral health workforce, including paraprofessionals. Grants are awarded to eligible institutions of higher education, training programs, and other organizations involved in training specified behavioral health service professionals in fields such as psychiatry, psychology, psychiatric nursing, social work, and occupational therapy, among others. Codified by the Cures Act in 2016,[126] the program authorization was subsequently amended by the SUPPORT Act in 2018,[127] which added language specifying that providers trained in trauma-informed care are eligible to participate.

---

[126] Cures Act §9021 (42 U.S.C. §294e-1).

[127] SUPPORT Act §7073.

PHSA Section 756 previously authorized $50 million to be appropriated for each of FY2019- FY2023.

PHSA Section 760 ("Training Demonstration Program") requires the Secretary to establish a demonstration program that awards grants to eligible entities to (1) support training for psychiatry residents and fellows, nurse practitioners, physician assistants, and social workers in underserved community-based settings integrating primary care and mental and substance use disorder treatment, and (2) support academic units or programs that provide training for students or faculty in the ability to recognize, diagnose, and treat mental and substance use disorders or develop evidence-based practices or recommendations for curricula content standards. Originally added by the Cures Act in 2016,[128] PHSA Section 760 specifies acceptable use of grant funds, eligible entities, granting priority, and required studies and reports.

PHSA Section 760 previously authorized $10 million to be appropriated annually for each of FY2018-FY2022.

Provision

Section 1311 amends PHSA Section 756 to specify that occupational therapy master's or doctoral level programs are grant eligible. The provision also adds trauma-informed training for paraprofessionals to allowable uses of funds.

Section 1311 extends the authorization of appropriations for the BHWET program. PHSA Section 756 now authorizes $50 million to be appropriated for each of FY2023-FY2027 (with specified allocations for each activity).

Section 1311 amends PHSA Section 760 by making technical corrections to language related to mental health disorders and by specifying that individuals completing clinical training requirements for licensure are eligible for training. It also adds counselors and nurses to the list of eligible professionals, as well as programs that focus on pediatric populations or trauma-informed care to the eligibility list. It adds health service psychologists, nurses, counselors, and physician assistants to the prioritized eligible grantees.

Section 1311 extends authorizations of appropriations for the Training Demonstration program, authorizing $31.7 million to be appropriated for each of FY2023-FY2027.

---

[128] Cures Act §9022 (42 U.S.C. §294k).

Section 1312. Reauthorization of Minority Fellowship Program

Background

PHSA Section 597 ("Fellowships") requires the Secretary to maintain a "Minority Fellowship Program" to award fellowships, which may include stipends, for post-baccalaureate training for mental health professionals in the fields of psychiatry, nursing, social work, marriage and family therapy, mental health counseling, and substance use disorder and addiction counseling. The SAMHSA-administered Minority Fellowship Program provides grants to professional associations (e.g., the American Psychiatric Association and the American Nurses Association) to offer stipends to minority doctoral students who are studying for degrees in a mental or behavioral health profession.[129]

PHSA Section 597 previously authorized $12.7 million (rounded) to be appropriated for each of FY2018-FY2022.[130]

Chapter 3—Eliminating the Opt-Out for Nonfederal Governmental Health Plans

Section 1321. Eliminating the Opt-Out for Nonfederal Governmental Health Plans

Background

Private health insurance—offered by private-sector insurance companies or sponsored by employers and other entities, such as unions—is the most common form of health coverage in the United States. Both private-sector employers and governmental employers may offer private health insurance to their employees and their dependents.

A nonfederal governmental plan is a governmental group health plan that is sponsored by entities such as states, counties, school districts, and

---

[129] Of note, the Health Resources and Services Administration (HRSA) within HHS also provides workforce development programming for behavioral health providers. See, for instance, *HRSA; Grants; Behavioral Health* at https://bhw.hrsa.gov/grants/behavioral-health.

[130] 42 U.S.C. §290ll(c).

municipalities.[131] Like private employers, sponsors of nonfederal governmental plans can choose to offer self-insured or fully insured plans.[132]

Per PHSA Section 2722, if a sponsor of a nonfederal governmental plan offers a self-insured plan, the sponsor may elect to exempt the plan from certain federal requirements that otherwise apply to self-insured group health plans. The exemption for self-insured, nonfederal governmental plans was established in the PHSA under the Health Insurance Portability and Accountability Act (HIPAA; P.L. 104-191) and later modified by the Patient Protection and Affordable Care Act (ACA; P.L. 111-148, as amended).[133] Per the ACA, self-insured, nonfederal plans may opt out of some or all of the following federal requirements:

- Coverage of Minimum Hospital Stay After Childbirth (42 U.S.C. §300gg-25);
- Mental Health Parity (42 U.S.C. §300gg-26);
- Coverage of Reconstruction After Mastectomy (42 U.S.C. §300gg-27); and
- Coverage for Students Who Take a Medically Necessary Leave of Absence (42 U.S.C. §300gg-28).[134]

Federal mental health parity law does not require applicable plans to cover mental health and substance use disorder (MH/SUD) benefits when such coverage is not otherwise required by federal or state law.[135] However, when a plan does cover both MH/SUD benefits and medical/surgical (M/S) benefits,

---

131 *Nonfederal governmental plan* is defined at 42 U.S.C. §300gg-91(d)(8)(C) and uses the definition of governmental plan at 29 U.S.C. §1002(32).

132 When group plan sponsors purchase coverage from insurers and offer it to their employees or other groups, these plans are referred to as *fully insured*. When group plan sponsors provide health benefits directly (instead of purchasing coverage from an insurer), these plans are referred to as *self-insured* or self-funded. For more information, see "Federal and State Regulation of Private Health Insurance" in CRS Report R47507, *Private Health Insurance: A Primer*.

133 For additional background on the exemption for self-insured, nonfederal governmental plans, see the relevant section in CRS Report R46003, *Applicability of Federal Requirements to Selected Health Coverage Arrangements*.

134 For discussions of these and other provisions, see CRS Report R45146, *Federal Requirements on Private Health Insurance Plans*.

135 Federal mental health parity law includes the Paul Wellstone and Pete Domenici Mental Health Parity and Addiction Equity Act of 2008 (MHPAEA; P.L. 110-343), as it amended prior parity law and has since been amended. For more information, see CRS Report R47402, *Mental Health Parity and Coverage in Private Health Insurance: Federal Requirements*.

parity law generally prohibits the imposition of more restrictive limitations on the MH/SUD as compared with the M/S benefits.

Provision

Section 1312 amends PHSA Section 597 to reauthorize SAMHSA's Minority Fellowship Program. PHSA Section 597 now authorizes $25 million to be appropriated for each of FY2023- 2027.

In 2021, almost 13 million state and local government employees were enrolled through their employer's health plan (i.e., a nonfederal governmental plan).[136] Among those employees enrolled, 64.4% (or approximately 8.3 million) were in a self-insured plan. For reference, approximately 62.2 million private-sector employees were enrolled through their employer's health plan in 2021, and among those enrollees, an estimated 57.9% (or about 36 million) were in a self-insured plan.

According to data published by the Center for Consumer Information & Insurance Oversight (CCIIO), as of June 2019, at least 174 nonfederal governmental entities across 35 states had elected to exempt at least one self-insured plan they offer from one or more of the four requirements above.[137] Nearly all of the 174 entities offered at least one plan that was exempt from the mental health parity requirement; significantly fewer entities offered plans that were exempt from each of the other three requirements. Overall, it is unclear how many nonfederal governmental entities offered plans that covered MH/SUD benefits at that time, nor is it clear how many such self-insured plans had not opted out of parity requirements.

---

[136] Estimates in this paragraph are based on Congressional Research Service (CRS) analysis of Medical Expenditure Panel Survey (MEPS) Insurance Component (IC) data from the U.S. Agency for Healthcare Research and Quality (AHRQ). See "Employee" data in the "Public Sector" and "Private Sector – National" tabs and accompanying tables B.1, B.2., B.2.b, and B.2.b(1) at https://datatools.ahrq.gov/meps-ic/. The MEPS-IC public sector data (available through 2021 at the time of this report) include state and local governmental entities. The MEPS-IC private sector data (available through 2022, but 2021 data used for comparison) include nongovernmental employers, the self-employed with employees, and the incorporated, self-employed with no employees. While employers may offer coverage to employees and their dependents, the MEPS-IC enrollment data include covered *employees* only. See "covered persons" in the glossary at the MEPS-IC webpage linked in this footnote.

[137] Centers for Medicare & Medicaid Services (CMS), Center for Consumer Information and Insurance Oversight (CCIIO), "List of HIPAA Opt-Out Elections for Self-Funded Non-Federal Governmental Plans," June 21, 2019, at https://www.cms.gov/CCIIO/Resources/Forms-Reports-and-Other-Resources/Downloads/HIPAAOptOuts.pdf.

Provision

Section 1321 amends PHSA Section 2722 to provide that self-insured, nonfederal governmental plans can no longer opt out of mental health parity requirements.[138] Such plans may not elect this exemption on or after the date of enactment (i.e., December 29, 2022), and they may not renew a mental health parity exemption that expires on or after 180 days after enactment (i.e., June 27, 2023).

There is an exception in Section 1321 for certain collectively bargained plans. As explained in subsequent guidance regarding this provision:

> Specifically, a self-funded, non-Federal governmental group health plan that is subject to multiple collective bargaining agreements (CBAs) of varying lengths and that has a MHPAEA opt-out election in effect on December 29, 2022, that expires on or after June 27, 2023, may extend such election until the date on which the term of the last collective bargaining agreement expires.[139]

Per CCIIO data updated as of July 2023 (i.e., after the enactment of this provision), at least 186 nonfederal governmental entities across 26 states had elected to exempt at least one self-insured plan they offer from one or more of the four requirements above—all but one of which included a parity exemption.[140] The details of all of these parity exemptions are not provided, but some of the plans were elected prior to December 29, 2022, and some are indicated as collectively bargained plans.[141]

---

138 42 U.S.C. §300gg-21(a)(2)(F).

139 CMS, CCIIO, "Insurance Standards Bulletin Series – Information: Sunset of MHPAEA opt-out provision for self- funded, non-Federal governmental group health plans," June 7, 2023, at https://www.cms.gov/files/document/hipaa- opt-out-bulletin.pdf. MHPAEA refers to the Paul Wellstone and Pete Domenici Mental Health Parity and Addiction Equity Act of 2008 (P.L. 110-343).

140 CMS, CCIIO, "HIPAA Opt-Out Elections for Self-Funded Non-Federal Governmental Plans," July 31, 2023, at https://www.cms.gov/files/document/hipaaoptouts03182021.pdf. (The document itself indicates it has been updated, but the URL retains a prior date.)

141 In August 2023, a proposed federal rule on mental health parity topics included proposed amendments to existing regulations as related to implementation of Section 1321. See Internal Revenue Service (IRS), Department of the Treasury; Employee Benefits Security Administration (EBSA), Department of Labor (DOL); CMS, Department of Health and Human Services (HHS), "Requirements Related to the Mental Health Parity and Addiction Equity Act," August 3, 2023, at 88 *Federal Register* 51552.

Chapter 4—Mental Health and Substance Use Disorder Parity Implementation

Section 1331. Grants to Support Mental Health and Substance Use Disorder Parity Implementation

Background

Both the federal and state governments regulate private health insurance.[142] Federal health insurance requirements typically follow the model of federalism: federal law establishes standards, and states are primarily responsible for monitoring compliance with and enforcement of those standards. States may impose additional requirements on insurers and the plans they offer (i.e., fully insured group and nongroup plans), provided the state requirements neither conflict with federal law nor prevent the implementation of federal requirements. In general, self- insured group plans are regulated by the federal government but not by state governments.

Per federal mental health parity law, applicable plans are generally prohibited from imposing more restrictive coverage limits, including nonquantitative treatment limitations (NQTLs), on their mental health and substance use disorder (MH/SUD) benefits as compared with their medical/surgical (M/S) benefits.[143] NQTLs include nonnumeric coverage restrictions or plan attributes, such as prior authorization requirements.

Per mental health parity provisions in the Consolidated Appropriations Act, 2021 (CAA, 2021; P.L. 116-260), plans also are required to "perform and document comparative analyses of the design and application of NQTLs" and to make such analyses available to applicable federal agencies or state authority, upon request.[144] The Secretaries of HHS, Labor, and the Treasury must annually request and review at least 20 of the NQTL analyses described above from plans that "involve potential [parity] violations" or complaints of noncompliance, or in "any other instances in which the Secretary determines

---

[142] See "Federal and State Regulation of Private Health Insurance" in CRS Report R47507, *Private Health Insurance: A Primer*.

[143] See "Parity Requirements Related to Coverage Limits and Benefit Classifications" in CRS Report R47402, *Mental Health Parity and Coverage in Private Health Insurance: Federal Requirements*.

[144] Consolidated Appropriations Act, 2021 (CAA, 2021; P.L. 116-260), Division BB, Title II, Section 203. Also see "NQTL Comparative Analyses" in CRS Report R47402, *Mental Health Parity and Coverage in Private Health Insurance: Federal Requirements*.

appropriate."[145] States are not required to request and review the NQTL analyses.

Separately, Section 1003 of the ACA added a new PHSA Section 2794 (42 U.S.C. §300gg-94), establishing a $250 million grant program, to be awarded during the five-year period beginning with FY2010, to assist states in carrying out premium rate review activities and related activities as specified.[146] ACA Section 1003 further specified that if there were remaining funds at the end of FY2014, those funds were available to the Secretary for additional grants to states for "planning and implementing the insurance reforms and consumer protections under part A" (of Title XXVII of the PHSA).

Separately, Section 6603 of the ACA also added PHSA Section 2794, "Uniform fraud and abuse referral format." It was codified at Title 42, Section 300gg-95, of the U.S. Code.

Provision

Section 1331 amends PHSA Section 2794 to establish new grants for states "to enforce and ensure compliance with" mental health parity requirements.[147] To be eligible for the grants, states must agree to request and review (an unspecified number of) the NQTL comparative analyses required of group and individual health insurance issuers. The Secretary is otherwise required to specify the timing, manner, and information requirements for state applications for the grants.

The amended PHSA Section 2794 authorizes $10 million to be appropriated for each of the first five fiscal years beginning after the date of enactment (i.e., December 29, 2022), to remain available until expended, for purposes of awarding these grants.

Section 1331 also includes a technical amendment regarding the PHSA Section 2794 that was added by ACA Section 6603. This provision is redesignated as PHSA Section 2795.[148]

---

[145] Ibid.

[146] See 42 U.S.C. §300gg-94(c)(1-2) regarding the initial premium rate review grants and the additional grants. The premium rate review requirements are at 42 U.S.C. 300gg-94(a-b). Regarding premium rate review requirements, see "Rate Review" in CRS Report R45146, *Federal Requirements on Private Health Insurance Plans*.

[147] 42 U.S.C. §300gg-94(c)(3).

[148] 42 U.S.C. §300gg-95.

Subtitle D—Children and Youth: Chapter 1—Supporting Children's Mental Health Care Access

Section 1401. Technical Assistance for School-Based Health Centers

Background

PHSA Section 399Z-1 ("School-Based Health Centers") requires the Secretary to award grants for the operating costs of school-based health centers (SBHCs). School-based health centers are health clinics located in schools that provide primary health services to children.[149] The section's authorization of appropriation was extended in P.L. 116-260 in 2020, which authorized to be appropriated such sums as necessary for each of FY2022-FY2026. Prior to the law's enactment in 2020, authorizations of appropriations had lapsed in FY2014.

Grants have never been explicitly awarded under the PHSA Section 399Z-1 authority since the section was enacted in 2010. Instead, HRSA has awarded grants to health centers authorized under PHSA Section 330 to establish school sites. Funding for this purpose has been made available in annual appropriations act. For example, the part of this law—the Consolidated Appropriations Act, 2023 (P.L. 117-328)—that provided appropriations for HRSA (in Division H) included $55 million for school-based health centers as part of the funds made available for the general Health Center program.

Provision

Section 1401 amends PHSA Section 399Z-1 by adding a new subsection requiring the Secretary to provide technical assistance to SBHCs by grants or contracts to private, nonprofit entities with expertise in school-based health centers. New subsection (l) specifies the purpose and requirements for such technical assistance, including support for program operations and implementation of evidence-based or evidence-informed best practices.

149 For complete definition, see Social Security Act Section 2110(c)(9)(A) (42 U.S.C. 1397jj(c)(9)(A)).

Section 1402. Infant and Early Childhood Mental Health Promotion, Intervention, and Treatment

Background

PHSA Section 399Z-2 ("Infant and Early Childhood Mental Health Promotion, Intervention, and Treatment") authorizes SAMHSA's Infant Early Childhood Mental Health grant program.

Originally added by the Cures Act,[150] PHSA Section 399Z-2 authorizes grants to support programs for infant and early childhood mental health promotion, intervention, and treatment. The program targets children up to age 12 who are at risk for, show early signs of, or have been diagnosed with a serious mental illness (including a serious emotional disturbance) and who would benefit from specified programs. Eligible entities are human services agencies or nonprofit institutions meeting specified criteria.

PHSA Section 399Z-2 previously authorized $20 million to be appropriated for the period FY2018-FY2022 to carry out the grant program.

Provision

Section 1402 amends PHSA Section 399Z-2 by adding a new subsection allowing the Secretary (directly or via grants or contracts) to provide technical assistance to eligible entities to provide mental health services for children, training for health care professionals, and consultation to early child care and education programs.

Section 1402 reauthorizes the Infant Early Childhood Mental Health grant program. PHSA Section 399Z-2 now authorizes $50 million to be appropriated for the period of FY2023-FY2027.

Section 1403. Co-Occurring Chronic Conditions and Mental Health in Youth Study

Background

Research has found that children with chronic health conditions exhibit symptoms of mental health disorders at higher rates than their healthier peers.[151] Previous HHS studies investigating mental and physical health

---

[150] Cures Act §10006.

[151] See Ann Marie Brady, Jessica Deighton, and Stephen Stansfeld, "Chronic Illness in Childhood and Early Adolescence: A Longitudinal Exploration of Co-Occurring Mental Illness,"

issues, such as suicidal ideation in medical populations, have focused primarily on adults.[152]

Provision

Section 1403 requires the Secretary to complete a study on the rates of suicidal behaviors among youth with chronic medical illnesses no later than 12 months after enactment (i.e., December 29, 2023). The provision requires the Secretary to submit a report to Congress on the results of the study, including recommendations for early intervention, dissemination of best practices, and strategies to reduce suicidal behaviors.

Section 1404. Best Practices for Behavioral and Mental Health Intervention Teams

Background

The federal government supports state and local efforts in promoting school safety and security.[153] For example, the U.S. Secret Service National Threat Assessment Center (NTAC) published an operational guide identifying how schools can enhance their safety using a threat assessment model.[154] School threat assessment interventions seek to identify students at risk of violence to self or others, assess their risk for engaging in violence or other harmful activities, and identify strategies to manage that risk.[155] According to NTAC, the first step in a targeted violence prevention plan is establishing a threat assessment team, sometimes referred to as a behavioral intervention team.[156]

Development and Psychopathology, vol. 33, no. 3 (May 4, 2020), pp. 885-898; and Andrew J. Barnes, Marla E. Eisenberg, and Michaal Resnick, "Suicide and Self-Injury Among Children and Youth with Chronic Health Conditions," *Pediatrics*, vol. 124, no. 5 (May 2010), pp. 889-895.

152 For example, Pamela L. Owens, Kevin Heslin, Kathryn Fingar, et al., "Co-occurrence of Physical Health Conditions and Mental Health and Substance Use Conditions Among Adult Inpatient Stays, 2010 Versus 2014," Agency for Healthcare Research and Quality, Statistical Brief #240, Rockville, MD, June 2018, https://hcup-us.ahrq.gov/reports/statbriefs/sb240-Co-occurring-Physical-Mental-Substance-Conditions-Hospital-Stays.jsp.

153 For more information, see CRS Report R46872, *Federal Support for School Safety and Security*.

154 U.S. Department of Homeland Security, United States Secret Service, National Threat Assessment Center, *Enhancing School Safety Using a Threat Assessment Model: An Operational Guide for* , July 2018, https://www.cisa.gov/sites/default/files/publications/18_0711_USSS_NTAC-Enhancing-School-Safety-Guide.pdf.

155 Ibid., p. 1.

156 Ibid., p. 3.

Composed of personnel in a variety of disciplines—including mental health professionals—behavioral intervention teams receive reports about students of concern, gather additional information, assess the risk posed to the school community, and develop strategies to mitigate any risk of harm.

Provision

Section 1404 adds a new PHSA Section 520H-1 ("Best Practices for Behavioral and Mental Health Intervention Teams") that requires the SAMHSA Assistant Secretary, in consultation with the U.S. Department of Education (ED), DOJ, and the Director of the NTAC, to submit to specified congressional committees a report on best practices for using school-based behavioral and mental health intervention teams. The provision defines a behavioral and mental health intervention team as a multidisciplinary team of trained individuals who can assess the behavioral health needs of youth, connect at-risk youth with appropriate services, and implement evidence-based interventions to mitigate threats of harm and support safe, supportive learning environments in K-12 and higher education settings.

Chapter 2—Continuing Systems of Care for Children

Section 1411. Comprehensive Community Mental Health Services for Children with Serious Emotional Disturbances

Background

PHSA Title V, Part E (Sections 561-565), authorizes SAMHSA's Children's Mental Health Services. PHSA Title V, Part E, requires the Secretary to award grants to support "comprehensive community mental health services for children with a serious emotional disturbance."[157] Reauthorized by the Cures Act,[158] the authorization specifies reporting requirements, technical assistance requirements, and the ages of children to be served, among other things. PHSA Section 565 ("General Provisions") provides definitions for terms used in the Title V, Part E, authorizations and includes the authorization of appropriations, among other things.

PHSA Section 565 previously authorized $119 million (rounded) to be appropriated for each of FY2018-FY2022.

---

[157] 42 U.S.C. §290ff.

[158] Cures Act §10001.

Provision

Section 1411 amends PHSA Section by adding "kinship caregivers" to the definition of "family" and reauthorizing SAMHSA's Children's Mental Health Services.

PHSA Section 565 now authorizes $125 million to be appropriated for each of FY2023-FY2027.

Section. 1412. Substance Use Disorder Treatment and Early Intervention Services for Children and Adolescents

Background

PHSA Section 514 ("Substance Use Disorder Treatment and Early Intervention Services for Children, Adolescents, and Young Adults") authorizes SAMHSA's Children and Families program. PHSA Section 514 requires the Secretary to award grants, contracts, or cooperative agreements to support substance use disorder services for children and adolescents. Eligible entities include public and private nonprofit entities, including Native Alaskan entities and Indian Tribes and Tribal organizations. PHSA Section 514 requires the Secretary to give priority to applicants meeting specified criteria (e.g., providing gender-specific and culturally appropriate treatment). The Cures Act reauthorized the activities in this provision in 2016, further specifying definitions for Indian Tribes or Tribal Organizations and Indian Health Service facilities, among other things.[159]

PHSA Section 514 previously authorized $29.6 million (rounded) to be appropriated for each of FY2018-FY2022.

Provision

Section 1412 amends PHSA Section 514 by making technical edits to Tribal terms and reauthorizing $29.6 million (rounded) for each of FY2023-2027 for SAMHSA's Children and Families program.

---

[159] Cures Act §10003.

Chapter 3—Garrett Lee Smith Memorial Reauthorization

Sections 1421-1424

Background

SAMHSA supports several suicide prevention initiatives, including the National Strategy for Suicide Prevention, a suicide prevention technical assistance center, and the Garrett Lee Smith (GLS) State and Campus suicide grant programs, among others. In 2004, the Garrett Lee Smith Memorial Act (P.L. 108-355) explicitly authorized three of these suicide prevention programs in PHSA Title V.

PHSA Section 520C ("Suicide Prevention Technical Assistance Center") authorizes the Garrett Lee Smith (GLS) Suicide Prevention Resource Center. Amended by the Cures Act,[160] PHSA Section 520C requires the Secretary, acting through the SAMHSA Assistant Secretary, to operate a technical assistance center focused on suicide prevention. The provision specifies the program's focus on suicide prevention across the lifespan and requires the Secretary to submit to Congress a report on the activities carried out by the center.

PHSA Section 520C previously authorized $6 million (rounded) to be appropriated annually for each of FY2018-FY2022 for the center.

PHSA Sections 520E ("Youth Suicide Early Intervention and Prevention Strategies") and 520E-2 ("Mental Health and Substance Use Disorder Services on Campus") authorize the Garrett Lee Smith (GLS) State and Campus suicide grant programs. The GLS State grant program—entitled the GLS State/Tribal Youth Suicide Prevention and Early Intervention grant program—awards grants to states to support comprehensive statewide youth suicide prevention and early intervention strategies. The GLS Campus Suicide Prevention grant program provides institutions of higher education with grants to implement an array of suicide prevention initiatives on campus.[161] Both authorizing provisions were previously amended by the Cures Act in 2016.[162]

PHSA Section 520E previously authorized $30 million for each of FY2018-FY2022. PHSA Section 520E-2 previously authorized $7 million for each of FY2018-FY2022.

---

[160] Cures Act §9008.

[161] SAMHSA *Justification of Estimates for Appropriations Committees, FY2024*.

[162] Cures Act §9008 and §9031.

Section 1421. Suicide Prevention Technical Assistance Center

Section 1421 amends PHSA Section 520C by making technical edits to Tribal terms and by requiring the Secretary to collaborate with DOD and VA when providing technical assistance to entities serving members of the Armed Forces and veterans. The provision amends the authorization for an annual report, requiring the Secretary to submit to Congress a report on the activities carried out by the center no later than two years after enactment (i.e., December 29, 2024).

Section 1421 reauthorizes the Suicide Prevention Technical Assistance Center. PHSA Section 520C now authorizes $9 million to be appropriated for each of FY2023-FY2027.

Section 1422. Youth Suicide Early Intervention and Prevention Strategies

Section 1422 amends PHSA Section 520E by adding pediatric health programs to the list of applicable service-delivery settings and adding Tribe-designated organizations to the list of eligible grantees. The provision adds pediatric health programs that provide families with supplies to securely store means commonly used in suicide to the list of service delivery settings receiving preference.

Section 1422 amends the requirement in PHSA Section 520E that no less than 85% of funds be used for "direct services," instead requiring no less than that amount to be used for "suicide prevention activities."[163] It also adds the Department of Education to the list of entities the Secretary is required to consult with in carrying out this program. It extends the deadline for grantees to submit an evaluation of grant-funded activities to 24 months (from 18 months). It amends the date the Secretary must submit a report to congressional committees on the effectiveness of program activities to December 31, 2025. The provision makes technical edits to Tribal terms and amends the definition of "youth" to include individuals younger than 10 years old and up to 24 years old.

Section 1422 reauthorizes the GLS State/Tribal Youth Suicide Prevention and Early Intervention Grant Program. PHSA Section 520E now authorizes $40 million to be appropriated for each of FY2023-2027.

---

[163] 42 U.S.C. §290bb-36(d).

Section 1423. Mental Health and Substance Use Disorder Services for Students in Higher Education

Section 1423 amends PHSA Section 520E-2 by changing the title to "Mental Health and Substance Use Disorder Services for Students in Higher Education." The provision adds promoting resiliency to the goals of the program and adds providing resources (in addition to services) to allowable uses of funds. The provision makes other technical changes to language related to mental health promotion and service provision. It also specifies the congressional committees to receive the program's annual report to Congress, and requires the report to include a needs assessment of the population served by grant recipients.

Section 1423 amends PHSA Section 520E-2 by reauthorizing $7 million for each of FY2023- FY2027 for the GLS Campus Suicide Prevention grant program.

Section 1424. Mental and Behavioral Health Outreach and Education at Institutions of Higher Education

Background

PHSA Section 549 ("Mental and Behavioral Health Outreach and Education on College Campuses") requires the Secretary, acting through the SAMHSA Assistant Secretary in collaboration with the CDC Director, to convene an interagency, public-private sector working group composed of representatives of certain specified groups. The working group is required to plan, establish, and coordinate a public education campaign, as specified, focused on mental and behavioral health on the campuses of institutions of higher education, as defined. Originally added by the Cures Act in 2016,[164] PHSA Section 549 specifies the elements required in the working group's plan.

PHSA Section 549 previously authorized $1 million to be appropriated for the period of FY2018- FY2022.

Provision

Section 1424 amends PHSA Section 549 by changing the heading to "Mental and Behavioral Health Outreach and Education at Institutions of Higher

---

164 Cures Act §9033.

Education" and adding representatives of minority-serving institutions and community colleges to the working group authorized in the section.[165]

Section 1424 amends PHSA Section 549 by reauthorizing $1 million for the period of FY2023- FY2027 for the national public education campaign.

Chapter 4—Media and Mental Health

Background

Emerging research suggests that smartphone and social media use may pose risks of harm to youth and adolescents.[166] For example, some studies have shown smartphone and social media use is associated with increases in depression, anxiety, and suicidality (among other mental and behavioral issues) for youth and adolescents, particularly girls.[167] Other studies suggest only moderate negative effects,[168] or even possible benefits of social media use.[169] A greater understanding of the range of possible health effects of smartphone and social media on youth and adolescents awaits further research.

---

[165] For more information on minority-serving institutions, see CRS Report R43237, *Programs for Minority-Serving Institutions Under the Higher Education Act*.

[166] See, for example, Kira E. Riehm, Kenneth A. Feder, and Kayla N. Tormohlen, et al., "Associations Between Time Spent Using Social Media and Internalizing and Externalizing Problems Among US," *JAMA Psychiatry*, vol. 76, no. 12 (September 11, 2019), pp. 1266-1273; and Chirag Gupta, Sangita Jogdand, and Mayank Kumar, "Reviewing the Impact of Social Media on the Mental Health of Adolescents and Youth Adults," *Cureus*, vol. 14, no. 10 (October 2022), p. e30143.

[167] See, for example, Yvonne Kelly, Afshin Zilanawala, and Cara Booker, et al., "Social Media Use and Adolescent Mental Health: Findings from the UK Millenium Cohort Study," *eClinicalMedicine*, vol. 6 (2018), pp. 59-68; and Jean M. Twenge and Eric Farley, "Not All Screen Time Is Created Equal: Associations with Mental Health Vary by Activity and Gender," *Social Psychiatry and Psychiatric Epidemiology*, vol. 56 (2021), pp. 207-217.

[168] See, for example, Amy Orben and Andrew K. Przybylski, "The Association Between Adolescent Well-Being and Digital Technology Use," *Nature Human Behavior*, vol. 3 (2019), pp. 173-182.

[169] See, for instance, Yalda T. Uhls, Nicole B. Ellison, and Kavri Subrahmanyam, "Benefits and Costs of Social Media in Adolescence," *Pediatrics*, vol. 140 (November 1, 2017).

Section 1431. Study on the Effects of Smartphone and Social Media Use on Adolescents

Section 1431 allows the Secretary to conduct or support research on smartphone and social media use by adolescents and the effects of use on emotional, behavioral, and physical health and development, and mental health disparities. The provision requires the Secretary to submit a report to Congress on the findings of the research no later than five years after enactment (i.e., December 29, 2027).

Section 1432. Research on the Health and Development Effects of Media and Related Technology on Infants, Children, and Adolescents

Section 1432 requires the Secretary to conduct or support research related to the health and developmental effects of specified media and technology use on infant, children, and adolescents. The provision requires the Secretary, acting through Director of the National Institutes of Health (NIH), to develop a research agenda assessing the effects of media and technology use on the cognitive development, physical health, and mental health of infants, children, and adolescents. The provision requires the NIH Director to submit a report to specific congressional committees no later than two years after enactment (i.e., December 29, 2024) on the progress made on this research program and a summary of research projects funded under this section.

Subtitle E—Miscellaneous Provisions

Section 1501. Limitations on Authority

Section 1501 prohibits the Secretary from allocating funding to any program authorized or amended by the Restoring Hope for Mental Health and Well-Being Act without considering the incidence, prevalence, or determinants of behavioral health issues (unless otherwise required by law).

Appendix. Abbreviations Used in This Report

Abbreviation	Definition
ACA	Patient Protection and Affordable Care Act (P.L. 111-148)
ACT	Assertive Community Treatment
AOT	Assisted Outpatient Treatment
ASPE	Assistant Secretary for Planning and Evaluation
BHWET	Behavioral Health Workforce Education and Training
CAA	Consolidated Appropriations Act
CARA	Comprehensive Addiction and Recovery Act of 2016 (P.L. 114-198)
CBAs	Collective Bargaining Agreements
CCBHC	Certified Community Behavioral Health Clinic
CCIIO	Center for Consumer Information & Insurance Oversight
CDC	Centers for Disease Control and Prevention
C.F.R.	*Code of Federal Regulations*
CMS	Centers for Medicare & Medicaid Services
COVID-19	Coronavirus Disease 2019
CSA	Controlled Substances Act
Cures Act	21st Century Cures Act of 2016 (P.L. 114-244)
DATA	Drug Addiction Treatment Act of 2000 (P.L. 106-310)
DEA	Drug Enforcement Administration
DOJ	U.S. Department of Justice
DOL	U.S. Department of Labor
ED	U.S. Department of Education
FDA	U.S. Food and Drug Administration
FQHC	Federally Qualified Health Centers
GAO	Government Accountability Office
GLS	Garrett Lee Smith
HHS	U.S. Department of Health and Human Services
HIPAA	Health Insurance Portability and Accountability Act (P.L. 104-191)
HRSA	Health Resources and Services Administration
HUD	U.S. Department of Housing and Urban Development
IHS	Indian Health Service
MHBG	Community Mental Health Services Block Grant
MHPAEA	Paul Wellstone and Pete Domenici Mental Health Parity and Addiction Equity Act of 2008 (P.L. 110-343)
MH/SUD	Mental Health/Substance Use Disorder
MOUD	Medications for Opioid Use Disorder
M/S	Medical/Surgical
NASEM	National Academies of Sciences, Engineering, and Medicine
NCEED	National Center of Excellence for Eating Disorders

Appendix. (Continued)

Abbreviation	Definition
NIH	National Institutes of Health
NQTLs	Non-Quantitative Treatment Limitations
NTAC	National Threat Assessment Center
OTPs	Opioid Treatment Program
PATH	Projects for Assistance in Transition from Homelessness
PHSA	Public Health Service Act
PRNS	Programs of Regional and National Significance
SABG	Substance Use Prevention and Treatment Block Grant
SAMHSA	Substance Abuse and Mental Health Services Administration
SBIRT	Screening, Brief Intervention, and Referral to Treatment
SED	Serious Emotional Disturbance
SMI	Serious Mental Illness
SOR	State Opioid Response
STOP Act	Sober Truth on Preventing Underage Drinking Act (P.L. 109-422)
SUD	Substance Use Disorders
SUPPORT Act	Substance Use Disorder Prevention that Promotes Opioid Recovery and Treatment for Patients and Communities Act (P.L. 115-271)
SUPTRS	Substance Use Prevention, Treatment, and Recovery Services
ONDCP	Office of National Drug Control Policy
OUD	Opioid Use Disorder
U.S.C.	U.S. Code
VA	U.S. Department for Veterans Affairs

Source: CRS.

Chapter 8

Looking at My Genes: What Can They Tell Me About My Mental Health?*

National Institute of Mental Health

What Are Genes?

Genes are segments of deoxyribonucleic acid (DNA), the biological "blueprint" for proteins that form the building blocks of our cells. Your DNA is passed down from your biological parents and varies a little from person to person. These variations contribute to differences in appearance, personality, and health. Certain genes, along with biological and environmental factors, can be associated with mental disorders, which are health conditions that can affect how you think, feel, and cope with life.

How Do Genes Affect Your Mental Health?

Common mental disorders like depression and anxiety are likely the result of a combination of life experiences, environment, and genetic variation. These variations can impact how your genes are turned "on" and "off" throughout life and play a role in the onset of some diseases.

Most genetic variants don't directly cause mental disorders. However, in rare cases, some uncommon gene variants can increase the risk of developing

---

* This is an edited, reformatted and augmented version of The National Institute of Mental Health, NIH Publication No. 24-MH-4298, Revised 2024.

In: Healing Minds
Editor: Wilburn M. Conner
ISBN: 979-8-89530-893-6

mental disorders. If you or a relative has one of these rare variants, it's a good idea to talk to a health care provider about the risks.

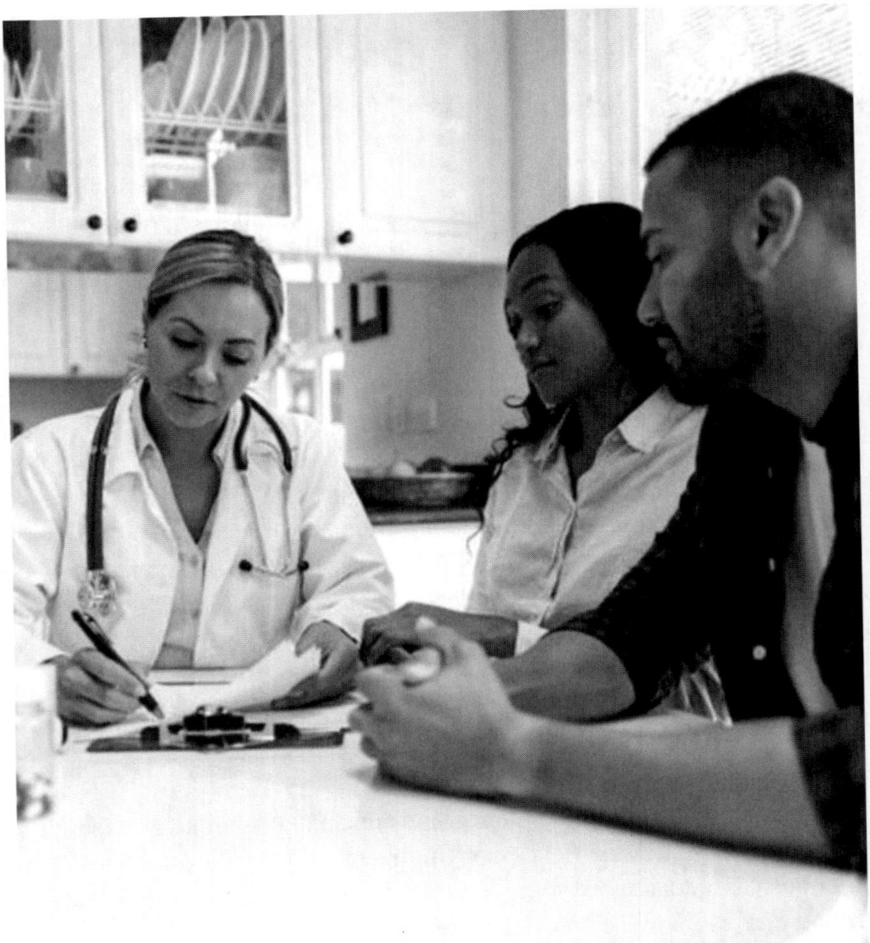

Should I Visit a Genetic Counselor?

Genetic counseling can give you information about how genetic conditions might affect you or your family. A geneticist or genetic counselor will collect your personal and family health history to determine how likely it is that you or a family member has a genetic condition. They can then help you decide whether a genetic test might be right for you or your relative. Genetic testing is often done before or during pregnancy, soon after birth, or if your health care provider suspects you may have a genetic disease.

To learn more about genetic counseling, visit the Genetic Counseling FAQ page of the National Human Genome Research Institute website at www.genome.gov/FAQ/Genetic-Counseling and the Centers for Disease Control and Prevention's Genetic Counseling webpage at www.cdc.gov/genomics/gtesting/genetic_counseling.htm.

Can Genetic Testing Help Predict My Risk of Developing a Mental Disorder?

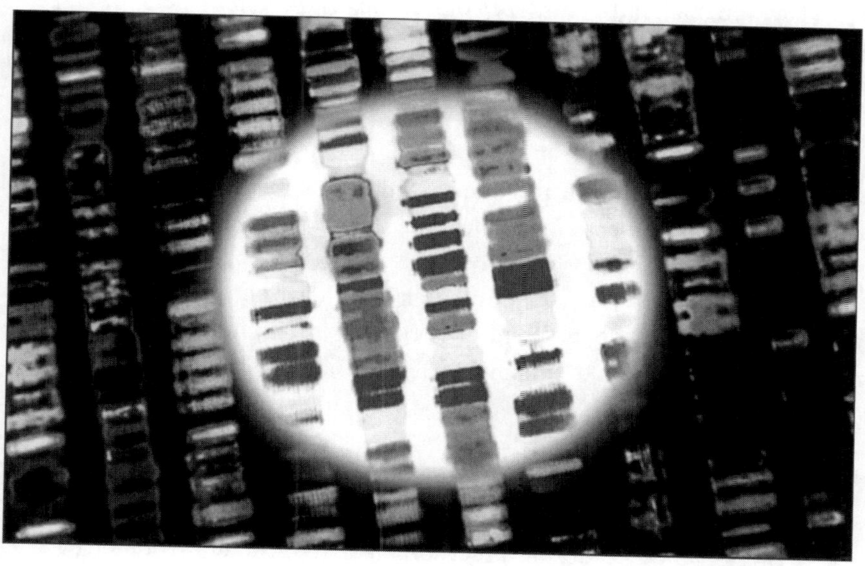

Currently, genetic tests cannot accurately predict your risk of developing a mental disorder. Although research is underway, researchers are still learning about the ways genes can contribute to mental disorders— or protect against them. Of those genes that are linked to mental disorders, most raise the risk by tiny amounts.

While recent studies have begun to identify the genetic markers associated with certain mental disorders and eventually may lead to better screening and more individualized treatment, it is still too early to use genetic tests to diagnose or treat mental disorders.

What Is the Difference Between Clinical Genetic Testing and Direct-to-Consumer Genetic Reports?

Clinical or Diagnostic Genetic Testing

Clinical genetic testing can help predict the risk of some diseases, such as cancer, but is not yet very useful for predicting the risk for mental disorders. Health care providers may order genetic testing for people who may have a high risk for rare genetic diseases. During testing, health care providers may search for a single gene or a few genes that are strongly associated with a specific disease.

There are many different types of genetic tests that may help to:

- Identify genetic variants that may increase the risk of developing a disease
- Diagnose disease
- Guide health care providers in deciding on the best medicine or treatment for certain people

If a disease runs in your family, your health care provider can tell you if it's detectable with genetic testing. For more information about clinical or genetic testing, visit www.genome.gov/FAQ/Genetic-Testing.

Direct-to-Consumer Genetic Reports

The purpose and audiences of direct-to-consumer genetic reports differ from clinical or diagnostic genetic testing.

For a fee, anyone can mail a saliva sample to companies that sell a direct-to-consumer genetic report. While advertisements may say that the company can provide information based on a person's genetic variation about their risks of developing specific diseases, these reports typically cannot help predict one's risk for developing mental disorders.

Because direct-to-consumer genetic reports for mental disorders are not accompanied by a health care provider's guidance, their results should be interpreted cautiously. These reports have varying levels of scientific support, may or may not be approved by the U.S. Food and Drug Administration, and can be misleading. If you decide to undergo direct-to-consumer genetic testing, the results should be discussed with your health care provider or genetic counselor before taking any action, such as changing your medications. For more information about direct-to-consumer tests, visit www.fda. gov/medical-devices/in-vitro-diagnostics/direct-consumer-tests.

How Can My Family Health History Help Me Understand My Health Risks?

Some mental disorders run in families, and your family's mental health history may be an important clue for determining your risk of developing a mental disorder. Having a close relative with a mental disorder could mean you are at a higher risk, but it doesn't necessarily mean you will develop that disorder. Many other factors play a role.

Knowing your family's mental health history can help you and your health care provider look for early warning signs and help your health care provider recommend ways to reduce your risk.

Talk to Your Relatives

The first step in creating a family health history is to talk to your relatives. The most helpful information comes from "first-degree" relatives—parents, brothers, sisters, and children. Health histories from "second- degree" relatives—such as nieces, nephews, half- brothers, half-sisters, grandparents, aunts, and uncles— also can be helpful but are less informative for your own risk.

Don't worry if you can't get complete information for every relative. Some people may not want to talk, and others may be unable to remember information accurately. That's okay. Whatever information you can collect will be helpful.

Keep a Record of Your Family History

Free programs like the Surgeon General's "My Family Health Portrait" can help you create a family health history. You can use the program to record information about your family's health and share it with your health care provider or family members. You can find the program at https://cbiit.github.io/FHH/html.

New or updated information can be added as a family grows or family members are diagnosed with health conditions. It may take a little time and effort, but this record can improve your family's health for generations.

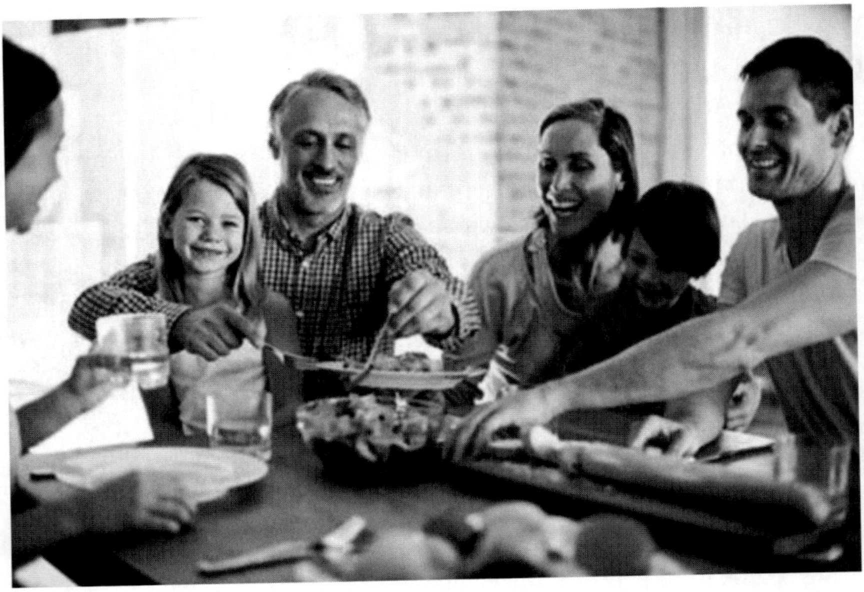

Talk With a Mental Health Professional

If mental disorders run in your family, consider talking with a mental health professional who can help you understand the illness' risk and ways to prevent or treat it. Asking questions and providing information to your health care provider can improve your care and results and increase safety and satisfaction. For tips and information about speaking with your health care provider, visit www.nimh.nih.gov/talkingtips and the Agency for Healthcare Research Quality at www.ahrq.gov/questions.

What Research Is NIMH Doing on Genetics?

The National Institute of Mental Health (NIMH) funds and conducts research to help answer important scientific questions about mental disorders. NIMH is currently studying and supporting research on the human genetic variations that contribute to the risk of different mental disorders. These include but are not limited to the following:

- Eating disorders, such as anorexia nervosa, binge eating disorders, and bulimia nervosa
- Mood disorders, such as anxiety disorders, bipolar disorder, and depression
- Neurodevelopmental disorders, such as autism spectrum disorder and intellectual disability
- Obsessive-compulsive disorder
- Post-traumatic stress disorder
- Psychosis and schizophrenia

Research investigating these topics will help the field take steps toward better screening and personalized treatment. Basic research efforts enhance our understanding of the underlying causes of disease and might result in improved clinical treatments.

You can learn more about ongoing research efforts by visiting www.nimh.nih.gov/news/science-news/ science-news-about-genetics.

Where Can I Find More Information About Genetics?

For information about how genes affect your risk for developing a disease or disorder, visit:

- Centers for Disease Control and Prevention: Family Health History: www.cdc.gov/genomics/famhistory
- National Human Genome Research Institute:
- www.genome.gov/health
- MedlinePlus: Genetics:
- https://medlineplus.gov/genetics

How Can I Find Help for Mental Disorders?

NIMH has information on ways to get help and find a health care provider or access treatment at www.nimh.nih.gov/findhelp. In addition, the Substance Abuse and Mental Health Services Administration has an online tool at https://findtreatment.gov to help you find mental health services in your area.

What Are Clinical Trials and Why Are They Important?

Clinical trials are research studies that look at new ways to prevent, detect, or treat diseases and conditions. These studies help researchers determine if a new treatment is safe and effective in people. The main purpose of a clinical trial is to gain new scientific knowledge so that others may be better helped in the future.

People volunteer for clinical trials for many reasons. Some people join clinical trials to help doctors and researchers learn more about a disease and improve health care. Other people, such as those with health conditions, join to try new or advanced treatments that aren't widely available.

NIMH supports clinical trials at the National Institutes of Health campus in Bethesda, Maryland, and across the United States. Talk to a health care provider about clinical trials, their benefits and risks, and whether one is right for you. For more information, visit www.nimh.nih.gov/clinicaltrials.

For More Information

Learn more at www.nimh.nih.gov/ health. For information about various health topics, visit the National Library of Medicine's MedlinePlus resource at https://medlineplus.gov.

National Institute of Mental Health

Office of Science Policy, Planning, and Communications
6001 Executive Boulevard, MSC 9663
Bethesda, MD 20892-9663
Phone: 1-866-615-6464

Email: nimhinfo@nih.gov
Website: www.nimh.nih.gov

Reprints

The information in this publication is in the public domain and may be reused or copied without permission. However, you may not reuse or copy images. Please cite the National Institute of Mental Health as a source. Read our copyright policy to learn more about our guidelines for reusing NIMH content at www.nimh.nih.gov/copyright.

Index

A

B

C

D

Q

R

S

T

U

V

W

Y